A Primer of Drug Action

A Primer of Drug Action

Fifth Edition

Robert M. Julien

St. Vincent Hospital and Medical Center
Portland, Oregon

W. H. FREEMAN AND COMPANY
New York

Library of Congress Cataloging-in-Publication Data

Julien, Robert M.
  A primer of drug action.
  (A series of books in psychology)
  Bibliography: p.
  Includes index.
  1. Psychotropic drugs.   2. Psychopharmacology.
I. Title. II. Series.
RM315.J75   1988   615'.78   87-36596
ISBN 0-7167-1962-2
ISBN 0-7167-1963-0 (pbk.)

Printed in the United States of America

34567890 VB 654321089

To my wife, Judi,

for her understanding and support

To my sons, Robert, Jr., and Scott,

for all their help in preparing this manuscript

Contents

Preface

In the 14 years since the first edition of *A Primer of Drug Action* was published, awareness of drug use and abuse has increased throughout all segments of society. People know more about the health consequences of both licit drugs, such as cigarettes and alcohol, and illicit ones, such as cocaine, marijuana, "designer" narcotics, and psychedelics. Yet neither the pharmacological actions of psychoactive drugs nor the goals of this text have changed. These drugs all act in a predictable fashion; each has inherent benefits, uses, risks, side effects, toxicities, and societal consequences. The objective of this book is still to transmit information about drugs from writer to reader in clear language.

Public awareness of drug risks and toxicities has also increased significantly during the last 14 years. This awareness is evidenced by the proliferation of rehabilitation and treatment programs, the recognition of drug dependence as a medical problem, the willingness of insurance programs to pay for drug rehabilitation, the increased enforcement of drug laws, and the public intolerance of certain types of drug users (e.g., cigarette smokers and intoxicated drivers).

Despite this increased awareness there is much about drug use that is still distressing: Hundreds of thousands of people still fall victim to cigarette and alcohol toxicities; cocaine use is seriously damaging an increasing number of users; marijuana has become a deeply ingrained cultural habit; experimentation with various psychedelic drugs continues; and drug use by minors continues to be a problem. Drug-abuse education as part of a national priority to decrease drug use continues to play a central role, although the limits of such education are well documented. Hence, the emphasis of

A Primer of Drug Action remains on those drugs that primarily affect people's thought and behavior.

Along with wanting reliable information about those drugs that are prone to abuse, many people seem to want more information about an increasing variety of drugs. Thus, the expansion of this edition includes information about drugs that are used to treat affective disorders and the various neurological drugs. These new chapters, combined with other updated information, increase the usefulness of this edition in those situations where a broad coverage of neuropsychopharmacology is desired. This text can also be coupled with my companion text, *Drugs and the Body* (New York: W. H. Freeman and Company, 1988), to provide a comprehensive introduction to the science of pharmacology.

Features of the Fifth Edition

Two totally new chapters have been added to this edition. Chapter 6, Antidepressants and Lithium: Drugs Used in Affective Disorders, explores the major causes of affective disorders and their treatment with tricyclic antidepressants, the second-generation antidepressants, the MAO inhibitors, electroconvulsive therapy, and lithium. Chapter 11, Neurological Drugs, presents those drugs used to treat Parkinson's disease, epilepsy, spasticity, and pain (nonnarcotic analgesics and local anesthetics).

This edition also contains updates on the benzodiazepine tranquilizers, "designer" drugs, cocaine, opiate and benzodiazepine receptors, contraceptives, urine testing for drugs of abuse, and the mechanisms of action of the major psychoactive drugs. Special emphasis is placed on the toxicities and consequences that result from the widespread use of alcohol and cigarettes as well as the episodic emergence of potent psychedelic drugs (e.g., cocaine and "designer" narcotics).

Robert M. Julien
January 1988

Preface to the First Edition

In this age of science and discovery, when we seem to be uncovering vast amounts of information about distant planets, the origin of the universe, the origin of man, the secrets of nature, and the boundless potentials of man's abilities, it seems strange that many of us know very little about our own bodies, especially about the responses of our bodies to drugs. Perhaps this is because we take drugs so casually, but perhaps it is also because those who are not trained in medical or biological science have neither sought nor received information about drugs that is scientifically correct yet comprehensible and relevant to their lives. Many books have been written about drugs, but how have these been written and for what audience are they intended? There are the standard textbooks of pharmacology (pharmacology being that branch of science that deals with the study of drugs and their actions), which are intended for students of medicine, pharmacy, dentistry, and other professional and paramedical fields. These books are written with the assumption that the reader has an understanding of anatomy, physiology, biochemistry, and organic chemistry, for much of the material they contain would otherwise be incomprehensible. Most of the other pharmacology texts are reference books written for the graduate student in pharmacology and for the professional pharmacologist. These are usually intensive treatises delving in great detail into specific areas of pharmacology. These latter texts presume a level of knowledge comparable at least to that of a student who has completed the first two years of graduate or medical education. This is not to say that there are no popular books on drugs written for the layman. A multitude of popular books dealing with various aspects of drug abuse have appeared. These books have generally been intended to frighten their readers; they emphasize the moral, social, and physical degradation thought to result from the use of drugs and are generously sprinkled with misinformation. Such books have been used in drug education programs in an effort to discourage young people from experimenting with illegal drugs. What they lack in factual content they make up for in enthusiasm.

It is now becoming more widely recognized that, if drug education is to make any impression on increasingly sophisticated audiences in the community, it must be accurate, factual, and completely consistent. It appears that a new sort of text is needed; one patterned after the classical pharmacology textbooks (those used in medical schools) but written for individuals with little or no scientific background. Too often, professionals tend to hide their knowledge in jargon so that it is relatively inaccessible to individuals outside their own profession. Information about drugs should, I feel, be presented without the jargon that usually accompanies it. This, then, is the overall objective of this book: the transmission of information about drugs from writer to reader in classical pharmacologic style and in language that is intelligible to readers who may lack scientific background in medical physiology, anatomy, biochemistry, and related subjects.

Robert M. Julien
October 1974

CHAPTER 1

Principles of Drug Action

How Drugs Affect the Body

When you seek relief from headache with an aspirin, social relaxation with alcohol, or any other drug-induced alteration of your physical or psychological state, the drug you use must somehow get from the external world into your body and ultimately to the specific site within the body where it can exert its effect.

Simple though this may sound, transporting a drug from outside the body to its ultimate site of action is a complex process. The taking of a drug involves the absorption of that drug into the bloodstream, the distribution of the drug by the circulating blood to all regions of the body, the action of the drug itself, the eventual breakdown of the drug into an inactive compound, and finally the excretion of the drug (Figure 1.1). *Pharmacokinetics* is the term applied to that area of pharmacology in which the factors that influence the absorption, distribution, tissue binding, metabolism, and excretion of drugs are elucidated.[1,2] Indeed, the principles apply whenever *any* drug is taken, whether for medical or recreational purposes. Thus, let us consider briefly the physiological and biochemical processes involved.

Drug Administration and Absorption

The terms *drug administration* and *drug absorption* refer to those mechanisms by which drugs are transported from the point of entry—stomach, intestine, or lungs—into the bloodstream. When administering any drug, one must be able to select a *route* of administration, a *dose* of the drug, and a *dosage form* (liquid, tablet, capsule, injection) that will place the drug at its site of action in a

Figure 1.1

Schematic representation of the fate of a drug in the body. (IV = intravenous; IN = intranasal; SM = smoked). [from C. N. Chiang and R. L. Hawks, "Implications of Drug Levels in Body Fluids: Basic Concepts," in R. L. Hawks and C. N. Chiang, eds., *Urine Testing for Drugs of Abuse*, NIDA Research Monograph No. 73 (Rockville, Md.: National Institute on Drug Abuse, 1986), p. 63.]

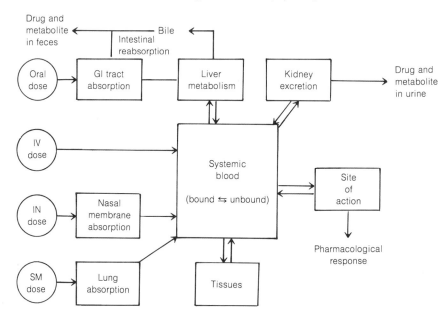

pharmacologically effective concentration and maintain this concentration for an adequate period of time.

Drugs are most commonly administered in four ways: *orally* (through the mouth), *rectally* (into the rectum), *parenterally* (by injection), and by *inhalation* through the lungs. Occasionally, drugs, such as nasal decongestants and antiasthma drugs, are administered through the *membranes of the mouth or nose.* A heart patient taking nitroglycerine, for instance, places the tablet under the tongue and the drug is absorbed into the bloodstream directly from the mouth. Cocaine, when sniffed, is absorbed through the nose, because the powdered drug adheres to the membranes on the inside of the nose and is absorbed directly into the bloodstream. Let us consider these methods of administration and absorption in more detail.

Absorption by Mouth

Drugs are most commonly taken by mouth. To be administered orally, the drug must be soluble in stomach fluid, be carried to the intestine, penetrate the lining of the intestine, and pass into the bloodstream. Indeed, the degree to which a drug can be absorbed depends on its solubility (in stomach fluid) and permeability (through the lining of the intestine).

Although alcohol is taken by mouth, it is absorbed slightly differently. Some is absorbed directly through the stomach into the bloodstream (a faster rate of absorption, because the stomach contents need not first be emptied into the intestine). If one drinks on an empty stomach, the effects of the alcohol may be felt very rapidly. If one drinks on a full stomach, the drug may pass into the intestine with the ingested food (into which it can dissolve), absorption is delayed, and its effects are slower to appear.

Drugs administered in liquid form, being already in solution, tend to be more rapidly absorbed than those given in tablet or capsule form. In solid form, the rate at which the drug dissolves becomes a limiting factor in its absorption. Occasionally, drugs are poorly manufactured and may fail to dissolve in the stomach. They may then pass through the intestine and be excreted in the feces without being absorbed into the body.

The dissolving and subsequent absorption of drugs into the bloodstream are fairly simple processes. The passage of a drug across the stomach lining, however, is more complicated (the process is explained in Appendix IV).

Although oral administration of drugs is widely used, it does have disadvantages. First, it may lead to occasional vomiting and stomach distress. Second, although the amount of a drug that is put into a tablet or capsule can be calculated, how much of it will be absorbed into the blood cannot always be predicted accurately owing to unexplained differences between individuals or differences in the manufacture of the drug. (Indeed, different brands of the same drug may be absorbed at widely differing rates.) Third, some drugs, such as procaine and insulin, when administered orally, are destroyed by the acid of the stomach before they are absorbed. To be effective, such drugs must be administered by injection.

Absorption through the Rectum

Although the primary route of drug administration is oral, some drugs are administered rectally (usually in a suppository) if the patient is vomiting, unconscious, or cannot swallow. However, absorption is often irregular, unpredictable, and incomplete, and many drugs irritate the membranes that line the rectum.

Absorption through the Lungs

Administration by inhalation or injection are the more frequently used alternatives to oral administration and both methods bypass the gastrointestinal tract.

Drugs administered as gases penetrate the cell linings of the respiratory tract easily and rapidly. Anesthetic gases (such as nitrous oxide or ether) have small molecular sizes and high fat solubility. Therefore, these gases pass through the membranes of the lungs nearly as fast as they are inhaled. They are absorbed promptly because of the close contact between the blood and the membranes of the lung. With very volatile substances (such as anesthetic gases), inhalation produces effects almost as fast as intravenous administration.

Despite our knowledge about the rapid absorption of gases, very little is known about the pulmonary absorption of other, non-gaseous drugs. Cigarettes and marijuana are examples, because their active ingredients are not gases but particles carried in the smoke. Although many drugs *appear* to be absorbed readily when inhaled as sprays, aerosols, smoke, or dust, knowledge of the extent and rate of absorption is incomplete. However, from hundreds of years of experience with nicotine, opium, and marijuana it is clear that inhalation is an effective mode of administration.

It is also well known that inhalation of substances that are not volatile, such as tars, which are abundant in inhaled cigarette smoke, can injure the sensitive tissues of the lung. Lung cancer, which can be induced by long-term inhalation of cigarette smoke, is thought to be fatal in over 90 percent of cases and is estimated to result in 72,000 deaths a year in the United States. It is not yet clear what will be the untoward effects produced by long-term inhalation of smoke obtained from marijuana.

Absorption by Injection

Administration of drugs by injection can be *intravenous* (directly into a vein), *intramuscular* (directly into a muscle), or *subcutaneous* (just under the skin). Each of these avenues has its advantages and disadvantages (Table 1.1), but some features are shared by all. In general, administration by injection produces a more prompt response than is obtainable by oral administration because absorption is more rapid after injection. More accurate dosage is attained with injection because the destruction of the drug in the gastrointestinal tract is avoided and the unpredictable process of absorption through the stomach lining is bypassed.

Administration by injection, however, has several drawbacks. First, because of the rapid rate of absorption (because the absorption processes through the stomach and intestine are bypassed), there is often little time to respond to an unexpected drug reaction or accidental overdose. Second, administration by injection requires sterile conditions. The current AIDS crisis is a vivid example of an

Table 1.1

Some characteristics of drug administration by injection.

Route	Absorption pattern	Special utility	Limitations and precautions
Intravenous	Absorption circumvented Potentially immediate effects	Valuable for emergency use Permits titration of dosage Suitable for large volumes and for irritating substances, when diluted	Increased risk of adverse effects Must inject solutions *slowly*, as a rule Not suitable for oily solutions or insoluble substances
Subcutaneous	Prompt, from aqueous solution Slow and sustained from repository preparations	Suitable for some insoluble suspensions and for implantation of solid pellets	Not suitable for large volumes Possible pain or necrosis from irritating substances
Intramuscular	Prompt, from aqueous solution Slow and sustained, from repository preparations	Suitable for moderate volumes, oily vehicles, and some irritating substances	Precluded during antigoagulant medicine May interfere with interpretation of certain diagnostic tests (e.g., creatine phosphokinase)

Modified from L. Z. Benet and L. B. Sheiner,[1] p. 6.

untoward result of unsterile injection techniques. Third, once a drug is administered it cannot be recalled.

An overdose of an orally administered drug may be counteracted by the induction of vomiting if the drug has not yet been completely absorbed into the bloodstream. In a hospital emergency room, a conscious patient who has ingested a large dose of barbiturates in a suicide attempt may be induced to vomit any undissolved tablets or capsules or any unabsorbed (although dissolved) drug. If the patient is *unconscious*, however, vomiting is usually *not* induced because the vomitus may be inhaled into the lungs, so a tube is passed into the stomach and the drug is washed out.

Intravenous Administration   In an intravenous (abbreviated i.v.) injection, a drug is introduced directly into the bloodstream. This technique avoids all the variables of oral absorption, and the drug is placed in the circulation with minimum delay. In addition, the dose of the drug can be controlled. The injection can be made slowly and it can be stopped instantaneously if untoward effects develop. Finally, the intravenous route permits the greatest accuracy in dosage, allows one to give large volumes of solution over a long period of time, and enables one to administer solutions that could irritate the veins if they were not given slowly, so they can be diluted in a large volume of fluid (the blood).

The intravenous route has several important drawbacks, however. First, it is the most dangerous of all avenues of drug administration because of the speed of onset of pharmacological action, which is faster than that of intramuscular or subcutaneous injection. Second, if a normally safe dose is given too rapidly, catastrophic and life-threatening effects (such as collapse of respiration or of heart function) may result. Third, allergic reactions to the drug may be mild when the drug is administered orally but may be extremely severe when the same drug is administered intravenously. Fourth, drugs that are not soluble in the blood or drugs dissolved in oily liquids may not be given intravenously because of the danger of blood clots forming. Finally, infection by bacterial contaminants is a continuous danger, and infectious diseases or abscesses may be induced unless sterile techniques are employed.

Intramuscular Administration   Drugs injected into skeletal muscle (usually in the arm or the buttocks) are generally absorbed fairly rapidly. Absorption of a drug from muscle is more rapid than absorption of the same drug from the stomach but is slower than when the drug is administered intravenously. The absolute rate of absorption of a drug from muscle depends on the rate of the blood flow to that muscle, the solubility of the drug, and the volume of the injection.

In general, most of the precautions that apply to intravenous administration apply to intramuscular injection. However, drugs intended for intramuscular administration should not usually be given intravenously, and one must be careful to avoid hitting a blood vessel when inserting a needle into muscle. Such an accident would result in inadvertent i.v. injection.

Subcutaneous Administration   Absorption of drugs that have been injected under the skin (subcutaneously) is quite rapid. The exact rate depends mainly on the ease with which the drugs penetrate the walls of the blood vessels and the rate of the blood flow through the skin. Irritating drugs should not be injected subcutaneously because they may cause severe pain and local tissue damage. The usual precautions to maintain sterility apply.

Self-administration of any drug by injection is to be discouraged except in certain circumstances (such as the injection of insulin by a diabetic) where oral administration is ineffective or when the drug is being taken therapeutically under a physician's direction. The risks associated with injection of a drug (risks of infection, overdose, allergic responses, and so forth) are often far greater than those associated with the oral administration of the same drug.

Distribution of Drugs throughout the Body

Once it is absorbed into the bloodstream, a drug is distributed throughout the body by the circulating blood. However, even after the drug reaches the bloodstream, it must still pass across various barriers in order to reach its site of action. Only a very small portion of the total amount of a drug in the body at any one time is in direct contact with the specific cells ("receptors") that produce the pharmacological action of the drug. Most of the drug is to be found in areas of the body remote from the drug's site of action. In the case of psychoactive drugs [drugs that alter mood or behavior as a result of their effect on the central nervous system (CNS)], most of the drug is located outside the brain and, therefore, does not contribute directly to the pharmacological effect.

Most discussions on psychoactive drugs cover only the amount of a drug in the brain that actively produces the pharmacological and psychological effects. Yet it is the total amount of a drug in the body that (1) governs the movements of the drug through the tissues and its ultimate elimination and (2) determines both the length of time and the intensity of the drug's effect.

Distribution of Drugs by Blood

Each minute the heart pumps approximately 5 liters (1 liter = 2.1 pints) of blood. Because the total amount of blood in the circulatory system is only about 6 liters, the entire blood volume circulates in the body about once per minute. Once a drug is absorbed into the blood, it is quite rapidly (usually within this 1-minute circulation time) distributed throughout the circulatory system.

A schematic diagram of the circulatory system is presented in Figure 1.2. Blood returning to the heart through the veins is first pumped into the pulmonary (lung) circulation system where carbon dioxide is removed and replaced by oxygen. The oxygenated blood then returns to the heart and is pumped into the great artery (the aorta). From there, blood flows into the smaller arteries and finally into the capillaries, where nutrients (and drugs) are exchanged between the blood and the cells of the body.

To perform this exchange, the body has an estimated 10 billion capillaries having a total surface area of more than 200 square meters. Probably no single functioning cell of the body is more than

Figure 1.2

The heart and circulatory system. Blood returning from the body tissues to the heart via the veins passes through the right atrium into the right ventricle and, with the contraction of the heart, is pumped into the arteries leading to the lungs. In the lungs, carbon dioxide (CO_2) is lost and replaced by oxygen (O_2). This oxygenated blood returns to the heart through the left atrium, is pumped out of the left ventricle into the aorta, and is carried to the body tissues, where oxygen and nutrients are exchanged in the capillary beds. Oxygen and nutrients are supplied to the body tissues through the walls of the capillaries; CO_2 and other waste products are returned to the blood. The CO_2 is eliminated through the lungs, and the other waste products are excreted through the kidneys.

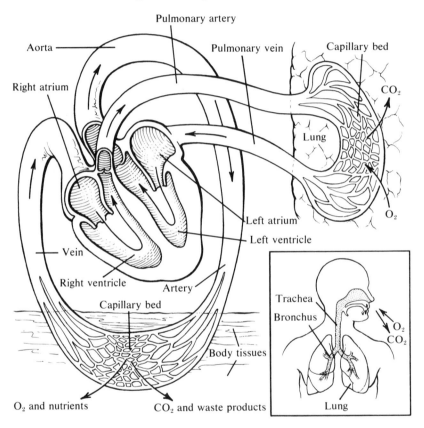

20 to 30 micrometers away from a capillary (1 micrometer = 0.0004 inch). A discussion of the structure and function of the capillary is presented in the following discussion. After blood passes through the capillaries, it is collected by the veins and returned to the heart to circulate again.

Thus, drugs are fairly evenly distributed in the blood. A normal, lean 150-pound man, however, contains approximately 41 liters of water (58 percent of the total body weight is composed of water). Therefore, if 41 liters represents the total body water and 6 liters of this represents the volume of the circulating blood, the remaining 35 liters of water must be in the body tissues. However, this water is not isolated from the blood, for fluids (and drugs) are transferred between the blood and the body fluids in and around the cells of the body. Thus, drugs are diluted not only by the blood but also by body water, because virtually all drugs can move out of the bloodstream and into the fluid that closely surrounds the cells of the body tissues. If the drug is capable of penetrating the cells, it will be further diluted by the intracellular fluids.

In addition to solubility, there is another factor that often limits the distribution of a drug in the body. Large amounts of many drugs may actually become bound firmly to proteins contained in the blood. Because blood proteins (albumin, for example) are quite large and thus are unable to leave the bloodstream, a drug that is bound to protein is confined within the blood vessels. Unable to leave the bloodstream, such a drug is prevented from reaching the cells of the body tissues. The confinement of a drug within the blood vessels might appear to render it useless. Indeed, if the drug's site of action is outside the blood vessels (in the brain, for example), its binding to blood proteins decreases its effectiveness. The more common situation, however, is that only small amounts of a drug are bound to blood proteins and the distribution of a drug may be more general, that is, throughout the body. Alcohol, for example, eventually can be found in equal concentrations throughout all the body water.

Unequal distribution among body water compartments is illustrated for three drugs in Figure 1.3. After absorption from the stomach into the bloodstream, drug 1 is bound almost completely to protein and is confined to the bloodstream. Drug 2 is not bound to blood proteins and passes easily out of the bloodstream into tissue fluid, but it is unable to pass into cells and therefore does not have access to the fluid inside them. Drug 3 is a compound that passes easily from the bloodstream and readily penetrates cell membranes into the fluid inside. An example of this last drug is thiopental (Pentothal), a commonly used anesthetic that induces anesthesia within a matter of seconds after i.v. injection. Thiopental is extremely soluble in the fat of cell membranes, so it can rapidly leave the bloodstream and pass into brain cells where it quickly depresses the brain and abolishes consciousness.

Body Membranes That Affect Drug Distribution

The absorption and distribution of drugs are affected by various types of membranes in the body. The four types of membranes most per-

Figure 1.3

Distribution of three hypothetical drugs into different body compartments. *Drug 1* is bound to blood proteins; *drug 2* is unbound, soluble in water but insoluble in fat; *drug 3* is unbound and soluble in both water and fat. Note that *drug 1* is largely restricted to the bloodstream, *drug 2* is distributed in the blood and in the fluid outside the body cells, and *drug 3* is distributed through all the body compartments and readily passes into the brain, easily crossing the blood-brain barrier.

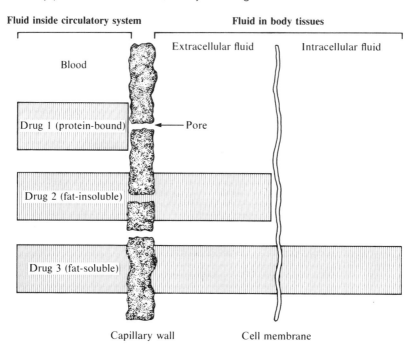

tinent to this discussion are those of (1) the cell walls, (2) the walls of the capillary vessels of the circulatory system, (3) the blood-brain barrier (a barrier that affects the passage of drugs into the brain), and (4) the placental barrier. Let us consider each of these.

Cell Membranes   To be absorbed from the intestine or to gain access to the interior of a cell, a drug must penetrate the cell membranes. What, then, is known of the structure and properties of such membranes that determine their permeability to drugs? The generalized picture that has emerged from chemical, physiological, and electron micrograph studies is represented in Figure 1.4. In this figure, the two layers of circles represent the protein head groups of complex protein-lipid molecules called phospholipids. These protein heads form a rather continuous layer on both the inside and outside of the cell membrane. The wavy lines that extend from the

Figure 1.4

Structure of the cell membrane. The inner and outer layers of the cell membrane are represented by circles and chemically are the protein groups of complex protein-fat molecules called phospholipids. The central core of the membrane is represented by wavy lines. This core consists of the fatty portions of the phospholipid molecules. The large globular structures represent large protein molecules located on the surface of the membrane and extending into or completely through the membrane. [After S. J. Singer and G. L. Nicolson, "The Fluid Mosaic Model of the Structure of Cell Membranes," *Science* 175 (1972): 720. Copyright © 1972 by the American Association for the Advancement of Science.]

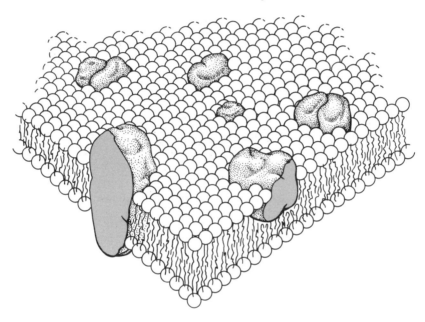

protein heads into the central core of the membrane are the lipid chains of the phospholipid molecules. Therefore, for our present purposes, the interior of the cell membrane can be considered to consist of a sea of liquid lipid in which large proteins float. This has been termed the *fluid mosaic model.*

Notice in Figure 1.4 that there appear to be several large globules situated on the outer layer of the membrane that extend either into or, in some cases, through the three layers of the membrane. These globules represent very large protein structures. The total thickness of this membrane is about 80 angstroms. (The angstrom, which is abbreviated Å, is equal to 0.0001 micrometer or 0.00000004 inch.) This membrane, consisting of protein and fat, provides a barrier that is permeable to some drug molecules and impermeable to others. From this model, it is not surprising that penetration through the membrane and thus into a cell by a drug molecule correlates with the solubility of that drug in oil (since oil is a fat and the core of this membrane consists of fat molecules).

In addition to this layered structure of protein and fat, the membrane appears to contain small holes or pores (about 8 Å in diameter) that permit the passage of small water-soluble molecules, such as alcohol and water itself. These cellular barriers (as hindrances to the absorption and distribution of drugs) are important for the passage of drugs from the stomach and intestine into the bloodstream, from the fluid that closely surrounds tissue cells to the interior of cells, from the interior of cells back into the body water, and from the kidneys back into the bloodstream. Most drugs are too large to penetrate the small pores and, thus, most water-soluble, fat-insoluble drugs cannot pass through the cellular barriers. (Appendix IV offers an expanded discussion of the properties of drugs that determine their relative solubilities in cell membranes.)

Blood Capillaries   As we have already discussed, drug molecules are distributed throughout the body by means of the circulating blood. Within a minute or so after a drug enters the bloodstream, it is distributed fairly evenly through the bloodstream. However, most drugs are not confined to the bloodstream because they are exchanged back and forth across the blood capillaries.

Figure 1.5 is a cross-sectional diagram of a capillary. Capillaries

Figure 1.5

Cross section of a blood capillary. Within the capillary are the fluids, proteins, and cells of the blood, including the red blood cells. The capillary itself is made up of cells that completely surround and define the central cylinder (or lumen) of the capillary. Water-filled pores form channels allowing communication between the lumen and the fluid outside the capillaries.

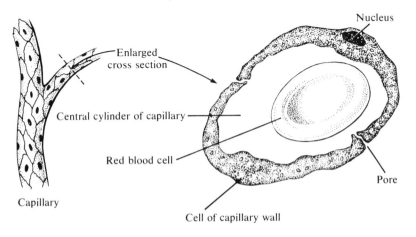

are tiny cylindrical tubes with walls formed by a thin, unicellular layer of cells tightly packed together and surrounded (for structural rigidity) by a thin "basement" membrane. Between the cells are minute passageways (pores) connecting the interior of the tube (the capillary) with the exterior (the body tissues). These pores have a diameter of between 90 and 150 Å and are larger than most drug molecules. Because it is only in the capillaries that drugs are exchanged between blood and body cells, the capillaries must be small (to bring water and essential body nutrients into close contact with the surrounding cells) and numerous (10 billion, it has been estimated).

Because most drug molecules are smaller than the pores, drugs are able to pass out of the capillaries into surrounding tissue with only minimal difficulty. As a result, most drugs reach the cells of most body tissues within a fairly short time, limited primarily by the rate of blood flow to the tissue. Therefore, in the transport of drug molecules out of blood capillaries and into tissues (and conversely from tissues back into the blood through the capillaries), it does not matter whether a drug is soluble in fat because the membrane pores are large enough for even fat-insoluble drug molecules to penetrate. These drug molecules traverse the capillary membrane at a rate roughly proportional to the difference in concentration of the drug on either side of the capillary membrane; that is, the higher the concentration of the drug in the blood and the lower the concentration in the tissues, the faster the drug diffuses out of the capillary.

These pores in the capillary membrane, however, are sufficiently small that the red blood cells and the blood proteins are largely confined to the bloodstream. Thus, the only drugs that do not readily penetrate capillary membranes are those rare drugs that are proteins and those that are bound to blood proteins. Because significant amounts of many drugs may be bound to blood protein and these proteins do not readily diffuse across the capillary membrane, this bound fraction of a drug is essentially trapped in the bloodstream and will not diffuse from the blood into the tissues. If a drug is capable of leaving the capillaries readily, its concentration in the blood will decline extremely rapidly and the drug might have both a rapid onset and a short duration of action.

The rate at which drug molecules enter specific body tissues depends upon two factors: the rate of blood flow through the tissue, and the ease with which drug molecules pass through the capillary membranes. Because blood flow is greatest to the brain and much poorer to the bones, joints, and fat deposits, drug distribution, everything else being equal, should follow a similar pattern. However, some capillaries (such as those in the brain) have special structural properties that may further limit the diffusion of a drug into the brain.

The Blood-Brain Barrier   The brain requires a protected environment to function normally, and the *blood-brain barrier* plays a key role in maintaining it.[3] This structural barrier involves specialized cells in the brain that affect nearly all its blood capillaries (see Figure 1.6). In most of the rest of the body, pores are present in the capillary membranes; in the brain, however, the capillaries are tightly joined together and covered on the outside by a fatty barrier called the glial sheath that arises from nearby astrocyte cells.

Figure 1.6

The blood-brain barrier. Blood and brain are separated both by capillary cells packed tightly together and by a fatty barrier called the glial sheath, which is made up of extensions (glial feet) from nearby astrocyte cells (*see inset*). A drug diffusing from blood to brain must move through the cells of the capillary wall because there are tight junctions rather than pores between the cells, and it must then move through the fatty glial sheath.

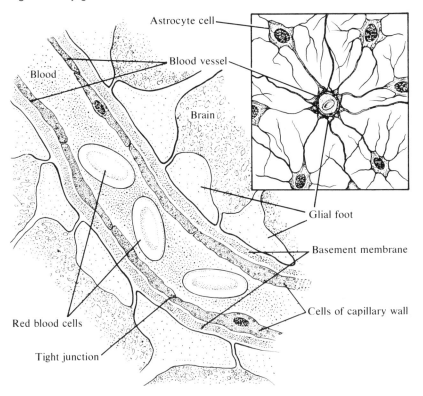

Thus, a drug leaving the capillaries in the brain has to traverse both the capillary cell wall itself (because there are no pores to pass through) and the membranes of the astrocyte cells in order to reach the cells in the brain. Passage of certain drugs (penicillin, for example) as well as ions and blood components is greatly restricted and so these drugs are unevenly distributed between blood and brain tissue. This decreased permeability of the capillaries in the brain to some substances is frequently described by the term blood-brain barrier. This term is very common and is useful for distinguishing drugs that can penetrate the brain from those that cannot.

The Placental Barrier   Among all the membrane systems of the body, the placenta is unique. It separates two distinct human beings with differing genetic compositions, physiological responses, and sensitivities to drugs. The fetus obtains essential nutrients and eliminates metabolic waste products through the placenta without depending on its own organs, many of which are not yet functioning. This dependence of the fetus on the mother, however, places the fetus at the mercy of the placenta when foreign substances (such as drugs) appear in the mother's blood.

Pregnant women in the United States regularly take an average of four prescription drugs and many other drugs purchased without prescriptions, and they have an undetermined exposure to potentially toxic substances in food, cosmetics, household chemicals, and the general environment. The extent to which these latter substances affect the fetus is not yet known. The consequences of maternal alcohol ingestion and cigarette smoking on fetal growth and development are now well documented and will be discussed in Chapters 4 and 5.

The effects of drugs on the fetus are of two major types. First, early in pregnancy, when the limbs and organ systems are forming, drugs may induce structural abnormalities (teratogenesis). Thalidomide was the most dramatic example of a teratogenic compound. This tranquilizer was marketed in several countries in the early 1960s, and, when given to women in the fifth through seventh weeks of pregnancy, produced a high incidence of abnormal growth of the limbs in the fetus. Second, later in pregnancy and during delivery, drugs may induce respiratory depression in the newborn baby because the baby is unable to metabolize or excrete them.

Schematic representations of the placental network, which transfers substances between mother and fetus, are shown in Figures 1.7 and 1.8. In general, the mature placenta consists of a network of vessels and pools of maternal blood into which protrude treelike or fingerlike villi (projections) containing the blood capillaries of the fetus (Figure 1.8). Oxygen and nutrients move from the mother's

Figure 1.7

Placenta, embryo, and section through part of uterus. [Redrawn from W. J. Hamilton, J. D. Boyd, and H. W. Mossman, *Human Embryology: Prenatal Development of Form and Function* (Baltimore: Williams & Wilkins, 1962), fig. 86, p. 85. Courtesy of Professors Hamilton, Boyd, and Mossman and Mr. Heffer.]

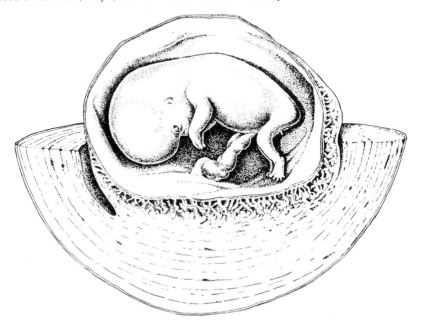

blood to that of the fetus, while carbon dioxide and other waste products move from the fetal to the maternal blood.

The membranes separating fetal blood from maternal blood in the intervillous space resemble, in their general permeability, cell membranes found elsewhere in the body. Fat-soluble substances diffuse across readily, while fat-insoluble substances diffuse less well. This is of interest because late in pregnancy and at the time of delivery most anesthetic liquids and gases and most pain-relieving agents penetrate both the blood-brain barrier and placenta very readily.

Anesthetics and narcotic analgesics may be found in fairly high concentrations in the newborn infant. There are numerous instances of withdrawal symptoms in infants born of addicted mothers, proving that morphine and other narcotics have free access to, and will affect, the fetus during pregnancy. Tranquilizing and sedating drugs also cross the placenta quite readily. The blood levels of a barbiturate administered intravenously to mothers in labor are plotted in Figure 1.9. The blood concentrations of the drug were determined in both

Figure 1.8

Placental network separating the blood of mother and fetus. [From C. M. Goss, ed., *Gray's Anatomy of the Human Body,* 29th ed. (Philadelphia: Lea & Febiger, 1973, fig. 2.51, p. 40.]

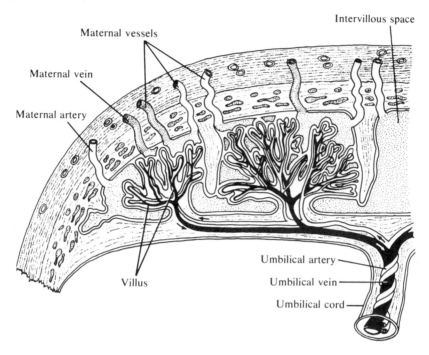

maternal and fetal blood. One can see from this figure that significant amounts of the barbiturate are distributed to the infant and that blood levels in the mother and the newborn baby are almost identical about 10 minutes after injection.

Data are not currently available about a possible relation between the extent of drug use at delivery and overall infant mortality. It is clear, however, that infants of mothers who are delivered under deep anesthesia are often less active than those delivered without benefit of drugs or with only small doses of depressants or narcotics and are physically and mentally depressed for the next 24 hours. The situation is further compounded by the fact that newborn babies, especially premature infants, have a very limited capacity to metabolize and excrete the drugs after delivery. Until more extensive details of drug effects are known, the fetus will continue to be treated with its mother in a rather haphazard manner, often inappropriately and sometimes with tragic results. The effects of drugs on the fetus are further discussed later in this chapter.

Figure 1.9

Effect of barbiturate on mothers in labor. Blood levels of secobarbital in mothers and their newborn infants after intravenous administration of the drug to the mothers. Each point represents one subject (*circles*, mothers; *asterisks*, infants). [From B. Root, E. Eichner, and I. Sunshine, "Blood Secobarbital Levels and Their Clinical Correlation in Mothers and Newborn Infants," *American Journal of Obstetrics and Gynecology* 81 (1961): 948.]

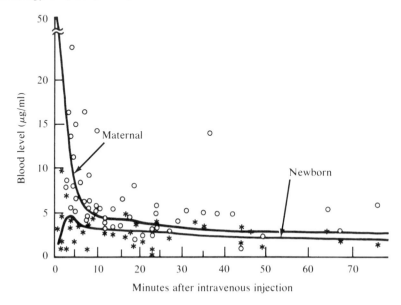

The Drug Receptor and the Myth of the "Magic Bullet"

Before producing a change in the functioning of a cell, which then leads to a change in body function or behavior, a drug must physically interact with one or more constituents of the cell. The cell component directly involved in this initial action of a drug is usually termed its *receptive substance* or, more simply, the drug *receptor*. It has been concluded from many years of pharmacological research that drugs attach to specific receptors on the cell membrane and such occupation of a receptor by a drug leads to a change of the functional properties of the cell.

A characteristic of the drug receptor is its high (but not absolute) degree of specificity for a drug molecule. What may appear to be a slight or insignificant variation in the chemical structure of a drug may greatly alter the intensity of the cell's response to it. For example, amphetamine and methamphetamine are both powerful stimulants of the central nervous system. They differ chemically only very slightly, but the change is such that methamphetamine is much more potent and, at equal doses of both drugs, produces much greater behavioral stimulation. Both drugs probably affect the same receptor in the brain but, for some reason, methamphetamine exerts a much more powerful action on it.

The drug molecule with the "best fit" to the receptor will elicit the most response from the cell. Thus, methamphetamine might "fit" the receptor better than amphetamine does. It is currently thought that the cellular response that follows the attachment of a drug to the receptor is followed by a change in the conformation of the cell membrane—a change that is thought to alter the cellular behavior and ultimately brain or body function.

In television cartoon advertisements for analgesic tablets, we see the compound being taken orally, dissolving in the stomach, being absorbed into the bloodstream, and then being rapidly (some more rapidly than others, according to the commercial message) distributed exclusively to the receptors (with hammers, pistons, lightning bolts, and so on) in the brain, which are immediately depressed so that the headache magically disappears. Thus, even in this day and age, a drug is often promoted as being some type of "magic bullet," which, upon being swallowed, immediately knows where its receptor is, streaks to that receptor, and in some mysterious way exerts its effect.

This idea of a drug's being selectively distributed to a very small area of the body is, of course, false. Subject to the physical and chemical factors discussed in this chapter, drugs are distributed through the body fairly evenly. There is no such thing as a magic bullet that somehow affects a specific target organ. Selectivity of drug action is more a function of the location of the drug receptors, the strength of the drug's attachment to the receptor, and the consequences of the interaction between drug and receptor than it is a property of selective distribution of the drug.

Termination of Drug Action

Drug action may terminate even though the drug is still present in the body. For example, the anesthetic agent thiopental, because of its high fat solubility, penetrates the brain and produces unconsciousness within a few seconds. The duration of unconsciousness is quite short (the patient awakens within 5 or 10 minutes) because thiopental (being so soluble in fat) is rapidly removed from the brain and transported to fatty deposits in the body. Even though the patient is awake, he or she is not completely "normal," because small amounts of thiopental are still present in the blood and brain. Most of the drug is stored in muscle and fat awaiting metabolism and excretion.

Another example of a drug whose action is reduced by redistribution before it is metabolized is fentanyl (Sublimaze), a narcotic widely used in anesthesia and known on the street as "China White." Fentanyl produces rapid and intense pain relief and euphoria. When it is administered intravenously, these effects disappear within about 15 minutes, although the drug remains in the body for several hours (see The Time Course of Drug Distribution and Elimination, below). The redistribution of fentanyl from the brain, the site of the analgesic and euphoriant actions, to muscle and fatty deposits results in the termination of the effects. Because the amount of a drug present in the blood reflects the amount stored in body tissues, low levels of fentanyl being released by the muscles and fatty deposits for elimination will appear in the blood over a time course of several hours. The ultimate rate of elimination of a drug from the body is usually determined by the rate at which it is metabolized by the liver and its waste products are excreted by the kidneys. Thus, to complete our discussion of the body's response to drugs, we should describe those processes by which drugs are eliminated from the body.

Elimination of Drugs by the Kidneys

The kidneys are the main excretory organs of the body. There are three other channels for excreting waste substances and drugs—the lungs, the skin, and the intestine—but these are less important. (They are discussed briefly later in this chapter.)

Physiologically, the kidneys perform two major functions: first, they excrete most of the products of body metabolism (including drugs), and second, they closely regulate the levels of most of the substances found in body fluids. The kidneys are a pair of bean-shaped organs (see Figure 1.10), each a little smaller than a fist and weighing about a quarter of a pound. They lie at the rear of the abdominal cavity at the level of the lower ribs.

The outer portion of the kidney is made up of some two million functional units called nephrons (Figure 1.11). Each unit consists of a knot of capillaries (the glomerulus) through which blood flows from the renal artery to the renal vein. This glomerulus is surrounded by the opening of the nephron (Bowman's capsule) into which fluid flows as it filters out of the capillaries. Pressure of the blood in the glomerulus causes fluid to leave the capillaries and flow into Bowman's capsule, from which it flows through the tubules of the kidney and finally into a duct that collects fluid from several

Figure 1.10

The architecture of the kidneys.

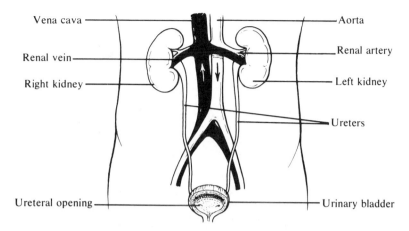

Vena cava — Aorta
Renal vein — Renal artery
Right kidney — Left kidney
Ureters
Ureteral opening — Urinary bladder

nephrons. This fluid from the collecting ducts is eventually passed through the ureters and into the urinary bladder, which is emptied periodically.

The basic function of the kidney is to maintain a proper internal environment and, in doing so, rid the blood of unwanted substances as they pass through. Substances that must be excreted include the products of body metabolism and sodium, potassium, and chloride, which accumulate in the body in excessive amounts. The kidney must also conserve water, sugar, and the necessary quantities of sodium, potassium, and chloride. The kidney rids the blood of un-wanted substances and retains ingredients essential to the body, as follows: First, a large portion of the blood, usually about one-fifth of it, is filtered into the tubules of the kidney. Left behind in the bloodstream are blood cells, proteins, and a small amount of fluid. As the filtered fluid flows through the kidney tubules, the unwanted substances fail to be reabsorbed into the bloodstream through the walls of the cells lining the tubules and pass into the urinary bladder for excretion later. Substances to be conserved are reabsorbed from the kidney into the bloodstream when they pass through the walls of the cells lining the tubules.

Because drugs are small particles dissolved in the blood, they, too, are usually filtered into the kidneys and then reabsorbed back into the bloodstream. Water is reabsorbed from the tubules into the bloodstream to a much greater extent than are most drugs, so the drugs become more concentrated inside the nephrons than they are in the blood. Because substances tend to move from areas of high concentration to areas of low concentration, drugs move out of the

Figure 1.11

A nephron within a kidney. Note the complexity of the structure and the intimate relation between the blood supply and the nephron. Each kidney is composed of more than a million such nephrons.

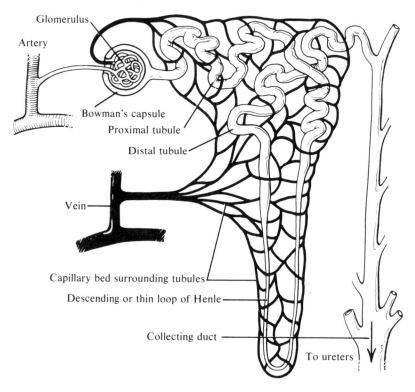

kidney back into the bloodstream. Thus, the kidney, by itself, is simply insufficient for the task of eliminating drugs from the body.

How, then, is the kidney able to function in the elimination of drugs from the body? In order for the body to hasten the urinary excretion of a drug, its reabsorption from the urine into the bloodstream must somehow be prevented. The drug must be changed by metabolic processes in the body into a compound that is less fat soluble and therefore less capable of being reabsorbed. This process of converting fat-soluble drugs into water-soluble metabolites that can be excreted by the kidney is carried out by the liver (Figure 1.12).

Free "unbound" drug in plasma is carried to the liver (by the hepatic artery and portal vein) and a portion is "cleared" from the blood by the liver cells and biotransformed (metabolized) to by-products (metabolites), which are returned to the bloodstream (see Figure 1.1). These metabolites are then transported in blood to the kidneys (Figure 1.12) for excretion.

Figure 1.12

How liver and kidneys eliminate drugs from the body. Drug may be filtered into the kidney, reabsorbed into the bloodstream, and carried to the liver for metabolic transformation to a more water-soluble compound that, having been filtered into the kidney, cannot be reabsorbed and is therefore excreted in urine.

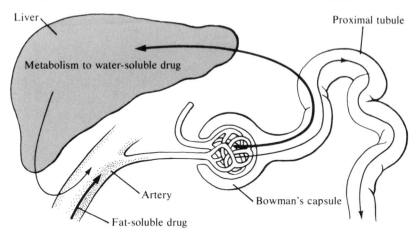

Usually (but not always) this process of metabolism also *decreases* the pharmacological activity of the drug. Thus, even though a metabolite might persist in the body (awaiting excretion), it would usually be pharmacologically inactive and would not produce the effects of the parent drug.

The exact mechanisms in the liver that result in the chemical alteration of a drug's structure are beyond the scope of our discussion, but suffice it to state that the reactions are carried out by a special system of enzymes in the liver cells. Many psychoactive drugs have the ability to *increase* the *rate* at which this enzyme system metabolizes a variety of such drugs, including themselves, thereby increasing the speed with which the drugs are eliminated. The drugs induce an increase both in enzyme activity of these cells and in the total amount of drug-metabolizing enzymes in the liver. Because these enzymes have a low specificity for drugs (that is, one enzyme may metabolize many different types of drugs), an increase in the metabolizing enzymes induced by one drug will increase the enzymes' rate of metabolizing that particular drug and a variety of others. This process will be elaborated upon later in this chapter, but it is important to note here that this enzyme-induction process is one mechanism for producing pharmacological *tolerance*, so that increasing doses of a drug must be administered in order to produce the same effect that smaller doses produced earlier.

Earlier, we discussed the processes of distribution of drugs from the mother to the fetus via the placenta. While the fetus is attached to the mother, drugs may be excreted through the umbilical cord back into the bloodstream of the mother. The mother can then eliminate the drug through her liver and kidneys. After delivery, however, the newborn baby must get rid of the drug by itself. Unfortunately, the newborn (especially the premature infant) has few drug-metabolizing enzymes in the liver, and the kidneys may not yet be fully functional. Therefore, the infant has great difficulty metabolizing and excreting drugs. If it has received a high concentration of depressants (anesthetics, narcotics, and so on) from the mother, the infant may be depressed for a long time after delivery.

Elimination of Drugs in Bile

Although excretion of drugs in bile is much less important than excretion by the kidney, many drugs, such as the antiobiotics penicillin, streptomycin, and tetracycline, are excreted to a small extent in the bile. After one of these drugs has been metabolized by the liver, it is secreted by the liver cells into the bile and passes into the intestine. There, if it is fat soluble, it may be reabsorbed by the intestine into the bloodstream and excreted by the kidney. If it is highly water soluble, however, it will remain in the intestine and be excreted with the feces.

Excretion of Drugs by the Lungs

Certain drugs may be absorbed through the lungs, such as many anesthetics, nicotine from cigarettes, cannabinols from marijuana, and the narcotic agents in opium. Although they may be absorbed by this route, nicotine, cannabinols, and opiates are *not* excreted by the lungs. They are metabolized by the liver and excreted in the urine. Anesthetic gases, however, *are* excreted by the lungs. As soon as the anesthesiologist stops administering anesthetic to the patient, the concentration of the anesthetic in the lungs drops below that in blood and the anesthetic rapidly passes back into the lungs from the bloodstream. It is then exhaled in the patient's expired air, so that eventually anesthesia is terminated.

Elimination of Drugs in Body Secretions

Besides the kidneys, bile, and lungs, other possible routes for the excretion of drugs include sweat, saliva, and milk. Many drugs and drug metabolites may be found in these secretions, but their concentrations are usually quite low, and these routes are usually not considered to be among the primary paths of drug elimination. Occasionally, however, concern arises over the transfer of drugs (such as nicotine) from mothers to their breast-fed babies. Similarly, concern has been expressed about the secretion of antibiotics administered to cows into milk that is to be consumed by humans. These topics are of obvious importance to the pharmacologist and to the Food and Drug Administration, especially because guidelines for such uses of drugs must be drawn in order to minimize the possible danger to the public.

The Time Course of Drug Distribution and Elimination

Knowledge of the relation between the *concentration* of a drug in the body and the *time* after its administration is essential for predicting the optimal dosages and dose intervals needed to reach a therapeutic effect, maintain it for the desired time, and recover from it.

Figure 1.13 illustrates this time-concentration relationship for a drug administered intravenously. Note that at time 0 the drug concentration in plasma peaks and is followed by a rapid and then a slower fall in level. The rapid fall reflects drug distribution from blood and brain to other body components, such as extracellular water, fat, and muscle. Mathematically, this distribution phase is represented by a "distribution half-life" that reflects the time it takes for distribution to reduce drug levels in plasma by 50 percent. If the distribution process lowers the plasma drug level below that required for a pharmacological effect (dotted horizontal line), the therapeutic effect must be regained by the administration of additional drug.

The slower decrease represents the time course of drug elimination from the body as a result of its metabolism (by the liver) and excretion (by the kidneys). The calculated elimination half-life reflects this process and provides insight into how long the residual effects of the drug will persist.

Figure 1.13 shows that the peak levels of pain relief produced by fentanyl are reached within seconds after i.v. injection. Fentanyl, as we have seen, rapidly redistributes to muscle and fat, reducing blood concentrations in the process. The distribution half-life of the drug is only about 8 minutes, but its half-life for elimination is about 45 minutes. As shown in Table 1.2, it takes four half-lives for 90 percent of the drug to be eliminated by the body (3 hours), and six half-lives for 98 percent elimination (4.5 hours). At this point, the patient is for most practical purposes "drug-free." It is important to remember that even though the analgesia was lost at 2 hours, the

Figure 1.13

Plasma levels of a narcotic drug (fentanyl) injected intravenously to a rat in a single bolus dose of 50 micrograms per kilogram body weight. The distribution and elimination half-lives are shown as 7.9 and 44.6 minutes, respectively. The horizontal line drawn at 1 nanogram (billionths of a gram) per milliliter plasma concentration is the level needed for analgesic effect. Thus, analgesia would be lost about 130 minutes after drug injection. [Data from C. C. Hug, Jr., and M. R. Murphy, "Tissue Redistribution of Fentanyl and Termination of its Effects in Rats," *Anesthesiology* 55 (1981): 369–375.]

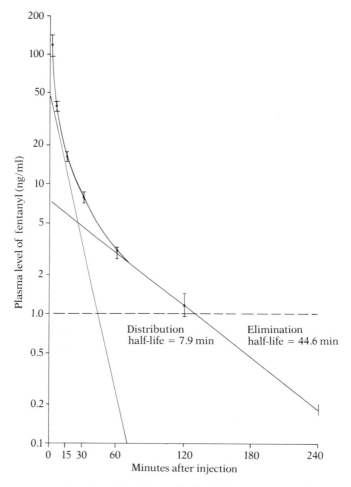

drug persisted at low levels in the body for up to 4.5 hours. The so-called drug hangover is a result of such prolonged elimination half-lives. Where appropriate throughout the text, drug half-lives will be used in referring to the duration of action of psychoactive drugs in the body. Some half-lives can be measured in days; thus, recovery from the drug may take a week or more.

Table 1.2

Half-life calculations.

Number of half-lives	Amount of drug in the body	
	% eliminated	% remaining
0	0	100
1	50	50
2	75	25
3	87.5	12.5
4	93.8	6.2
5	96.9	3.1
6	98.4	1.6

Tolerance and Dependence

Drug *tolerance* may be defined as a state of progressively decreasing responsiveness to a drug. A person who develops tolerance requires a larger dose of the drug in order to achieve the effect originally obtained by a smaller dose.

Physical dependence is an entirely different phenomenon, even though it is associated with drug tolerance in most cases. A person physically dependent on a drug needs it in order to function normally. The state of physical dependence is revealed by withdrawing the drug and noting the occurrence of withdrawal symptoms (abstinence syndrome) some time after the drug is withheld. The symptoms of withdrawal can be terminated by readministration of the drug.

Tolerance and physical dependence are thought to occur in the central nervous system, at the level of the nerve cell. However, *indirect* mechanisms may induce tolerance in the *absence* of physical dependence. For example, the administration of a barbiturate sedative may increase the amount of drug-metabolizing enzymes in the liver, with the result that some of the barbiturate would be metabolized faster and its sedative effect limited. Therefore, larger amounts of the drug will be needed to achieve an effect similar to that observed when the drug was administered for the first time if the tolerance is to be overcome.

A more specific example of this is presented in Table 1.3. In the experiment, rabbits were pretreated with three daily doses of pentobarbital (a short-acting barbiturate). The rabbits were then given a single challenging dose of pentobarbital. The length of time that

Table 1.3

Effect of pentobarbital pretreatment on the duration of pentobarbital action. Rabbits were pretreated with three daily doses of pentobarbital (60 mg/kg) subcutaneously, then given a single challenging dose of 60 mg/kg intravenously.

Pretreatment	Sleeping time (minutes)	Plasma level of pentobarbital on awakening (μg/ml)	Pentobarbital half-life in plasma (minutes)
None	67 ± 4	9.9 ± 1.4	79 ± 3
Pentobarbital	30 ± 7	7.9 ± 0.6	26 ± 2

SOURCE: H. Remmer, "Drugs as Activators of Drug Enzymes," in B. B. Brodie and E. G. Erdos, eds., *Metabolic Factors Controlling Duration of Drug Action* (*Proceedings of First International Pharmacological Meeting*), vol. 6. (New York: Macmillan, 1962), p. 235.

the rabbits slept and the amount of pentobarbital in the animals' bloodstreams at the time of awakening were measured and compared with the sleeping time and the blood levels of pentobarbital in rabbits that were not pretreated but that were given an identical dose of the drug. The data indicate that, although the pretreated animals slept less than half as long as the control rabbits, their blood levels of the drug upon awakening were approximately the same. Pretreatment had raised the animals' tolerance for the drug—not by affecting the "sleep center" in the brain, but by the induction of metabolizing enzymes in the liver that caused the drug to be metabolized and excreted more rapidly.

Such a mechanism of tolerance as the induction of drug-metabolizing enzymes does not, however, fully explain the tolerance and physical dependence that can develop with the use of many psychoactive drugs, for it accounts only for the necessity to increase the dosage to produce a drug effect. It is not uncommon to see alcoholics and people dependent on sedatives increase their dosages by factors of 10 and others dependent on narcotic analgesics increase their dosages by factors of between 10 and 20. Therefore, there must exist (and there do exist) other mechanisms in the body that are responsible for the induction of tolerance and for the withdrawal state seen when certain drugs are removed. Such mechanisms are situated within the brain and involve cellular adaptation to the continuous presence of drug at the receptors.

Drug Safety and Effectiveness

We have discussed the general principles of how the body handles a drug, but before we discuss specific drugs, we should describe briefly several other factors that influence the effects of drugs on the body.

Obviously the rates of absorption, distribution, metabolism, and excretion to a large extent determine the intensity and duration of a drug's action. Other factors contributing to the drug response include (1) the possibility that one drug will affect the body's response to another drug, (2) hypersensitivity to a drug, (3) allergy to a drug, and (4) individual sensitivity to a drug.[4] Drug toxicity—both the side effects invariably associated with a drug and the more serious toxicities, including those that may be fatal—must always be considered.

Psychoactive drugs are usually classified according to their most prominent behavioral effect. Thus, drugs are classified as depressants, stimulants, hallucinogens, narcotics, and so on. However, for a true evaluation of a drug to be made, its effects should be related to the dosage administered.

The classification of a drug as a sedative does not adequately describe the actions of the compound, at least not until one understands all that the term *sedative* implies. (The implications are discussed in Chapter 3.) At low doses, a sedative may exert little or no effect; at moderate doses, the compound may induce sedation; at higher doses, it may put the patient to sleep; at extremely high doses, it may cause death. Thus, on the basis of dosage, this drug might be classified as a placebo (a compound that exerts no real effect), a sleep-inducing agent, or a lethal substance.

The time course of drug action may be characterized by the latency of onset, the time taken to each maximum effect, and the duration of the action. These characteristics are largely determined by the rates of absorption, distribution, metabolism, and excretion of the drug. A drug that is slowly absorbed will have a long latency of onset, whereas a drug administered intravenously may have an almost instantaneous onset of action. The time needed for the drug to reach peak effect is often determined by its distribution in the body. Psychoactive drugs that cross the blood-brain barrier rapidly and reach nerve tissue quickly usually take a shorter time to reach maximum effect than do drugs that only slowly gain access to the brain. For example, both thiopental and pentobarbital (Nembutal) are sleep-inducing agents. Thiopental is more far soluble than pentobarbital and crosses the blood-brain barrier within an extremely short time (usually a few seconds). Pentobarbital, because it has some difficulty passing through the blood-brain barrier, may take many minutes to build up concentrations in the brain sufficient to induce sleep.

Similarly, rates of redistribution of a drug in the body, metabolism to inactive products, and excretion of the metabolized product determine the duration of drug action. Thiopental, with its high solubility in fat, rapidly leaves brain tissue and is carried to the muscles and fatty areas of the body. Thus, the blood levels of thiopental are quite low, so the patient awakens (the drug having left the brain, although not the body), and the drug is then slowly metabolized and excreted. Pentobarbital, being less soluble in fat, is not redistributed to the fatty areas, so the blood levels of the drug are much higher, with the result that the patient is sedated for a prolonged time—until the drug is metabolized and excreted. In order for the sedative action of pentobarbital to be terminated, the drug must be metabolized by the liver and excreted in urine. As the dosage of the drug is increased, drug effects are usually perceived earlier and the duration of action is prolonged.

Drug Interactions

It is widely appreciated that the effects of one drug can be modified by the concurrent administration of another drug. For example, alcohol, taken after a sleeping pill or a tranquilizer (discussed in Chapter 3), will increase sedation and the loss of coordination. This may be of little consequence if the dosages of each drug are low (one or two tablets and only one or two drinks), but higher dosages of either or both drugs can be dangerous both to the user and to others. If a person can normally ingest a limited amount of alcohol and still drive a car without significant loss of control or coordination, the concurrent ingestion of a tranquilizer may profoundly affect his or her driving performance, endangering driver, passengers, and other motorists. Literally hundreds of other examples could be given, and one should be aware of the danger of significant interactions occurring when more than one drug is taken at the same time.

We have already discussed two of the primary factors contributing to drug interactions. First, many drugs are bound to plasma proteins and this binding serves as a reservoir of inactive drugs. If a second drug displaces a drug already bound to the protein (by competing for the same protein), more of the previously bound drug will be able to pass out of the bloodstream and be available to the receptor and thus a more intense effect may be produced: the displacing drug would increase the effects or the toxicity (or both) of the displaced drug.

Second, in our discussion of tolerance we stated that a drug that is metabolized by the liver may induce new enzymes, which can then metabolize any of a variety of other drugs. Thus, an enzyme-inducing drug such as pentobarbital (see Table 1.3) will decrease the activity of other drugs metabolized in the liver by increasing their rates of metabolism. As can be seen, a wide variety of factors influence a drug's action in the body, making the use of more than one drug at a time risky, whether they are used separately or mixed in one concoction. Mixtures often complicate therapy because it often has not been established that more than one drug is needed, and if toxic effects should occur, it may be difficult to determine which drug is responsible.

Drug Toxicity

No drug is free of toxic effects, and while often they may be trivial, occasionally they are serious. As we mentioned earlier, no drug exerts a single effect; usually several different body functions are altered. These multiple effects of drugs occur despite the fact that one is usually interested in obtaining a single or perhaps a small number of the drug's many possible effects. The desired effect is usually considered to be the *main effect*, while the unwanted responses are labeled the *side effects*. To achieve the main effect, the side effects must be tolerated, which is possible if they are minor but may be limiting if they are more serious. The distinction between main and side effects is relative and depends on the purpose of the drug. What may be one person's side effect may be the main effect sought by another person. With morphine, for example, the pain-relieving properties may be sought, but the intestinal constipation induced is an undesired side effect and must be tolerated. However, morphine may also be used to treat diarrhea, so that the constipation induced is considered the main effect and any relief of pain a side effect.

In addition to side effects that are merely irritating, drugs may occasionally induce more serious toxic manifestations, perhaps due to allergy or hypersensitivity to the drug. Serious blood disorders, toxicity to the liver or the kidney, or abnormal fetal development (teratogenesis) may be induced. The incidence of all these serious toxic effects is fortunately quite low. Allergies to drugs may take many forms, from mild skin rashes to fatal shock caused by such drugs as penicillin. Allergy differs from normal side effects that may often be eliminated, or at least made tolerable, by a simple reduction in dosage. A reduction in the dose may be *useless* for a drug allergy because exposure to *any* amount of the drug is hazardous and possibly catastrophic.

Because drugs are concentrated, metabolized, and excreted by the liver and kidney, damage to these organs by drugs is not uncommon. An example of *drug-induced* liver damage is that caused by alcohol. Similarly, a class of major tranquilizers called the phenothiazines, of which chlorpromazine (Thorazine) is an example, may induce jaundice by increasing the viscosity of bile in the liver.

Finally, infectious hepatitis or AIDS may accompany drug injection if strict sterility is not observed.

The thalidomide tragedy dramatically illustrated how drugs may adversely influence fetal development. Much controversy has also arisen over the possible effects of LSD on fetal development. The seriousness of the problem of drug action on the fetus and the wide range of possible consequences was noted as early as 1968:

> It is clear that the risks of chemical teratogenesis . . . are accentuated during the first trimester of pregnancy. Until much more information becomes available, the very diversity of known teratogens and mutagens (drugs that alter the structure of chromosomes in the cell) should dictate caution. . . . A woman who is known to be pregnant should not be exposed to drugs at all during the first trimester unless the need is pressing. At least until experimental or statistical investigations show them to be harmless, caffeine, nicotine, and alcohol, to which people are so frequently exposed, should be regarded as possibly hazardous to the fetus during the first three months of pregnancy.[5]

The considerable data compiled since 1968 quite clearly delineate the adverse effects of nicotine and ethyl alcohol on the fetus. Indeed, these two drugs are thought to be the two major preventable health hazards in the country today. More will be said about the toxicity of these drugs in Chapters 4 and 5.

Placebo Effects

Pharmacology is concerned with the actions of drugs on biological mechanisms. The term *placebo*, however, refers to a pharmacologically *inert* substance that elicits a significant reaction. Because this action is independent of any chemical property of the drug, it arises largely because of what the individual expects, desires, or was told would happen. This placebo response seems to arise from a person's mental set or from the entire environmental situation or setting in which the drug is taken. In certain predisposed individuals, a placebo may produce extremely strong reactions with far-reaching consequences.

Even more remarkable is the demonstration that placebos may evoke patterns of altered behavior that are similar and as long lasting as those observed when a pharmacologically active drug is ingested. Thus, in discussing the pharmacology of a psychoactive agent, we must pay particular attention to the set, the setting, and the predisposition of the subjects taking it if we are to describe the pharmacological effects of a drug accurately.

Responses closely mimicking those produced by pharmacologically active drugs can be learned without drug or placebo. For instance, meditation techniques can produce states that closely resemble those produced by drugs, especially altered states of consciousness. It may, for example, be possible to use meditation to alter activity in certain centers of the brain in much the same way that a drug would alter the activity. Indeed, the placebo effect is a powerful element of drug-induced responses.

Development of New Drugs

To complete our discussion of the effects of drugs in the body, let us describe briefly the processes and procedures through which new drugs are developed and evaluated before they are released for public use.

The earliest medicinal products were usually natural in origin: crude powders of leaves or roots, or extracts from a variety of plants or animals. One of the great advances of the twentieth century was the development of organic chemistry, which has made practical the synthesis of new drug molecules that, it is hoped, offer more promise than many products obtained from natural sources. Although new drugs are occasionally discovered by accident, they usually result from systematic and tedious laboratory investigation and careful scientific observation.

The development and marketing of new drugs in the United States is rigidly controlled by the federal government through the Food and Drug Administration (FDA). Before it is marketed for general clinical use, a new drug is subjected to thorough laboratory and clinical pharmacological studies that demonstrate the usefulness and safety of the compound. Before studies in humans are permitted, the pharmacology of a new drug must be extensively delineated in animals. These studies include the establishment of the range of effective doses, the doses at which side effects occur, and the lethal doses in various animals. The studies on the safety and toxicity of the drug are evaluated after administration of single doses and during long-term use. From all these studies, a risk/benefit ratio is determined. Because of differences between species of animals, these studies must usually be carried out in at least three different species. In this preliminary testing on animals, neither the mechanism of the drug's action nor the range of its possible clinical usefulness need be completely described, although the absorption, distribution, metabolism, and excretion of the drug are carefully delineated.

Having been found safe to use in animals, the compound may be taken into initial clinical trial (phase 1), which is usually conducted on normal volunteer subjects, as well as on patients, and is aimed at establishing the drug's safety, dose range, and possible prob-

Figure 1.14

The phases of drug development in the United States. [Adapted from E. M. Ross and A. G. Gilman, "Pharmacodynamics: Mechanism of Drug Action and the Relationship between Drug Concentration and Effect," in A. G. Gilman, L. S. Goodman, T. W. Rall, and F. Murad, eds., *Goodman and Gilman's The Pharmacological Basis of Therapeutics,* 7th ed. (New York: Macmillan, 1985), p. 59.]

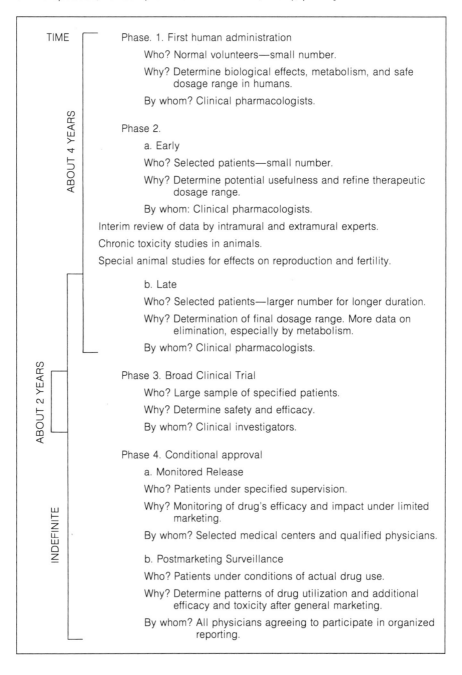

TIME

Phase. 1. First human administration

Who? Normal volunteers—small number.

Why? Determine biological effects, metabolism, and safe dosage range in humans.

By whom? Clinical pharmacologists.

Phase 2.

a. Early

Who? Selected patients—small number.

Why? Determine potential usefulness and refine therapeutic dosage range.

By whom: Clinical pharmacologists.

Interim review of data by intramural and extramural experts.

Chronic toxicity studies in animals.

Special animal studies for effects on reproduction and fertility.

b. Late

Who? Selected patients—larger number for longer duration.

Why? Determination of final dosage range. More data on elimination, especially by metabolism.

By whom? Clinical pharmacologists.

Phase 3. Broad Clinical Trial

Who? Large sample of specified patients.

Why? Determine safety and efficacy.

By whom? Clinical investigators.

Phase 4. Conditional approval

a. Monitored Release

Who? Patients under specified supervision.

Why? Monitoring of drug's efficacy and impact under limited marketing.

By whom? Selected medical centers and qualified physicians.

b. Postmarketing Surveillance

Who? Patients under conditions of actual drug use.

Why? Determine patterns of drug utilization and additional efficacy and toxicity after general marketing.

By whom? All physicians agreeing to participate in organized reporting.

ABOUT 4 YEARS

ABOUT 2 YEARS

INDEFINITE

lems requiring further study (Figure 1.14). If phase 1 studies indicate safety, the drug may be subjected to a thorough clinical pharmacological evaluation (phase 2). These studies of necessity are closely controlled to eliminate such variables as placebo response and investigator bias. Statistical validation is of paramount importance. Finally, if a drug still looks promising, it will enter phase 3 of the human studies, a period of extended clinical evaluation. In this phase, the compound is made available to investigators throughout the country for use in a variety of clinical situations. This is done in order to elicit information about the drug's safety, efficacy, side effects, dosage, variability of response, and so on.

If a drug passes all of these trials, it may receive conditional approval by the FDA for broad use by physicians and medical centers who agree to a procedure of organized reporting of therapeutic results, limitations, and problems.

Currently, it costs a pharmaceutical manufacturer more than 25 million dollars to take a new compound through laboratory and clinical testing to the marketing stage. Although this attention to detail may seem excessive, it works to the benefit of the public. Most drugs currently on the legitimate market have reasonable risk/benefit ratios; though none is completely without risk, most are relatively safe.

Notes

1. L. Z. Benet and L. B. Sheiner, "Pharmacokinetics: The Dynamics Of Drug Absorption, Distribution and Elimination," in A. G. Gilman, L. S. Goodman, T. W. Rall, and F. Murad, eds., *Goodman and Gilman's The Pharmacological Basis of Therapeutics*, 7th ed. (New York: Macmillan, 1985), pp. 3–34.
2. R. R. Levine, *Pharmacology: Drug Actions and Reactions*, 3d ed. (Boston: Little, Brown, 1983), pp. 211–247.
3. M. W. B. Bradbury, "The Structure and Function of the Blood-Brain Barrier," *Federation Proceedings* 43 (1984): 186–190.
4. R. R. Levine, *Pharmacology: Drug Actions and Reactions*, 3d ed. (Boston: Little, Brown, 1983), pp. 249–273.
5. A. Goldstein, L. Aronow, and S. M. Kalman, *Principles of Drug Action*, (New York: Harper & Row, 1968), p. 733.

CHAPTER 2

Classification of Psychoactive Drugs

A Starting Point for Understanding

Coherent discussion of psychoactive drugs requires some method of classifying them. At least three methods of classification come readily to mind, but each has its limitations. Probably the most useful method would be to classify the drugs according to their mechanisms of action, but our knowledge of the brain's physiology is too limited for this method to be comprehensive. A second method would be to identify similarities in chemical structure, on the assumption that drugs of similar chemical structure may be expected to exert similar effects. There are, however, too many drugs of apparently similar structure whose pharmacological activity is different, and too many drugs of apparently dissimilar chemical structure whose pharmacological activity is nearly identical with other drugs. A third method would be to divorce our classification entirely from scientific investigation and classify drugs according to their legality, popularity, potential for misuse, or whatever social concern is currently in vogue. The most realistic classification thus is behavioral: How does each drug affect its user's behavior? Table 2.1 presents such a classification.

Assumptions about the Classification

There are five qualifications to be aware of regarding the usefulness of this table.

First, it should be noted that the action of psychoactive drugs

Table 2.1

Classification of drugs that alter mood or behavior or that are useful in treating neurologic diseases. Only representative agents from each class of drug are listed.

1. Sedative-Hypnotic Compounds: CNS Depressants
   Barbiturates
      Long-acting: phenobarbital (Luminal)
      Intermediate-acting: amobarbital (Amytal)
      Short-acting: pentobarbital (Nembutal); secobarbital (Seconal)
      Ultrashort-acting: pentothal (Thiopental)
   Nonbarbiturate hypnotics
      Glutelthimide (Doriden)
      Methyprylon (Noludar)
      Methaqualone
   Antianxiety agents
      Meprobamate (Miltown, Equanil)
      Chlordiazepoxide (Librium)
      Diazepam (Valium)
   Others
      Ethyl alcohol; bromide; paraldehyde; chloral hydrate; anesthetic gases and liquids: ether, halothane, chloroform, etc.

2. Behavioral Stimulants and Convulsants
   Amphetamines: (Benzedrine; Dexedrine; Methedrine)
   Clinical antidepressants
      Monoamine oxidase (MAO) inhibitors; (Parnate)
      Tricyclic compounds (Tofranil; Elavil)
   Cocaine
   Convulsants: strychnine; (Metrazol; Pictrotoxin)
   Caffeine
   Nicotine

3. Narcotic Analgesics: Opiates
   Opium; heroin; morphine; codeine; (Numorphan; Dilaudid; Percodan; Demerol)

4. Antipsychotic Agents
   Phenothiazines: chlorpromazine (Thorazine)
   Reserpine (Serpasil)
   Butyrophenones: haloperidol (Haldol); droperidol (Inapsine)
   Lithium

5. Psychedelics and Hallucinogens
   LSD (lysergic acid diethylamide)
   Mescaline
   Psilocybin
   Substituted amphetamines: DOM (STP); MDA; MMDA; TMA
   Tryptamine derivatives; DMT; DET; bufotenin
   Phencyclidine (Sernyl)
   Cannabis; marijuana; hashish; tetrahydrocannabinol

6. Neurological Drugs
   Antiepileptic drugs: phenytoin (Dilantin); carbamazepine (Tegretol); valproic acid (Depakene); clonazepam (Clonopin)
   Antiparkinsonian drugs: Levodopa; amantadine (Symmetrel); bromocriptine (Parlodel)
   Drugs for Spasticity: baclofen (Lioresal); dantrolene (Dantrium)
   Nonnarcotic analgesics; aspirin; acetaminophen (Tylenol); Ibuprofen (Advil, Motrin.); indomethacin (Indocin); phenylbutazone (Butazolidin)
   Local anesthetics: procaine (Novacain); lidocaine (Xylocaine)

generally is not restricted to any one functional or anatomical sub-division of the brain. There are exceptions, of course (such as the use of l-dopa for the treatment of Parkinson's disease), but usually a psychoactive drug will affect a variety of processes simultaneously. This complicates the classification of drugs because, at different doses, different behavioral actions may predominate. Some compromises must therefore be made.

Second, the ultimate action of any given psychoactive drug may be explained by alterations in the synthesis, release, action, metabolism, and so on, of a specific neurotransmitter chemical. (The neurochemical processes that mediate transmission of information between neurons are discussed at some length in Appendix II.) However, that neurotransmitter chemical may be involved in many different activities of the brain (norepinephrine, for example, may be involved in temperature regulation, arousal, satiety, rage, and so on). Thus, although a psychoactive drug might ultimately be found to exert a single effect on a specific neurotransmitter chemical, a variety of behavioral effects would be expected because this neurotransmitter is involved in many different functions.

Third, it is important to understand that psychoactive drugs do not create *new* behavioral or physiological responses; they simply *modify* ongoing processes. Current thought holds that the behavioral effects that psychoactive drugs exert are secondary to their blocking or modifying biochemical and/or physiological processes, particularly the various steps of synaptic transmission in the brain.

Fourth, the classification of psychoactive drugs in Table 2.1 is not rigid. Different behavioral responses are observed at different doses. Alcohol, for example, is classified as a general depressant compound, despite the fact that, at low doses, behavioral excitation may be observed. Thus, classification alone does not clearly describe the pharmacology of a drug. Classification, however, serves as a starting point from which several compounds may be compared and contrasted.

Finally, in the use of centrally acting drugs, certain factors that may lead to compulsive misuse of the drug must be considered. Such factors include physiological and psychological dependence and tolerance. Psychoactive drugs differ in their potential to induce such hazards. It should be apparent, however, that any drug that is capable of favorably altering mood or behavior or of creating a pleasurable state of consciousness is capable of inducing psychological dependence—that is, a compulsion to use the drug for a favorable effect. This is not to state, however, that the use of a drug for recreation or to achieve pleasure is necessarily wrong.

The Future Discussion

In subsequent chapters we will describe specific agents within each of the classes of psychoactive agents listed in the table. Alcohol and marijuana are discussed separately (in Chapters 4 and 10). Although both agents might well be included in the chapter on sedative-hypnotic compounds (Chapter 3), because of their wide range of use, ready availability, and social and legal implications they deserve separate presentation.

Chapter 12 discusses the effects of body hormones on the brain and on behavior—for example, oral contraceptives and fertility agents. Although these are not directly related to psychoactive drugs, the chapter has been included because of the wide interest in such drugs. Because the limbic system, hypothalamus, and pituitary gland are thought to be important sites of action of these compounds, a discussion of their physiological, pharmacological, behavioral, and sociological effects seems pertinent.

Finally, two new chapters have been added to this edition. Chapter 6 presents an expanded discussion of drugs used to treat the affective disorders (mania and depression). These drugs (the antidepressants and lithium) have become widely used, and their unique properties clearly separate them from the behavioral stimulants (Chapter 5).

The drugs discussed in Chapter 11 (neurologic drugs) are totally new to this edition. Their usefulness in treating epilepsy, parkinsonism, and spasticity as well as their usefulness as nonnarcotic analgesics, anti-inflammatory agents, and local anesthetics is stressed. Chapter 11 is included to complete the presentation of centrally acting drugs and make this text more useful for comprehensive coverage of neuropsychopharmacology.

Let us now consider the first category in the table: sedative-hypnotic compounds.

CHAPTER 3

Sedative-Hypnotic Compounds

Drugs That Depress the Central Nervous System

The sedative-hypnotic compounds are drugs of diverse chemical structure capable of inducing varying degrees of behavioral depression. They are divided somewhat arbitrarily into (1) the barbiturates, (2) the nonbarbiturate hypnotics, (3) the antianxiety agents, and (4) a group of miscellaneous compounds not structurally related to those mentioned—alcohol, bromide, the general anesthetics, paraldehyde, and so on (see Table 2.1).

The classification of these compounds as sedative-hypnotics may be somewhat misleading. They are capable of inducing not only behavioral sedation or hypnosis (sleep) but also behavioral alterations, ranging from (at low doses) relief from anxiety, to sedation, release from inhibition, sleep, general anesthesia, coma, and finally (at high doses) death as a result of the depression of the respiratory centers in the medulla. (See Appendix II for a discussion of the anatomy of the brain.) This gradation of action is illustrated in Figure 3.1.

Virtually all of the sedative-hypnotic compounds discussed in this chapter are capable of inducing *any* of the states of behavioral depression depicted in the figure. Thus, while the terms sedative or tranquilizer refer to a drug that diminishes environmental awareness, spontaneity, and physical activity, higher doses produce drowsiness and lethargy and even higher doses produce sleep and unconsciousness.

Depending on the dose, therefore, any sedative-hypnotic com-

Figure 3.1

Continuum of behavioral sedation. How increasing doses of sedative-hypnotic drugs affect behavior.

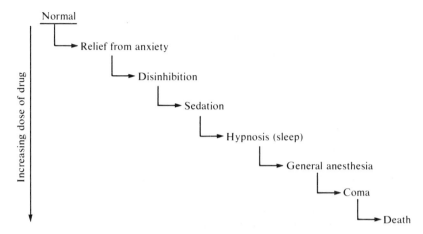

pound may be classified as a *sedative*, a *tranquilizer*, a *hypnotic*, or an *anesthetic*. The compounds do not differ from one another in their sites of actions, uses, or abilities to induce various stages of depression but, rather, in their individual potency and in the chemical differences that cause them to be handled differently by the body.

For example, a much smaller amount of secobarbital (a barbiturate) than of meprobamate (a dicarbamate) may be required to induce sleep. Secobarbital, therefore, is said to be more *potent*. But comparison by potency is rather meaningless, because such factors as safety and efficacy may be more important in determining a compound's usefulness. (The dose-response relationship is discussed in Appendix V.)

Five Principles of CNS Depressants

Because the sedative-hypnotic drugs are similar pharmacologically, let us use the barbiturates as a prototype and compare the other compounds with them. Also, because all CNS depressants are so similar in their actions, five general principles that apply fairly uniformly to all the CNS depressants can be summarized.

First, the effects of CNS depressants are *additive* with one another and with the behavioral state of the user. For example, alcohol will exaggerate the depression induced by barbiturates. Barbiturates will intensify the impairment of driving ability induced by alcohol.

Similarly, a person who is depressed or physically tired may be profoundly affected by a dose of depressant drug that would only slightly affect a person who feels normal or excited. Sedative drugs are also frequently *supra-additive* in their depressant effects. Thus, the observed depression is greater than what one would predict by calculating the depression caused by each drug individually. It may be said that the whole is greater than the sum of its parts. Such intense depression is often unpredictable and unexpected, and it can lead to dangerous or even fatal consequences. Depressant drugs should not be used in combination except with the advice and guidance of a physician, especially if one of the drugs is ethyl alcohol (Chapter 4).

Second, *antagonism* occurs between the CNS depressants and the behavioral stimulants. Such antagonism is usually nonspecific; that is, when a person is profoundly depressed by a sedative drug, the administration of a stimulant will seldom *specifically* block the action of that depressant and return the patient to normal, although the stimulant may temporarily arouse the patient. In fact, the stimulant may do more harm than good, because when it wears off, the patient will become even more depressed. What is needed clinically is a specific antagonist to CNS depressants, a drug that actually displaces the depressant from its receptors in the brain, thus immediately terminating the action of the depressant. Such a drug might save thousands of lives each year if it were used, for example, to treat individuals who had attempted suicide with CNS depressants (sleeping pills). Treatment of these individuals is at present difficult.

Third, clinical experience indicates that general depressants exert a depressant action upon all neurons within the brain and all tissues of the body. However, it is well known that low doses of these compounds induce behavioral excitement, a state that is often sought when a person wants to "get loaded" or "get drunk." The excitement is thought to be due to a depression of inhibitory neurons within the brain, which leaves one in a state of *disinhibition*. Because alcohol often induces euphoria, one occasionally finds alcohol classified mistakenly as a stimulant rather than as a depressant. It is believed that, at low doses of alcohol (or other depressant), inhibitory synapses in the brain are depressed slightly earlier than are excitatory synapses. If inhibition is depressed, behavioral excitation would be observed, because all neurons within the brain are held in a close balance between excitation and inhibition, and this would appear to account for the euphoria induced by low doses of sedative-hypnotic drugs. At higher doses, however, excitatory synapses also are depressed and sleep follows.

Methaqualone (the "love drug," see the following discussion) provides another example of the misclassification of a depressant drug. Methaqualone is a sedative-hypnotic agent of moderately low potency that, like all depressant drugs, is capable of inducing a state of disinhibition or euphoria at certain doses. During such disinhibition one might certainly feel more euphoric about sexual experiences, but such feelings are limited by at least two factors: (1) while sensation may be increased, performance may be decreased, and (2) because the effect depends on the dose, overdoses induce sleep or (with higher doses) deeper levels of behavioral depression.

Fourth, in general, behavioral depression induced by a single dose of depressant drug is seldom followed by a period of either mental or behavioral hyperexcitability after the drug action is terminated. As the drug is metabolized and excreted, the individual slowly reverts from a depressed state to a normal one. However, if large doses of depressants are *repeatedly* administered over a prolonged period of time, the depression induced *is* followed by a period of hyperexcitability which, upon withdrawal of the drug, may be quite severe and might even lead to convulsions and death. These agents, therefore, are capable of inducing physiological dependency.

Fifth, use of the sedative-hypnotic compounds has the inherent capability of inducing psychological dependence and tolerance as well. The tolerance is secondary both to the induction of drug-metabolizing enzymes in the liver (so that the drug is metabolized more rapidly) and to the adaptation of cells in the brain that enables them to function in the presence of the drug. In such instances neurons become tolerant of the presence of the drug and larger doses must be administered in order to obtain a given behavioral effect.

In addition, a remarkable degree of *cross-tolerance* may occur. This is a condition in which tolerance to one drug results in a lessened response to another drug. *Cross-dependence*, too, may be exhibited. This is a condition in which one drug can prevent withdrawal symptoms associated with physical dependence on a different drug. Essentially, any sedative-hypnotic drug can substitute for any other in the same class, regardless of chemical structure.

Historical Background

The use of depressants is as old as history. Alcohol is the oldest of these agents and in earlier days was held to be a remedy for practically all diseases and problems. In fact, in the Middle Ages alcohol was believed to be the long-sought elixir of life. More recent history of depressant drugs began with the discovery of nitrous oxide (laughing gas) by Joseph Priestley in 1772. However, nitrous oxide did not become widely used in medicine as an anesthetic for approximately

100 years and was then soon followed by other anesthetic agents, including ether and chloroform.

Although barbituric acid was first prepared in 1864, it was not until 1903 that the first barbiturate derivative was introduced into medicine as a sedative drug. This was followed in 1912 by the commercial introduction of phenobarbital. Since that time, more than 2500 barbiturates have been synthesized and approximately 50 have been marketed.

These agents (together with other depressant compounds such as bromide and paraldehyde) were the only general depressants available until the early 1950s when meprobamate (Equanil) was introduced as a "minor tranquilizer." (In reality, meprobamate appears to be pharmacologically very similar to the barbiturates introduced many years earlier, and the term "minor tranquilizer" is more a sales gimmick than a pharmacological description.) Then in about 1960, chlordiazepoxide (Librium) became the first available benzodiazepine tranquilizer. This compound and its derivative, diazepam (Valium), share many of the characteristics of the general depressants. However, they also exert specific effects on inhibitory neurotransmission (discussed in the following section), independent of the nonspecific depression that is observed at higher doses.

Site and Mechanism of Action

The barbiturates, nonbarbiturate hypnotics, ethyl alcohol, bromide, paraldehyde, chloral hydrate, and the general anesthetics are all general depressants of the central nervous system. In addition, they reduce the rate of metabolism in a variety of tissues throughout the body, depressing any system that uses energy. Most of these depressant effects, however, require high concentrations of the drug. In *normal doses,* the sedative-hypnotic compounds appear to be selective depressants of certain pathways within the brain that are involved in wakefulness. More specifically, the behavioral-depressant action of these compounds appears to result from an action on the arousal centers within the brain: the ascending reticular activating system (the ARAS) and the diffuse thalamic projection system. As we shall discuss in Chapter 5, these two centers within the brainstem and midbrain are important for the maintenance of behavioral arousal.

Depression of synaptic transmission processes within these centers appears to account for the various stages of behavioral depression induced by the sedative-hypnotic drugs. The processes of synaptic transmission are much more sensitive to these drugs than is the process of conduction along axons. Because these compounds depress synaptic transmission, one would expect that pathways with many synapses would be especially susceptible to drug-induced depression. In fact, physiological studies have demonstrated that the ARAS and the diffuse thalamic projection system are composed of multitudes of such polysynaptic pathways, which accounts for the unusual sensitivity of these areas to depressant drugs.

Because sedative-hypnotic drugs produce widespread depression of the CNS, it is not surprising to find that they are useful for a variety of purposes. Therefore, these drugs are used as sedatives, hypnotics (sleep-inducing agents), antiepileptic agents (Chapter 11), muscle relaxants, amnesics, general anesthetics, and antianxiety drugs. It should be noted, however, that the diffuse action of these agents limits their clinical usefulness for any one specific purpose, and a continuing search exists for drugs that can be used in specific situations (for example, antianxiety agents) without the same degree of generalized CNS depression.

Regarding antianxiety agents, the benzodiazepines that were once thought to be nonspecific CNS depressants have now been shown, both clinically and experimentally, to possess high antianxiety effectiveness with lower incidences of nonspecific depression. These drugs have thus become drugs of choice for the treatment of anxiety (see the following discussion). The benzodiazepines appear to be specific facilitators of synaptic transmission, which is mediated by the inhibitory neurotransmitter gamma-aminobutyric acid (GABA) (discussed in Appendix II). Benzodiazepines appear to bind to a specific receptor adjacent to GABA receptors, potentiating the actions of GABA on neurons throughout the brain. Therefore, the antianxiety, antiepileptic, sedative, and hypnotic actions of benzodiazepines appear to result from interactions with GABA and not from nonspecific CNS depression.

Drug-Induced "Brain Syndrome"

In certain psychiatric and neurological disorders, such as the dementias, a behavioral pattern characteristic of depressed nerve function is observed. To diagnose this and other psychiatric disorders, a mental status examination is performed that encompasses 12 areas of mental function (Table 3.1).

Different psychiatric disorders manifest with differing deficits in this examination. Schizophrenics, for example, have an intact sensorium, adequate memory and behavior, are cooperative, and may speak with a normal stream of talk. Their mental status examination is characterized by disturbed thought processes with absence of logic and, frequently, with misperceptions of reality. (The

Table 3.1

The mental status examination. Twelve areas of mental function.

1. General appearance
2. Sensorium:
   a. orientation to time, place, and person
   b. clear vs. clouded
3. Behavior and mannerisms
4. Stream of talk
5. Cooperativeness
6. Mood: inner feelings
7. Affect: surface expression of feelings
8. Perception
   a. illusions: misperception of reality
   b. hallucinations: not present in reality
9. Thought processes: logical vs. strange or bizarre
10. Mental content: fund of knowledge
11. Intellectual functions: ability to reason and interpret
12. Insight and judgment

pathological processes possibly involved in schizophrenia are further discussed in Chapter 7.)

In instances where neurons are reversibly depressed (as in intoxication with alcohol or other sedative-hypnotic drugs) or irreversibly damaged (as in dementia), five of the functions of the mental status examination are particularly altered: sensorium, affect, mental content, intellectual function, and insight and judgment. When a person is intoxicated with alcohol or barbiturates, for example, sensorium is clouded and the individual is disoriented as to time and place. Memory is impaired and there is frequently a retrograde amnesia with loss of short-term memory. The intellect is depressed and judgment is decreased. The individual's affect is shallow and labile; that is, he or she is very vulnerable to external stimuli and may be sullen and moody at one moment and exhibit a mock anger at the next. When such a mental status is seen, it is diagnosed as a "brain syndrome" secondary to depressed nerve-cell function.

Certain individuals (such as the elderly) who already have some natural loss of nerve-cell function are more likely to be adversely affected by these drugs. A person whose sensorium is partially clouded or who is somewhat disoriented will become even more so when these drugs are taken. The net result is increased disorientation and further clouding of consciousness. Frequently, this is manifested as a state of drug-induced "paradoxical excitement," characterized by a labile personality with marked anger, delusions, hallucinations, and confabulations. The treatment of such a drug-induced disorder is discontinuation of the sedative drug.

Uses of Sedative-Hypnotic Drugs

The major antianxiety and sedative-hypnotic drugs are listed in Table 3.2 along with their principal uses and elimination half-lives. Principal uses include relief from anxiety, treatment of insomnia, use in alcohol detoxification, prevention of epileptic seizures, and

Table 3.2

Sedative-hypnotic drugs: Principal uses and pharmacokinetic data.

Drug classification: generic (trade)	Antianxiety	Insomnia	Alcohol withdrawal	Antiepileptic	Anesthetic	Preanesthetic medication	Elimination half-life (hours)
Benzodiazepines							
Alprazolam (Xanax)	x						4–28
Chlordiazepoxide (Librium)	x		x			x	8–24
Clonazepam (Clonopin)				x			15–30
Clorazepate (Tranxene)	x		x	x			50–100
Diazepam (Valium)	x		x	x		x	20–90
Flurazepam (Dalmane)		x					50–100
Halazepam (Paxipam)	x						14–30
Lorazepam (Ativan)	x	x	x	x		x	10–20
Oxazepam (Serax)	x		x				10–25
Prazepam (Centrax)	x						20–100
Temazepam (Restoril)		x					10–20
Triazolam (Halcion)		x					2–5
Midazolam (Versed)					x	x	1–2
Quazepam (Dormalin)		x					35–40
Barbiturates							
Phenobarbital (Luminal)	x	x		x			24–140
Mephobarbital (Mebaral)				x			50–120
Amobarbital (Amytal)		x				x	10–40
Pentobarbital (Nembutal)		x					15–50
Secobarbital (Seconal)		x					15–40
Thiopental (Pentothal)					x		3–6
Methohexital (Brevital)					x		1–2
Miscellaneous Hypnotics							
Chloral hydrate (Noctec)		x					4–7
Ethchlorvynol (Placidyl)		x					10–25
Glutethimide (Doriden)		x					5–22
Methaqualone (Parest, Quaalude)[1]		x					19–41
Methyprylon (Noludar)		x					4–8
Meprobamate (Equanil)	x						10–24

[1] Removed from licit market, but widely available on illicit market.

as either a preanesthetic sedative or an agent to induce anesthesia. Of these, relief from anxiety is the most common use, although drug therapy should not be the first or the only form of treatment. Counseling by either a physician or a psychologist is the first choice and may be all that is required to resolve less severe forms of anxiety, especially situational anxiety, or anxiety that occurs secondary to another condition. For individuals with primary anxiety disorders, behavioral therapies aimed at relaxation and systematic desensitization may be useful.

For individuals who either refuse such treatment or do not adequately respond to it, antianxiety drugs may be useful. Intermittent administration during periods of greatest stress is the most rational form of therapy. Antianxiety drugs are also indicated in acute situational anxieties when suffering is genuine and normal daily activities are disrupted. The overuse of sedatives, however, may hinder the development of personal coping skills or the mobilization of social support systems in the family or the extended community. In situations where anxiety is accompanied by severe emotional depression, antidepressants (Chapter 5) are the treatment of choice, as sedatives may intensify the depression.

The essential functions of sleep are still unknown, although it is generally recognized to have a restorative quality and diminishes fatigue and dysphoria. There are several different sleep disorders, but insomnia is the most common. One-third of the U.S. population complains of poor sleep, and one-third of this group believes it to be a major problem. When a sedative-hypnotic is indicated, the choice of drug depends on the cause of insomnia.[1] If anxiety is paramount, a long-acting antianxiety drug (Table 3.2) taken at bedtime may be most appropriate. Insomnia that is caused by pain or depression may be best treated with an analgesic (Chapter 7) or antidepressant that has sedative side effects (Chapter 5). The widely used sedative-hypnotics marketed for insomnia, however, do not induce *normal* sleep as defined by electroencephalogram or eye movements (see below).

Some sedatives are also used to treat symptoms of alcohol withdrawal. In such instances a long-acting compound (note the elimination half-lives of these sedatives in Table 3.2) replaces alcohol, which has a short half-life, about 10 percent being metabolized per hour (Chapter 4). Such therapy provides a longer, often less traumatic withdrawal.

Since sedative-hypnotic drugs depress the functioning of the brain, all have antiepileptic properties. Eight of those listed in Table 3.2 are particularly useful in this regard. Finally, one agent (thiopental) is used solely as a rapid-acting anesthetic to produce unconsciousness after intravenous injection. Others produce sedation and relief from anxiety in patients about to go into surgery.

There are several limitations to the use of sedatives. These compounds are *not* analgesic and therefore they are *not* used for the relief of pain. In addition, their depressant action upon the brainstem can interfere fatally with respiration, especially when used intravenously or in suicide attempts. The other problems associated with these compounds (dependency, tolerance, and loss of coordination) will be discussed in the following section.

The Barbiturates

The barbiturates comprise a group of compounds that are capable of producing all degrees of behavioral depression, ranging from mild sedation, through anesthesia, to coma and death. The extent of the drug effect depends on several factors: the particular agent in question, the dose, the route of administration, the behavioral state of the individual when the drug is administered, and the rates of absorption, distribution, metabolism, and excretion. Thus, to describe the pharmacology of the barbiturates, we should distinguish the effects observed with the various types over a wide range of doses. Furthermore, the handling of the various types by the body should be compared and contrasted to determine the onset, intensity, and duration of the drug effect. Finally, the context in which barbiturates are taken must be carefully identified and evaluated in order to determine the effect of set and setting on the response.

Absorption, Distribution, Metabolism, and Excretion

Barbiturates traditionally have been subclassified into compounds of varying durations of action. As shown in Table 3.2, their half-lives can be quite short (5–10 minute redistribution half-life of thiopental), longer (24–48 hour half-lives for amobarbital, pentobarbital, and secobarbital), and very long (79–100 hours for butabarbital and phenobarbital). A drug's duration of action is determined by the rate it is absorbed, distributed, metabolized, and excreted.

For example, in the stomach barbiturates are in a fat-soluble form and thus are rapidly and completely absorbed into the bloodstream. As a result, they are usually administered by mouth. Occasionally, however, a short-acting barbiturate (that is, thiopental or methohexitol) is administered intravenously for use as a general anesthetic. The intravenous administration of barbiturates is a difficult technique and usually is not attempted except in emergencies or when adequate provisions are made for supporting respiration and circulation (and therefore life) in case of untoward reaction. Fatal accidents have resulted from the intravenous administration of barbiturates by inexperienced persons.

The barbiturates are well distributed to most body tissues. Thiopental and methohexitol are very soluble in fat and therefore penetrate the blood-brain barrier easily and rapidly. As a result, these compounds induce sleep very quickly (usually within seconds). The long-acting barbiturates, by contrast, exist in blood in a more water-soluble form and penetrate the blood-brain barrier with slightly more difficulty. Sleep induction with these long-acting compounds, therefore, is delayed. There is also a class of intermediate-acting barbiturates.

A barbiturate's duration of action is determined by its metabolism and excretion. Within a few minutes after thiopental or methohexitol is administered, the drug rapidly leaves the brain (so its action is cut short) and is redistributed to muscle and fat deposits such as adipose tissue. It is then slowly metabolized by the liver and excreted by the kidneys, which is why people who have been sedated or anesthetized with thiopental may, even though they awaken within a very few minutes, find that they are groggy for several hours afterward. This grogginess is the result of the low levels of the drug remaining in the blood while it is slowly metabolized and excreted. The drug is still present, but the concentration in the brain is not high enough to induce sleep or anesthesia.

Because the long-acting barbiturates (such as phenobarbital) exist in the blood primarily in a water-soluble form and are only slightly soluble in muscle and body fat, they circulate in the bloodstream in concentrations sufficient to keep the individual sedated or drowsy until they are either metabolized by the liver or excreted by the kidneys. The significant amounts of drug that persist in the bloodstream largely accounts for the hangover that lasts for several hours or even days after one of these agents has been ingested.

Urinalysis is being used more commonly to screen for the presence of barbiturates and other psychoactive drugs of use and abuse. Depending on the exact barbiturate taken, positive tests will be achieved over a period of time as short as 30 hours to as long as several weeks after drug ingestion. A positive screen for barbiturates necessitates more specific confirmation of the various barbiturates.

Thus, in summary, three processes are responsible for the termination of the depressant action of the barbiturates: *redistribution* to the muscle and fat, *metabolism* by the liver, and *excretion* by the kidneys. The process of redistribution is of primary importance in the termination of the hypnosis induced by thiopental, while excretion by the kidneys (usually following metabolism of the drug by the liver) is essential for the termination of the hypnotic action of the long-acting compounds.

Pharmacological Effects

At normal doses, the general depressant action of barbiturates is largely restricted to synapses in the CNS. The initial brain-wave alterations induced by the barbiturates resemble a high-voltage, low-frequency pattern characteristic of slow-wave sleep.

Normal sleep (not drug-induced) is a complex physiological process involving alternating episodes of rapid-eye-movement (REM) sleep and slow-wave sleep. Because barbiturate-induced sleep is characterized by slow waves, REM sleep is absent. Because dreaming occurs during REM sleep and is largely absent during slow-wave sleep, barbiturate-induced sleep differs from normal sleep in that the time spent in REM sleep is greatly reduced and dreaming is suppressed. In fact, some investigators think that this absence of REM sleep with loss of dreaming may be harmful and may even be capable of precipitating psychotic episodes. Individuals on barbiturates and deprived of REM sleep exhibit an increase in the proportion of time spent in REM sleep after they have stopped taking the drug—one example of a withdrawal effect following prolonged periods of barbiturate-induced depression.

Symptoms of drowsiness or a hangover may follow the use of a barbiturate. Such drowsiness, resulting from the presence of the drug in the body, may last for only a few hours, but more subtle alterations of judgment, motor skills, and behavior may persist for hours or days until the compound is completely eliminated. Such a hangover closely resembles that following intoxication by alcohol.

Other physiological effects of the barbiturates are relatively minor, except for the depressant effects on respiration, which are minimal at sedative doses but result in death when an overdose is taken. The barbiturates appear to have no significant effects on the cardiovascular system, the gastrointestinal tract, the kidneys, or other organs until toxic doses are reached. In the liver, however, barbiturates stimulate the synthesis of enzymes that metabolize barbiturates and some other drugs, an effect that produces a degree of tolerance to such drugs.

Psychological Effects

Many of the behavioral effects of the barbiturates are quite similar to those observed during alcohol-induced inebriation and may even be indistinguishable from them. Barbiturates may initially produce behavioral disinhibition, presumably by depressing the central inhibitory synapses. This disinhibition (coupled with the relief from anxiety that is produced by small amounts of sedation) may result in a mild state of euphoria. As with alcohol, however, an individual may react occasionally by withdrawing, becoming emotionally depressed, or by becoming aggressive and violent. Higher doses (or low doses combined with another depressant) lead to behavioral depression and sleep.

The individual's mental set and the physical or social setting in which the drug is ingested are important because they may largely determine whether a person experiences relief from anxiety or exhibits mental depression, aggression, or other unexpected or unpredictable responses.

An additional behavioral effect of consequence is the ataxia (staggering) and loss of motor coordination that may accompany use of depressant drugs. For instance, driving skills will be severely impaired by barbiturates and this should be considered a predictable consequence of their use. The effects of barbiturates are additive with the effects produced by any other depressant compound (including alcohol) that may be in the blood. Thus, the behavior of one who normally can tolerate a given dose of a barbiturate might be noticeably affected if alcohol or another depressant were present in the bloodstream. Such additive effects might be of little consequence if low doses of two drugs are ingested, but they might lead to more serious consequences if the individual tried to drive a car, for example. When relatively high doses of barbiturates are combined with relatively large amounts of alcohol, profound depression is induced. Numerous accidental overdoses, leading to respiratory failure and death, have resulted from such combinations.

Adverse Reactions

Side Effects and Toxicity   Drowsiness is one of the primary effects induced by the use of barbiturates. Obviously, such drowsiness is often the effect a person seeks. Quite frequently, however, when one is seeking a state of disinhibition or relief from anxiety drowsiness is a necessary side effect.

Another side effect is impaired performance and judgment. As one text puts it:

A person need not be rendered staggering drunk before his motor performance and, probably more important, his judgment are significantly impaired. The most common offending agent in this regard is alcohol. . . . At this time it should be emphasized that all sedatives are equivalent to alcohol in their effects; that all are additive in their effects with alcohol; and that their effects persist longer than might be predicted.[2]

Other side effects are usually minor and include such actions as slight decreases in blood pressure and heart rate (as occur during natural sleep), drug-induced hangover, and other effects on various systems of the body that are not significant enough to merit discussion here.

Tolerance   The barbiturates are capable of inducing at least two types of tolerance: (1) that following the induction of metabolizing enzymes in the liver, and (2) that following the adaptation of neurons in the brain to the presence of the drug. As we discussed in Chapter 1, many barbiturates are capable of inducing enzymes in the liver that metabolize the barbiturates and many other drugs that might be in the body at that time. Thus, subsequently, a higher dose would be required to maintain a given level of drug in the body. In other words, more of the drug would be needed to achieve the same concentration of the drug at the receptor and thus achieve the same effect—assuming that the receptor did not become insensitive to the drug.

It appears, however, that receptors within the brain are capable of adapting to the presence of barbiturates. Therefore, more of the drug would have to be presented to the receptor in order to stimulate it to the same level. The doses would have to be larger for two reasons: first, to maintain an adequate amount of the drug in the blood and, second, to raise the blood levels in order to stimulate the receptor to the same extent.

An individual does not necessarily develop tolerance to *all* the effects of the barbiturates. The tolerance we have described is primarily restricted to the sedative effects. The respiratory centers in the brainstem apparently *do not* become tolerant of the presence of barbiturates. If the patient tolerates the drug-induced euphoria and behavioral sedation but not the respiratory-depressant effects of the drugs, the risks associated with the use of the drug would progressively *increase* as that tolerance develops; in essence, the margin of safety in the use of the drug would decrease. Because the concentration of the drug in the blood that will produce respiratory failure remains approximately the same, the person using increasingly larger doses of barbiturates for social or recreational purposes risks taking a dose that may be severely toxic or even lethal.

Physical Dependence   Barbiturates induce physical dependence. Withdrawal symptoms appear when administration of the drug is stopped. Physical dependence on the barbiturates is in some respects similar to the physical dependence induced by the opiate narcotics (see Chapter 6) but differs in two important respects. First, the dose of barbiturate required to induce physical dependence is much higher than the dose usually required to induce sleep. For example, approximately 100 milligrams of pentobarbital (Nembutal) will induce sleep, and serious physical tolerance does not develop until, as tolerance builds, the patient reaches daily dosages of 800 milligrams or more. Also it is usually only after such large doses of the drug are reached that removal of the drug leads to *serious* and possibly lethal withdrawal symptoms. Opiate withdrawal may produce severe symptoms when even *normal* doses are discontinued. This is not to say, however, that normal doses of barbiturates may not produce some degree of physical dependence and symptoms of withdrawal when discontinued, but such symptoms at low doses are not usually serious or life-threatening. Among the symptoms is a rebound increase in REM sleep. Patients experiencing this rebound may find it difficult to sleep and may be quite irritable for days or weeks after the barbiturate is discontinued.

Second, barbiturate withdrawal also differs from opiate withdrawal in that the former may lead to life-threatening convulsions. Withdrawal from the opiate narcotics is not usually as dangerous. Periods of hallucination, restlessness, and disorientation may be associated with these withdrawal convulsions. Such withdrawal hyperexcitability is even more serious in an epileptic patient, who is more prone to severe convulsions. In such patients, serious withdrawal convulsions may be observed even when rather low doses of barbiturates are discontinued.

Psychological Dependence   Psychological dependence refers to a compulsion to use a drug for a pleasurable effect. All sedative-hypnotics are apt to be abused compulsively, the most abused being alcohol. The sedative-hypnotics are one of our most widely used classes of psychoactive drugs. Each year we ingest enough barbiturates such that if everybody were to consume his or her yearly allotted dose at one time, we would kill the entire population from respiratory depression three times over. Approximately 3000 deaths a year occur from overdoses. Such extensive use suggests that psychological dependence occurs in many individuals. Because they are capable of relieving anxiety, inducing sedation, and producing a state of euphoria, these drugs may be used to achieve a variety of psychological states. Many individuals in our society (especially older people) appear to be psychologically dependent upon the hypnotic effect of the barbiturates.

Nonbarbiturate Hypnotics

In the early 1950s, two nonbarbiturates, glutethimide (Doriden) and methyprylon (Noludar), were introduced as new drugs that produce sedation and sleep. Strictly speaking, these were not new drugs because their structures are virtually identical to those of the barbiturates except for one slight modification of the molecule (see Figure 3.2). The pharmaceutical industry frequently markets "new" drugs by making minor changes in old ones. This is not meant to confuse the reader but to demonstrate that what is sold as a "nonbarbiturate" is in reality so similar to the barbiturates that the receptors in the brain upon which barbiturates act probably cannot differentiate between them. Yet these nonbarbiturates may be promoted as something "new."

Other nonbarbiturate hypnotics include chloral hydrate, ethchlorvynol, and methaqualone (Table 3.2). Interest in methaqualone rose dramatically in recent years, and it became one of the leading drugs of abuse after marijuana and alcohol. Its popularity was due to its undeserved reputation as an aphrodisiac. This reputation created such illicit use that the manufacturer stopped its production and removed it from the market in 1984. Pharmacologically, however, methaqualone is similar to the barbiturates in its effects and is actually an *an*aphrodisiac. It appears that the effects of set, setting, and expectation are more potent than the drug's pharmacological effects.

It should be noted, however, that low doses of any sedative can induce relief from anxiety and promote euphoria. The side effects

---

Figure 3.2

Structural formulas of phenobarbital (a barbiturate) and two nonbarbiturate hypnotics. Note the close structural resemblance of the nonbarbiturate compounds to phenobarbital.

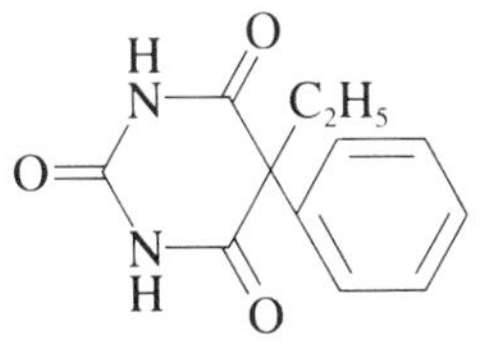

Phenobarbital

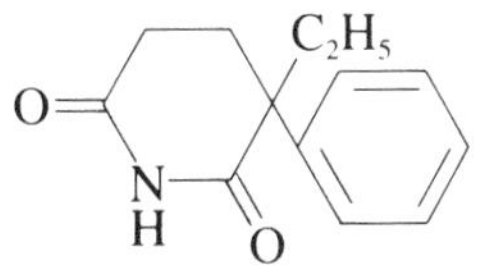

Glutethimide (Doriden)

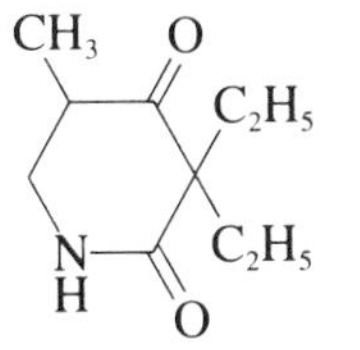

Methyprylon (Noludar)

and toxicity of methaqualone are similar to those associated with the barbiturates. Behavior and driving abilities are impaired and the possibility of tolerance and dependence should be considered. Methaqualone, far from being a "love drug," is merely one of several sedative-hypnotic compounds that may favorably affect the user when administered in the appropriate setting and with the proper mental set or expectations.[3]

Overdoses of methaqualone have been fatal. Death may occur from respiratory arrest, pulmonary edema (water in the lungs), or other causes. Street preparations purported to be methaqualone may consist of numerous other compounds, often psychedelics, such as PCP (Chapter 8), that can produce undesirable effects, especially if not anticipated by the user.[4]

Meprobamate

Meprobamate (Equanil, Miltown) was one of the first tranquilizers to be introduced in the United States. Physicians began using it in the early 1950s as an alternative sedative-hypnotic product to alcohol and the barbiturates. Somehow the term *tranquilizer* came to distinguish it from the barbiturates, a distinction that with meprobamate appears to be more theoretical than real. Low doses of barbiturates are effective as daytime sedatives and as antianxiety agents, while higher doses induce sleep. The same appears to be true for meprobamate. Doses between 200 and 400 milligrams produce long-lasting daytime sedation, euphoria, and relief from anxiety; higher doses induce sleep. Meprobamate appears to be less effective in relieving anxiety than the benzodiazepines.

Meprobamate is well absorbed orally and is not administered by injection. It is rapidly distributed to the brain and, because it is readily reabsorbed from the kidney, must be metabolized before excretion. Therefore, meprobamate has a long duration of action and the sedation it induces will last for 10 hours or longer.

In general, meprobamate and the barbiturates induce the same pharmacological and toxicological effects—tolerance, physical dependence, and psychological dependence can be induced to approximately the same extent. When chronic administration of high doses of meprobamate is abruptly stopped, withdrawal symptoms may include convulsions, coma, psychotic behavior, and even death. It is somewhat more difficult, however, to commit suicide with meprobamate than with the barbiturates because meprobamate is not as potent a respiratory depressant as the barbiturates are and thus its margin of safety is greater. Successful suicide following the ingestion of meprobamate is rare, probably owing to this rather low potency.

Benzodiazepines

Through the 1950s, the only sedative-hypnotic agents available were alcohol, the barbiturates, meprobamate, and the nonbarbiturate derivatives, glutethimide and methyprylon. In 1960, the first benzodiazepine, chlordiazepoxide (Librium), was introduced. To date, 14 benzodiazepines have been marketed (Table 3.2).

During the first 20 years of their availability, benzodiazepines were thought to resemble closely the barbiturates in their pharmacological action. However, these drugs facilitate GABA neurotransmission (discussed previously). Thus, they are considered to be superior to the barbiturates for most uses for which they are prescribed. Today, the benzodiazepines are generally considered to be the agents of first choice when an antianxiety, sedation, or hypnotic action is required. They are effective and safe and overdosage is less lethal than that of other sedatives. There are two caveats, however: (1) the additive effects of benzodiazepines and alcohol can lead to serious depression of respiration and reduced visual-motor and driving skills; and (2) benzodiazepines should not be used during pregnancy, especially in the first trimester (see the following discussion).

The popularity of these compounds is indicated by the fact that diazepam and chlordiazepoxide are currently two of the most widely prescribed drugs in the United States. More than 45 million prescriptions for diazepam (Valium) are filled each year, only slightly more than are filled for chlordiazepoxide. Such use also leads to extensive misuse. Diazepam is one of the primary drug-related reasons for visits to hospital emergency rooms across the nation. It is the first or second most abused drug in many cities, and it is mentioned in more than 54,000 episodes of drug abuse. Seventy percent of these episodes involved women, and suicide attempts were involved in 51 percent of all incidents.

Absorption, Distribution, Metabolism, and Excretion

All the benzodiazepines are lipid soluble, so they cross the blood-brain barrier readily. However, their disposition in the body varies greatly because the extent of solubility can vary by a factor of 50, depending on the specific agent. Most benzodiazepines are available for oral administration, with only midazolam excluded (it is available only in parenteral form). These drugs are completely absorbed orally, with the exception of clorazepate, which must first be converted (by enzymes in the stomach) to a metabolite that is completely absorbed and is pharmacologically active. The rate of absorption of benzodiazepines varies; some agents have a rapid onset while others take several hours to elicit significant effects. Triazolam is most rapidly absorbed, achieving peak levels within 1 hour, thus making it quite useful for inducing sleep. The slower onset, longer-acting agents (such as diazepam) are more useful when prolonged antianxiety effects are desired and when rapid onset and brief duration of action are less desirable.

All benzodiazepines are metabolized before excretion. In addition, many of their metabolites are pharmacologically active and contribute significantly to the pharmacological effects of the parent drug. Thus, the duration of clinical action may persist long beyond the time of metabolism of the parent compound because the metabolite may be as active or even more active than the originally administered drug. For example, the half-life of flurazepam in the body is about 3 hours, but its active metabolite persists for about 2 days.

In choosing a drug for a clinical effect, therefore, one needs to determine the desired rapidity of onset and duration of action. For example, antianxiety and antiepileptic effects are best achieved by choosing drugs with long durations of action, while induction of sleep is best treated with a rapid-onset, short-acting agent so that morning hangover is minimized.

Chlordiazepoxide, diazepam, lorazepam, and midazolam are available for use by injection. Indications for intravenous use of these drugs include the induction of general anesthesia, preanesthetic sedation, intraoperative sedation (such as by an oral surgeon), and the rapid control of seizures (status epilepticus).

The duration of action and elimination half-lives of the different benzodiazepines vary widely. The half-lives for major benzodiazepines are as follows: chlordiazepoxide, 5–10 hours; diazepam, 30–60 hours; oxazepam (Serax), 5–10 hours; flurazepam (Dalmane), 2–3 hours for the parent drug and 50–100 hours for active metabolites.

Because of the long elimination time for the benzodiazepines, an individual who has been using a drug for months or years may maintain detectable urinary concentrations of the drug for weeks to months after discontinuation of its use.

Adverse Reactions

Daytime sedation and drug hangover are the most common untoward effects of the benzodiazepines, but their incidence is somewhat lower than that seen with the barbiturates. Other side effects include dizziness, lassitude, prolonged physical and psychomotor reaction times, incoordination, staggering, interruption of thought and psychomotor function, confusion, and amnesia. Judgment and motor performance are significantly impaired because a drug-induced "brain syndrome" occurs in a manner similar to that seen in individuals taking barbiturates. Cumulative interaction with alcohol is of special significance and especially serious. In the elderly, drug action is prolonged and the magnitude of the "brain syndrome" is intensified.

Sleep patterns are disrupted; REM sleep is depressed; and REM rebound occurs upon drug discontinuation. However, it is usually less severe than that seen following cessation of barbiturate therapy because the duration of action of most benzodiazepines (and their active metabolites) is quite prolonged.

Despite these side effects, the benzodiazepines are remarkably safe compounds. Even when taken in huge amounts (as in suicide attempts), benzodiazepines are rarely fatal unless they are combined with other sedative drugs, such as alcohol. Cardiovascular and respiratory depression rarely occur.

Therapeutic Uses

As outlined previously and in Table 3.2, therapeutic uses of benzodiazepines include the treatment of anxiety, insomnia, seizures, and alcohol withdrawal. Some benzodiazepines also are used for the induction of anesthesia and as preanesthetic medication.

Benzodiazepines serve an important role in the treatment of generalized anxiety disorders when such treatment is combined with psychotherapy, counseling, and behavioral techniques such as meditation and relaxation therapy. In the treatment of acute situational anxieties, benzodiazepines are less frequently needed unless anxiety inhibits normal functioning. Counseling, supportive psychotherapy, and behavioral therapy may be more important.

In the treatment of panic and phobic disorders, benzodiazepines can play an important supportive role, although they are not usually drugs of first choice. One benzodiazepine (alprazolam) has been shown to be particularly effective in treating these disorders. Alprazolam differs from other benzodiazepines in that it may have some usefulness in the treatment of major depression; however, the effectiveness of such use is controversial. For the treatment of panic disorders, an antidepressant such as imipramine is usually the agent of first choice and alprazolam is added, if needed. Agents such as monoamine oxidase inhibitors, which are potentially more toxic, should not be tried unless treatment with the other agents has failed. Behavioral techniques may be beneficial as adjunctive therapy.

Tolerance and Dependence

Their pharmacological similarity to the barbiturates and the other sedative-hypnotic compounds makes it seem likely that the benzodiazepines would induce tolerance and dependence. Indeed, some degree of tolerance can be measured after repeated administration, but it does not appear to be as marked as that induced by the barbiturates. Physical dependence has been described. Finally, since these agents may produce relaxation and induce behavioral disinhibition, a feeling of well-being, and euphoria, some degree of psychological dependence would be expected. Excessive use of the benzodiazepines may produce undesirable behavior, including disorientation, confusion, rage, and other symptoms resembling those of drunkenness.

Because these compounds are sedative agents, their effects are additive with those of other sedative-hypnotic compounds. Thus, while a clinical dose of a benzodiazepine may not severely impair driving performance, the addition of alcohol may induce significant impairment—probably one of the greatest impediments to the social use of these agents. Although we seriously try to prevent individuals from driving while under the influence of alcohol, we are not yet serious about restraining individuals who ingest tranquilizers. Legal guidelines for what may be considered safe blood levels of sedatives have not yet been established and the public is unaware that tranquilizers *do* impair concentration. The influence of alcohol, by contrast, is widely publicized.

Use in Pregnancy

The use of benzodiazepines during early pregnancy has been associated with the development of cleft lip in newborns, but this observation remains controversial. These drugs do, however, readily cross the placental barrier and drug levels in the fetus approach those in the mother. As a general rule, therefore, it might be wise to avoid the use of benzodiazepines during pregnancy, especially during the first trimester. Withdrawal symptoms may occur in infants born to mothers who are physically dependent on benzodiazepines during their pregnancy. Finally, benzodiazepines can be detected in breast milk, so maternal intake and infant behavior should be carefully monitored during periods of breast-feeding.

General Anesthetics

General anesthesia, a behavioral state on the continuum of depression illustrated in Figure 3.1, is the most severe state of intentional drug-induced depression. Beyond general anesthesia there are only coma and death. Thus, the induction of general anesthesia with depressant drugs is a serious undertaking and should be performed only by competent persons.

The agents that are used to induce general anesthesia differ widely in physical properties and chemical structure. They range from gases (such as nitrous oxide), to volatile liquids (isoflurane, halothane, and enflurane), to drugs in solutions intended for intravenous administration (thiopental). The gases and volatile liquids are inhaled; the other anesthetics are usually injected directly into the bloodstream. All anesthetics are rapidly distributed to the brain, where anesthesia is thought to follow depression of synaptic transmission. The exact mechanisms, however, have not been delineated. It is thought that depression of the arousal center in the brainstem (the ARAS) may be involved in the loss of consciousness (see Appendix III).

General anesthetics (like the other sedative-hypnotics) produce a generalized, graded, dose-related depression of all functions of the central nervous system. Thus, their pharmacological effects are similar to those observed with the barbiturates: an initial period of sedation, relief from anxiety, and disinhibition, followed by onset of sleep. As anesthesia deepens, reflexes are progressively depressed and analgesia is induced. At this point, a patient is said to be anesthetized. Deepening of anesthesia results in loss of reflexes and depression of respiration and of brain excitability: a state of deep anesthesia.

Occasionally, certain anesthetic agents become misused drugs. Nitrous oxide is an example. A gas of low anesthetic potency, it is incapable of inducing deep levels of anesthesia if an adequate oxygen concentration is maintained. Nitrous oxide induces a state of behavioral disinhibition, analgesia, and euphoria. One of the problems occasionally encountered when nitrous oxide is used for recreational purposes is that, unless the compound is administered with at least 21 percent oxygen (room air is 21 percent oxygen) hypoxia (decreased oxygen content of the blood) can be induced. But in order to achieve high enough concentrations of nitrous oxide to get a good behavioral effect, concentrations of 50 percent or greater must be inhaled. If such concentrations are mixed with room air, inhaled oxygen concentrations drop to low levels and the hypoxia may result in irreversible brain damage.

Within the last few years other forms of recreational anesthesia with accompanying hypoxia induced by the inhalation of glue, gasoline, and so on have been encountered. The volatile hydrocarbons in these products are capable of inducing a general anesthesia similar to that produced by ether or the other anesthetics. Thus, when these products are administered by people who are unaware of the dangers, hypoxia or depression of respiration from too deep a level of anesthesia may occasionally result in death. The results of inhaling these volatile products, which are found throughout our society, are pharmacologically similar to inhaling or ingesting any other sedative-hypnotic compound.

Use of Sedative-Hypnotic Compounds in Pregnancy

As we pointed out in Chapter 1 (Figure 1.8), drugs are transferred from the mother to the fetus through the placenta. Because the sedative-hypnotic compounds are capable of depressing all body systems, their distribution through the placenta implies that they will also depress the fetus. Though information is constantly being gained about the effects of depressant drugs on the fetus, this is a serious problem that remains unresolved.

As stated previously, congenital malformations have been associated with the use of benzodiazepines during the first trimester; thus, they should not be used during that period. Mothers physically dependent on benzodiazepines while pregnant can expect to bear infants who exhibit drug withdrawal signs after delivery. The effects of these drugs when transmitted through breast milk to an infant are unknown. It is precisely because specific data are lacking that caution is necessary. It is known that when sedative-hypnotic agents are administered at the time of delivery, they are found in the newborn baby in significant concentrations, and because the newborn baby has limited metabolizing and excreting systems, it is frequently depressed for a long time after delivery. This often results in low Apgar scores and difficulties with feeding ("floppy infant syndrome"). It is pharmacologically and medically prudent to avoid the use of sedative-hypnotics either during pregnancy or at the time of delivery, unless the drugs are administered under the close supervision of a physician.

Notes

1. W. B. Mendelson, *The Use and Misuse of Sleeping Pills* (New York: Plenum, 1980).
2. F. H. Meyers, E. Jawetz, and A. Goldfien, *Review of Medical Pharmacology*, 3d ed. (Los Altos, Calif.: Lange Medical Publications, 1972), p. 219.

3. For a review of methaqualone, see D. R. Wesson and D. E. Smith, "Methaqualone: Just Another Downer," *Journal of Psychedelic Drugs* 5, no. 2 (Winter 1972): 167–169, and H. W. Elliott, ed., "Drugs of Abuse—1973," *Annual Review of Pharmacology* (1974), pp. 517–520.
4. C. V. Wetli, "Changing Patterns of Methaqualone Abuse," *Journal of the American Medical Association* 249 (1983): 621.
5. D. J. Greenblatt, D. R. Abernethy, M. Divoll, J. S. Harmatz, and R. I. Shader, "Pharmacokinetic Properties of Benzodiazepine Hypnotics," *Journal of Clinical Psychopharmacology* 3 (1983): 129.

CHAPTER 4

Alcohol

The Most Popular Drug

By alcohol we mean ethyl alcohol, a psychoactive drug that is quite as powerful as the more notorious drugs, but it is the only drug with which obvious self-induced intoxication is socially acceptable.[1]

Ethyl alcohol (alcohol, ethanol) is similar in most respects to the sedative-hypnotic compounds discussed in Chapter 3. Alcohol is classified pharmacologically as a general depressant and is capable of inducing a general, nonselective, reversible depression of the central nervous system. However, it differs from the compounds discussed in Chapter 3 in that it is used primarily for social or recreational, rather than medical, purposes. Being one of the most widely used of all drugs, alcohol has created special problems both for the individual user and for society in general. Thus, it deserves separate discussion.

How Alcohol Is Handled by the Body

Alcohol is absorbed, distributed, metabolized, and excreted in certain specific ways.

Absorption

Alcohol is rapidly and completely absorbed from the entire gastrointestinal tract. Already liquid, alcohol does not have to dissolve in the stomach as does a drug in tablet form. Alcohol is a small, fat-soluble molecule that readily penetrates body membranes. If it is vaporized, it can be absorbed readily through the lungs. Because it is so rapidly and completely absorbed when taken orally, the drug is seldom administered intravenously; indeed this might even be dangerous because of its potent depressant action on the nervous system. Fatalities have resulted from inhalation of alcohol through the lungs because the drug is so rapidly absorbed and distributed to the brain, causing a sudden depression of the respiratory control centers in the brainstem.

The rate of absorption can be modified in various ways. In a person with an empty stomach, approximately 20 percent of a single dose of alcohol is absorbed from the stomach, usually quite rapidly. If the stomach is full, absorption is delayed. The rate of absorption from the stomach also depends on the volume of fluid in which the alcohol is taken. In general, the more concentrated the alcohol in the stomach, the more rapid the absorption. Thus, diluted solutions (such as beer) are absorbed more slowly than are concentrated solutions (such as cocktails, which may contain between 10 and 50 percent alcohol).

Approximately 20 percent of the administered alcohol is absorbed from the stomach. The remaining 80 percent is absorbed rapidly and completely from the upper intestine, the limiting factor being the time the stomach takes to empty. Food in the stomach will slow absorption for two reasons: first, by diluting the alcohol and covering some of the stomach membranes through which alcohol would be absorbed, and, second, by prolonging the emptying time. Thus, blood levels of alcohol will increase much faster in an individual who has fasted than in someone who has just eaten a large meal. In either case, however, the alcohol will still be completely absorbed.

Distribution

Since alcohol is a small molecule soluble in both water and fat, it is evenly distributed throughout all body fluids and tissues, including those of the brain. Since vaporized alcohol may be absorbed through the lungs into the blood, the reverse also holds true: small amounts of alcohol are excreted from the body through the lungs. Indeed, most of us are familiar with the "alcohol breath" that results from exhalation of alcohol. Because alcohol diffuses into all muscle masses and fat deposits of the body, an obese or muscular person would have lower blood levels of alcohol than a lean individual to whom an identical dose of the drug was administered. In other words, the obese or muscular individual would have to ingest more drug than a slender individual would in order to achieve the same level of intoxication. However, because of the peculiar rate of metabolism of alcohol by the body (see the next section), a larger individual would retain the alcohol somewhat longer than would a slender person.

Alcohol also is freely distributed to the fetus. It crosses the placenta and the infant's blood-brain barrier easily. Fetal alcohol levels reach those of the drinking mother. It can be detected on the baby's breath at birth, in amniotic fluid during pregnancy, and in the baby's blood. Research on the impact of maternal alcohol consumption on human infants has demonstrated that "fetal alcohol syndrome," consisting of serious birth defects in 30 to 50 percent of newborns of alcoholic mothers, can result when it is ingested at critical times of embryonic development.[2] This syndrome is more completely discussed in the section on side effects and toxicities of alcohol.

Metabolism

Approximately 95 percent of the alcohol that enters the body is metabolized before it is excreted. Metabolism usually occurs in the liver, where alcohol is converted to carbon dioxide and water. The small amount (5 percent) that is not metabolized is excreted unchanged, primarily in the urine and through the lungs. Alcohol has little nutritional value and provides only calories when metabolized.

The rate of metabolism of most drugs in the liver depends on the concentration of the drug in the blood: the higher the concentration, the faster the rate of metabolism. Alcohol, however, differs in that the rate of metabolism is linear with time and is minimally affected by variations in blood concentration. In the adult, the metabolic rate is approximately 10 milliliters (one-third ounce) of 100 percent ethanol per hour. In other words, it would take an adult 1 hour to metabolize the alcohol contained in 1 ounce of 80–100 proof whiskey (about 40 percent ethanol), a 4-ounce glass of wine, or 12 ounces of beer. Alcohol is metabolized slowly, constantly, and independently of the amount ingested. Consumption of 4 ounces of wine, 12 ounces of beer, or 1 ounce of whiskey an hour would keep blood levels of alcohol fairly constant. Thus, if a person ingests more alcohol per hour than is metabolized, blood concentrations increase. This demonstrates that there is a limit to the amount of alcohol that can be consumed in an hour without a person's becoming drunk as a result of the accumulation of alcohol in the blood.

Factors that may alter the rate of metabolism of alcohol are many and varied but usually not of clinical significance. Alcohol is capable of inducing drug-metabolizing enzymes in the liver, however, thereby increasing its own rate of metabolism (inducing tolerance) and also the rate of metabolism of other compounds similarly metabolized by the liver (cross-tolerance). Although there have been many attempts to develop treatments that might hasten the elimination of alcohol (and therefore reduce the seriousness of acute alcohol intoxication), none has succeeded. There is at present no practical way of increasing the rate of metabolism of alcohol.

Mention should be made here of disulfiram (Antabuse), a drug frequently used to treat chronic alcoholism because it inhibits aldehyde dehydrogenase, an enzyme that carries out a specific step in alcohol metabolism (the metabolism of acetaldehyde to acetate). An earlier metabolic step is not blocked, however. Thus alcohol is still metabolized to acetaldehyde, which accumulates in the body, making the patient extremely uncomfortable with headache, nausea, vomiting, drowsiness, hangover, and so on. Disulfiram makes alcoholics feel so dreadful when they drink that they are discouraged from drinking. If they refuse to continue taking the drug, treatment often fails.

Excretion

Approximately 95 percent of the alcohol ingested is metabolized to products that eventually are converted to carbon dioxide and water. The remaining 5 percent is excreted unchanged by the kidneys and lungs. Thus, the treatment of acute alcohol intoxication by increasing the rate of urinary excretion is doomed to failure since so little is removed from the body by this route. It therefore appears that, once alcohol is in the body, the slow, steady rate of metabolism of the drug by the liver is the only way of detoxifying and removing the drug from the body.

Sites and Mechanisms of Action

Like the sedative-hypnotics, alcohol depresses all the neurons in the brain, producing disorientation, mental clouding, impaired memory, decreased judgment, and labile affect. Such a state, which is often misinterpreted as behavioral stimulation, is similar to the loss of inhibition and induction of euphoria characteristic of low doses of all sedative-hypnotic drugs. It is postulated that inhibitory synapses are depressed slightly earlier than are excitatory ones, thus inducing a state of disinhibition or mild euphoria.[3-4]

One explanation for drunken behavior is that the higher centers in the cerebral cortex are released from the inhibitory controls exerted upon them from the brainstem, resulting in impaired thought, organization, and motor processes. Low doses of alcohol may produce mild euphoria, but also loss of discrimination, fine movement, memory, concentration, control, and so on. There may be wide fluctuations in mood with frequent emotional outbursts. As the levels of alcohol in the brain are increased, the cerebral cortex is depressed and the state of disinhibition or euphoria is progressively lost. Objective testing has clearly demonstrated that alcohol does *not* increase or improve performance.

The mechanism by which alcohol exerts its depressant action is unclear. It may involve inhibition of the release of calcium-dependent neurotransmitters, which presumably interact at a site in the presynaptic nerve terminal.

Pharmacological Effects

The graded depression of synaptic transmission is the prime physiological effect of alcohol. Respiration, although transiently stimulated at low doses, is progressively depressed and, at very high blood concentrations, death may result. Like the other sedative-hypnotic compounds, alcohol slows EEG activity toward slow-wave sleep and depressed REM sleep, inhibiting dreaming.

Also like the other sedative-hypnotic compounds, alcohol is anticonvulsant and may suppress epileptic convulsions. When alcohol ingestion is stopped, however, this antiepileptic action may be followed by hyperexcitability that lasts for several days. An alcoholic (whether or not he or she is also epileptic) may have seizures when the drug is withdrawn, the seizures peaking approximately 8 to 12 hours after the last dose of the drug. Finally, it should be stressed that the effects of alcohol are additive with other sedative-hypnotic compounds, resulting in more sedation or greater impairment of driving or other performance than might be expected.

The minor tranquilizers (especially the benzodiazepines) and marijuana are the drugs most frequently combined with alcohol, and they increase its deleterious effects on the performance of motor and intellectual skills and on alertness. The combination of alcohol and tranquilizers may produce supra-additive effects that cause fatal depression of cardiac and respiratory functions. Thus, these combinations can be hazardous and occasionally are fatal. The combined use of alcohol and other sedatives during performance of tasks such as driving is extremely dangerous, especially when the hazards are not recognized.[5]

The effects of alcohol on the circulation and on the heart are becoming more appreciated. Alcohol dilates the blood vessels in the skin, producing a warm flush and a decrease in body temperature. Thus, alcohol taken to keep warm when one is exposed to cold weather is pointless and might even be dangerous if it is vital to conserve body heat. Long-term use of alcohol is also associated with diseases of the heart muscle, resulting in heart failure. Several reports have noted that despite the fact that low doses of alcohol consumed daily (up to 2.5 ounces) may reduce the risk of coronary artery disease, there is evidence that chronic ingestion of large quantities of alcohol predisposes to coronary artery disease and can produce angina pectoris (chest pain associated with decreased oxygen delivery to the heart). Irregularities in the heartbeat can occur both in patients with alcohol-related diseases and in other individuals during periods of alcoholic intoxication.[5]

The effects of alcohol on the liver are significant. Ethanol can produce irreversible changes in both its structure and function. The significance of alcohol-induced liver dysfunction is illustrated by the fact that 75 percent of all deaths attributed to alcoholism are due to cirrhosis of the liver,[6] and cirrhosis is the seventh most common cause of death in the United States.[7]

Alcohol exerts a diuretic effect by increasing the excretion of fluids by affecting the functioning of the kidney, by decreasing the action of the antidiuretic hormone, and by the diuretic action simply produced by the large quantities of fluid ordinarily ingested as alcoholic beverages. Alcohol, however, does not appear to harm either the structure or function of the kidney.

Alcohol (like methaqualone and the other sedative-hypnotic drugs) is not an aphrodisiac. In fact, while the behavioral disinhibition induced by low doses of alcohol may cause some loss of restraint, alcohol depresses body function and actually interferes with sexual performance; as Shakespeare wrote, "it provokes the desire, but it takes away the performance" (*Macbeth*).

Psychological Effects

The psychological and behavioral effects of alcohol are similar to those of other sedative-hypnotic agents. In general, the short-term effects are primarily restricted to the central nervous system. The behavioral reaction to disinhibition, occurring at low doses,[8] is unpredictable and is determined to a large extent by the individual, his or her mental set, and the setting in which the drinking occurs. In one setting a person may be relaxed and euphoric; in another, withdrawn or violent. Mental set and setting become progressively *less* important with increasing doses since sedation dominates and behavioral activity decreases. At low doses, a person may still function (although in less coordinated fashion) and attempt to drive or otherwise endanger himself and others. As the dose increases, he or she becomes progressively incapacitated. There is now convincing data that alcohol intoxication, with its resulting disinhibition, plays a major role in a large percentage of violent crimes. Indeed, over 50 percent of crimes and highway accidents are alcohol-related.[9]

Long-term effects may involve many different organs of the body, depending on whether drinking is *moderate* or *heavy*. It appears that long-term ingestion of moderate amounts of alcohol (approximately two martinis a day) produces few physiological, psychological, or behavioral changes in the individual. But long-term ingestion of larger amounts leads to a variety of disorders and discomforts affecting many parts of the body and brain. These disorders are included in the term *alcoholism*. Alcoholism is a multifaceted syndrome characterized by chronic excessive ingestion of alcohol, accompanied by the development of tolerance and dependency.

Alcohol is quite caloric but has little nutritional value. A person may survive for years on a diet of alcohol and not much else but suffer slowly developing vitamin deficiency and nutritional diseases, which may result in gradual physical deterioration. Indeed, alcohol abuse has been suggested as the most common cause of vitamin and trace element deficiency in adults.[7]

Tolerance and Dependence

The patterns and mechanisms of the development of tolerance to and physical and psychological dependence upon alcohol are similar to those of all the sedative-hypnotic compounds. The extent of tolerance depends upon the amount, pattern, and extent of alcohol ingestion. Individuals who ingest alcohol only intermittently (on sprees), or more regularly but in moderation, develop little or no tolerance; individuals who regularly ingest large amounts of alcohol develop marked tolerance.

The physical dependence that develops with chronic ingestion is such that withdrawal of the drug results in a period of rebound hyperexcitability that may lead to convulsions and even death. Concomitant with this hyperexcitability is a period of tremulousness, with hallucinations, psychomotor agitation, confusion and disorientation, sleep disorders, and a variety of associated discomforts— a syndrome sometimes referred to as *delirium tremens* (DTs, rum fits).

Psychological dependence on alcohol also occurs and, indeed, frequently appears to be socially acceptable. This psychological dependence appears to result from the state of disinhibition, relief from anxiety, and euphoria, so that the use of alcohol becomes a compulsive pleasure. Certainly, this psychological attraction to the drug is a major problem to be considered in the treatment of the alcoholic or, more widely, in attempts to discourage the recreational misuse of alcohol.

Side Effects and Toxicity

Many of the side effects and toxicities associated with alcohol have already been mentioned, but let us summarize them and expand upon them here. In the acute use of alcohol, behavior is altered as a result of depression of the function of the central nervous system, with the induction of a drug-induced "brain syndrome." This is manifested as a clouded sensorium with disorientation, impaired insight and judgment, amnesia ("blackouts"), and diminished intellectual capabilities. One's affect may be labile, with vulnerability to external stimuli and expressions of anger. In high doses, delusions, hallucinations, and confabulations may be present. Socially, these alterations result in an unpredictable state of disinhibition (drunkenness), alterations in driving performance, and uncoordinated motor behavior.

In chronic alcohol ingestion, a variety of chronic toxicities are observed. Whereas *acute* intoxication produces a *reversible* brain syndrome secondary to reversible depression of nerve cells, long-term alcohol ingestion may *irreversibly* destroy nerve cells, producing a permanent "brain syndrome" with dementia (Korsakoff's syndrome). The liver may become infiltrated with fat and over a period of time become cirrhotic (scarred). The digestive system is also affected and pancreatitis (inflammation of the pancreas) and chronic gastritis (inflammation of the stomach) with development of peptic ulcers may be seen. As mentioned previously, a variety of toxicities of the heart can occur, including weakness of the heart muscle, coronary artery disease, angina pectoris, and electrical abnormalities of heart function.[10]

There is now indisputable evidence that alcohol is one cause of cancer. Heavy drinking increases the risk of developing cancer of the tongue, mouth, throat, voice box, and liver. In the United States, these sites represent approximately 10 percent of all cancers. Alcohol also has a synergistic action with tobacco, further increasing the risk of cancer. For example, the risk of head and neck cancers for heavy drinkers who smoke is 6 to 15 times greater than for those who abstain from both. The risk of throat cancer is 44 times greater for heavy users of both alcohol and tobacco than for nonusers (Figure 4.1). While the mechanism of this carcinogenic action of alcohol is unclear, it may result from a decrease in body immunity secondary to alcohol ingestion.

Recently,[11,12] data have appeared that link minimal-to-moderate

Figure 4.1

Relative risks of esophageal cancer in relation to the daily consumption of alcohol and tobacco. The risk is 44.4 times greater for individuals consuming 20 grams or more of tobacco and 80 grams or more of alcohol per day (upper right block) than for individuals consuming little or none of either drug (lower left block). One ounce of ethyl alcohol is approximately 23.4 grams; thus 40 grams is 1.7 ounces or approximately equivalent to three drinks. [From *Third Special Report to the U.S. Congress on Alcohol and Health*, U.S. Department of Health, Education, and Welfare, June 1978. Data from A. J. Tuyns, G. Pequignot, and O. M. Jenson, "Le cancer de l'oesophage en Ille et Vilaine en fonction des niveaux de consommation d'alcool et de tabac: Des risques qui se multiplient," *Bulletin du Cancer* 65(1) (1977): 45–60.]

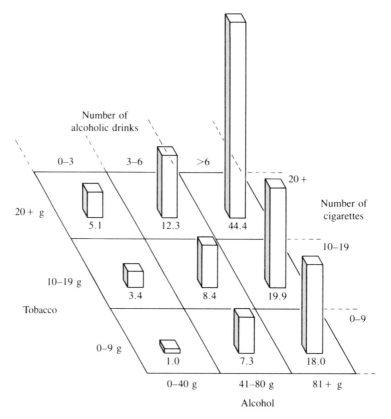

alcohol intake with significant increases in the incidence of breast cancer in women. Although these data are alarming, the topic is currently being debated, and additional verification is needed before the data can be accepted.

As mentioned earlier, fetal alcohol syndrome has been described in the offspring of mothers who demonstrated high blood levels of alcohol during critical stages of fetal development. In 1977, the National Institute on Alcohol Abuse and Alcoholism released the following statement relevant to this syndrome:

Recent reports indicate that heavy use of alcohol by women during pregnancy may result in a pattern of abnormalities in the offspring, termed the fetal alcohol syndrome, which consists of specific congenital and behavioral abnormalities. Studies undertaken in animals corroborate the initial observations in humans and also indicate an increased incidence of stillbirths, resorptions, and spontaneous abortions. Both the risk and the extent of abnormalities appear to be dose-related, increasing with higher alcohol intake during pregnancy. In human studies, alcohol is an unequivocal factor when the full pattern of the fetal alcohol syndrome is present. In cases where all of the characteristics are not present, the correlation between alcohol and the adverse effects is complicated by such factors as nutrition, smoking, caffeine, and other drug consumption.

Given the total evidence available at this time, pregnant women should be particularly conscious of the extent of their drinking. While safe levels of drinking are known, it appears that a risk is established with ingestion of 3 ounces of absolute alcohol or six drinks per day. Between 1 ounce and 3 ounces, there is uncertainty but caution is advised. Therefore, pregnant women and those likely to become pregnant should discuss their drinking habits and the potential dangers with their physicians.[5]

Information gathered since 1977 indicates that high blood alcohol levels during a critical time of embryonic development are probably necessary to produce fetal alcohol syndrome. The average daily alcohol consumption may not be as important as maximum concentrations obtained during binge drinking at critical periods. Infants born to moderately heavy drinkers, however, exhibit at least twice the incidence of congenital anomalies as infants born to nondrinking mothers. Alcohol ingestion during the first trimester is most apt to cause fetal maldevelopment; later in pregnancy it is most apt to adversely affect fetal nutrition and size. Mild-to-moderate mental retardation, increasingly recognized as a component of the syndrome, may be the result of brain malformation during fetal development. Thus, the fetal alcohol syndrome consists of intrauterine growth retardation (length, weight, head circumference), multiple congenital malformations, retarded brain maturation, and an undetermined degree of mental retardation.[13] Not all features are necessarily present in any given infant. At the present time the projected incidence of fetal alcohol syndrome makes it the third leading cause of birth defects with associated mental retardation— following only Down's syndrome and spina bifida—and the only one of the three that is preventable.

A recent study of over 31,000 pregnancies concludes that consuming only one or two drinks daily is associated with a substantially increased risk of producing a growth-retarded infant.[14] Less than one drink per day has minimal effect but could not be ruled as "safe."

The effects of *paternal* drinking or alcoholism on the fetus is unknown. Over 25 percent of moderate to heavy drinking pregnant women report heavy drinking on the part of the infant's father. This may or may not be significant.

Chronic Excessive Alcohol Ingestion

Of the 160 million Americans of drinking age, 112 million drink and 48 million do not.[15] As many as 11.5 million may have serious alcohol problems, and about half that number, 5.75 million, are identifiable alcoholics. The daily consumption of about ½ pint of 80-proof liquor a day is thought to place one's health at risk. Approximately 10 percent of the drinking population ingests this quantity of alcohol in the form of beer, wine, or "hard" liquor.

As stated by Jaffe[1]:

If cigarette smoking is excluded, alcoholism is by far the most serious drug problem in the United States and most other countries. Measured in terms of accidents, lost productivity, crime, death, or damaged health, the combined social costs of problem drinking in the United States were estimated for 1980 to exceed 89 billion dollars annually. The cost in broken homes, wasted lives, loss to society, and human misery is beyond calculation.

Effects of chronic alcoholism include psychological problems (anxiety, depression, loss of control over drinking), social problems (work, family life), and physiological problems (tremors, periods of amnesia and memory loss, poor motor control, liver disease, etc.).

In long-term alcoholism with malnutrition, chronic degeneration may be observed. This consists of a bloated look, flabby muscles, fine tremors, decreased physical capacity and stamina, and increased susceptibility to infections. This state of chronic degeneration is not present in the majority of alcoholics with adequate nutrition, though adequate nutrition does not fully protect the brain, the liver, or the digestive tract.

An extensive bibliography and review of the consequences of alcohol can be found in two recent government reports.[16,17]

To date, no effective drug is available to help persons decrease their alcohol intake. As stated previously, disulfiram (Antabuse), given prior to alcohol consumption, induces an adversive reaction that is presumed to deter further drinking. However, this approach to limiting drinking is not the treatment of choice, because the goal is total abstinence. Failure rates of treatment with disulfiram are high and clinical efficacy is low.

An alternative approach is to develop drugs that modulate ethanol intake, allowing a combined behavioral and pharmacological approach to limiting ethanol intake in persons with alcohol-related problems.[18] Citalopram is a possible drug for this purpose, because it is a selective inhibitor of the active reuptake of serotonin into the presynaptic nerve terminals from which it was released (discussed in Chapter 6 and Appendix II). In patients with early-stage drinking problems, the drug has been found to effectively decrease the numbers of drinks consumed and has increased the number of abstinent days.[19] Such effects appear to be independent of citalopram's antidepressant action. Although much additional research must be done in this area, this finding suggests that drug-induced reinforcement of serotonin neurotransmission may limit ethanol intake, providing a new pharmacological direction to the treatment of the problem drinker.[20] The first such serotonin uptake blocker, fluoxetine (Prozac), was released in the United States in early 1988.

Treatment of Alcoholism

In a text devoted to the basic principles of drug action, discussion of the treatment of drug problems is a secondary objective. However, because the use and abuse of alcohol are so widespread in our society it seems pertinent to delineate briefly some of the newer concepts relating to alcoholism and its treatment.

Prior to about 1960, alcoholism was seldom considered a medical problem. Individuals were routinely arrested for public drunkenness, denied medical services, and allowed to go through a withdrawal syndrome in the drunk tank of the local jail. It was not until the late 1950s that the American Medical Association (or a minority within that association) recognized the syndrome of alcoholism as an illness. In his book *The Disease Concept of Alcoholism*, (1960), E. M. Jellinek presented the hypothesis that alcoholism is a disease.[21] Such labeling served to reduce many of the social stigmata of alcoholism and formed the concept that the deficit in alcoholism lies in an individual who is unable to tolerate its effects. To be free of the disease, therefore, the person with this deficiency must totally abstain from alcohol. This concept also implies that no matter how they become alcoholic, all alcoholics are the same because they all have the same disease. This concept is the basis of nearly all alcoholism treatment programs today. As M. Mann puts it, "alcoholism is a disease which manifests itself chiefly by the uncontrollable drinking of the victim, who is known as an alcoholic."[22]

In contrast to this uniform concept, others postulate that no single entity can be defined as alcoholism and that alcoholism is not a unitary concept but a collection of various signs, symptoms, and behaviors.[23-27] Alcohol dependence is a health problem (rather than a disease) affecting five areas of life health: (1) drinking health, (2) emotional health, (3) vocational health, (4) social/family health, and (5) physical health. Not all alcohol-dependent persons are impaired in each area of life health nor does impairment in one area necessarily imply impairment in other areas.

For example, a person's drinking health may be severely impaired without much alteration in his or her physical or vocational health, as in the executive with adequate diet and social and family supports. On the other hand, in treatment, drinking health may be solved by total abstinence, yet other life areas such as social/family health and emotional health may not be remedied or may be even worsened. Therefore, different individuals with alcohol problems will exhibit different profiles of impairment in life health. As such, different prescriptions for treatment and different levels of expectation for success must be employed for each individual. For example, sobriety may be a reasonable expectation for an individual with minimally impaired life health, while attenuated drinking with modest improvements in health may be all that can be reasonably expected for a more severely impaired alcoholic.

Such individualism may be some distance off, however, since society has only recently begun to look less scornfully upon the alcoholic and is just beginning to recognize that each alcoholic should have an individual set of therapeutic objectives. The goal of future treatment programs may not *necessarily* be total abstinence from alcohol for every alcoholic but, rather, a reduction in life problems associated with drinking. It has been estimated that alcohol abuse and alcoholism cost various segments of the American economy some $90 billion per year. Business and industry sustain some $20 billion of that total in lost productivity.[25] More than 2400 organizations have functioning programs designed to identify employees with alcohol-related problems and provide them with counseling. The bibliography is intended to help the interested reader pursue these newer concepts of alcoholism and its treatment.

Notes

1. J. H. Jaffe, "Drug Addiction and Drug Abuse," in A. G. Gilman, L. S. Goodman, T. W. Rall, and F. Murad, eds., *Goodman and Gilman's The Pharmacological Basis of Therapeutics*, 7th ed. (New York: Macmillan, 1985), p. 548.

2. J. W. Hanson, K. L. Jones, and D. W. Smith, "Fetal Alcohol Syndrome," *Journal of the American Medical Association* 235 (5 April 1976): 1458–1460.

3. E. Majchrowicz and E. P. Noble (eds.), *Biochemistry and Pharmacology of Ethanol*, vols. 1–3 (New York: Plenum Press, 1979).

4. J. M. Ritchie, "The Aliphatic Alcohols," in A. G. Gilman, L. S. Goodman, T. W. Rall, and F. Murad, eds., *Goodman and Gilman's The Pharmacological Basis of Therapeutics*, 7th ed. (New York: Macmillan, 1985), pp. 372–373.

5. U.S. Department of Health, Education, and Welfare, *Alcohol and Health: Third Special Report to the U.S. Congress* (Washington, D.C.: U.S. Government Printing Office, 1978).

6. C. S. Lieber, "Alcoholism: Medical Implications," in *Research Developments in Drug and Alcohol Use. Annals of the New York Academy of Science* 362 (1981): 132–135.

7. M. J. Edkardt, T. C. Harford, C. T. Kaelber, et al., "Health Hazards Associated with Alcohol Consumption," *Journal of the American Medical Association* 246 (1981): 648–666.

8. National Institute on Alcohol Abuse and Alcoholism, "Alcohol and Disinhibition: Nature and Meaning of the Link," U.S. Department of Health and Human Services (Washington, D.C.: U.S. Government Printing Office, 1983).

9. R. G. Niven, "Alcoholism—A Problem in Perspective," *Journal of the American Medical Association* 252 (1984): 1912–1914.

10. B. M. Altura, "Cardiovascular Effects of Alcohol and Alcoholism—A Symposium," *Federation Proceedings* 41 (1982): 2437–2476.

11. A. Schatzkin, Y. Jones, R. W. Hoover, et al., "Alcohol Consumption and Breast Cancer in the Epidemiologic Follow-Up Study of the First National Health and Nutrition Examination Study," *New England Journal of Medicine* 316 (1987): 1169–1173.

12. W. C. Willett, M. J. Stampfer, G. A. Colditz, et al., "Moderate Alcohol Consumption and the Risks of Breast Cancer." *New England Journal of Medicine* 316 (1987): 1174–1180.

13. L. P. Finnegan, "The Effects of Narcotics and Alcohol on Pregnancy and the Newborn," in *Research Developments in Alcohol and Drug Use. Annals of the New York Academy of Science* 362 (1981): 136–157.

14. J. L. Mills, B. I. Granbard, E. E. Harley, et al., "Maternal Alcohol Consumption and Birth Weight," *Journal of the American Medical Association* 252 (1984): 1875–1879.

15. S. Blume, "National Patterns of Alcohol Use and Abuse," in *Research Developments in Drug and Alcohol Use. Annals of the New York Academy of Science* 362 (1981): 4–15.

16. *Report to the President and the Congress on Health Hazards Associated with Alcohol and Methods to Inform the General Public of These Hazards* (Washington, D.C.: U.S. Government Printing Office, 1980).

17. *Fifth Special Report to the U.S. Congress on Alcohol and Health.* U.S. Department of Health and Human Services (Washington, D.C.: U.S. Government Printing Office, 1984).

18. C. A. Naranjo, E. M. Sellers, and M. O. Lawrin, "Modulation of Ethanol Intake by Serotonin Uptake Inhibitors," *Journal of Clinical Psychiatry* 47 (1986): 4 (Suppl.), 16–22.

19. C. A. Naranjo, E. M. Sellers, J. T. Sullivan, D. W. Woodley, K. Kadler, and K. Sykora, "The Serotonin Uptake Inhibitor Citalopram Attenuates

Ethanol Intake," *Clinical Pharmacology and Therapeutics* 41 (1987): 266–274.

20. C. A. Naranjo and E. M. Sellers (eds.), "Research Advances in New Pharmacological Treatments for Alcoholism" (Amsterdam: Elsevier, 1985).

21. E. M. Jellinek, *The Disease Concept of Alcoholism* (New Haven, Conn.: Hillhouse Press, 1960).

22. M. Mann, *New Primer on Alcoholism*, 2d ed. (New York: Holt, 1968).

23. E. M. Pattison, L. Sobel, and L. C. Sobel, *Emerging Concepts of Alcohol Dependence* (New York: Springer-Verlag, 1977).

24. S. Cohen, *The Alcoholic Problem: Selected Issues* (New York: Haworth Press, 1983).

25. H. J. Harwood, D. M. Napolitano, P. L. Kristiansen, et al., *Economic Costs to Society of Alcohol, Drug Abuse, and Mental Illness* (Rockwell, Md.: Alcohol, Drug Abuse, and Mental Health Administration, June 1984).

26. J. E. Peachey and C. A. Naranjo, "Role of Drugs in Treatment of Alcoholism," *Drugs* 27 (1984): 171–182.

27. H. A. Skinner, "Primary Syndromes of Alcohol Abuse: Their Measurement and Correlates," *British Journal of Addiction* 76 (1981): 63–76.

CHAPTER 5

Central Stimulants

Amphetamine, Caffeine, Cocaine, and Nicotine

The compounds ordinarily classified as central stimulants are drugs that increase behavioral activity, thought processes, and alertness or elevate the mood of an individual. These drugs differ widely in their molecular structures and in their mechanisms of action. Thus, describing a drug as a *stimulant* does not adequately describe its pharmacology. By contrast, the term *nonselective general depressant* nicely characterizes the pharmacology of a large group of drugs that produce graded, nonselective depression of the central nervous system and the effects illustrated in Figure 3.1. No such generalization can be made about central stimulants. The convulsions induced by a stimulant such as strychnine, for example, are very different from the behavioral stimulation and psychomotor agitation induced by a stimulant such as amphetamine.

The drugs broadly classified as central stimulants may, however, be subdivided into several groups of agents that, because of similarities in sites and mechanisms of action, may be conveniently discussed together. These drugs are divided into four different classes, each classification being based on a different site or mechanism of action (see Table 5.1).

Classification

The first two groups of central stimulants—behavioral stimulants and clinical antidepressants—have as a common denominator the ability to augment the action of the chemical neurotransmitter nor-

Table 5.1

Classification of CNS stimulants.

Class	Mechanism of action	Examples
1. Behavioral stimulants	Augmentation of norepinephrine and dopamine neurotransmitter	Cocaine Amphetamines Methylphenidate (Ritalin) Pemoline (Cylert) Phenmetrazine (Preludin)
2. Clinical antidepressants	a. Blockade of norepinephrine reuptake b. Increased norepinephrine secondary to MAO inhibition	Imipramine (Tofranil) Amitriptyline (Elaval) Tranylcypromine (Parnate)
	c. Blockade of serotonin reuptake	Zimelidine* Fluvoxamine* Fluoxetine (Prozac)
3. Convulsants	Blockade of inhibitory synapses	Strychnine, picrotoxin, pentylenetetrazol (Metrazol) bicuculline
4. General cellular stimulants	a. Activation of intracellular metabolism b. Stimulation of certain acetylcholine synapses	Caffeine Nicotine (tobacco)

* Not available in the United States.

epinephrine. In general, the behavioral stimulants will elevate mood and stimulate behavior in normal individuals, whereas the clinical antidepressants are relatively devoid of behavioral activity in normal individuals, although they relieve depression and elevate mood in individuals who are psychologically depressed. Behavioral stimulants are discussed in this chapter, and clinical antidepressants are discussed in Chapter 6.

Examples of behavioral stimulants include cocaine, the many derivatives of amphetamine, methylphenidate (Ritalin), pemoline (Cylert), and phenmetrazine (Preludin). Cocaine and the amphetamines are commonly abused drugs. Methylphenidate and pemoline are employed in the treatment of hyperkinetic disorders of children. Phenmetrazine (as well as the amphetamines and methylphenidate) has been used widely as an appetite suppressant in the treatment of obesity.

The third group of CNS stimulants includes a number of compounds that produce convulsions, usually by blocking inhibitory synapses within the brain and spinal cord. Such convulsants include strychnine, picrotoxin, pentylenetetrazol (Metrazol), and bicuculline.

The fourth group of CNS stimulants consists of two widely used compounds. The first is caffeine, which acts inside nerve cells to increase their rates of cellular metabolism, not at the synapse between neurons. The second compound is nicotine, the principal ingredient in tobacco. Nicotine exerts its action secondary to stimulation of certain acetylcholine synapses both within the brain and in the peripheral nervous system.

Behavioral Stimulants

Cocaine and the amphetamines are generally classified as CNS, psychic, psychomotor, or behavioral stimulants. These compounds elevate mood, induce euphoria, increase alertness, reduce fatigue, provide a sense of increased energy and alertness, decrease appetite, improve task performance, and relieve boredom. Anxiety, insomnia, and irritability are common. At higher doses, irritability and anxiety become more intense and a pattern of psychotic behavior may appear. Despite their differences in chemical structure, cocaine and the amphetamines produce remarkably similar behavioral effects. Indeed, both animals and drug-dependent individuals have great difficulty differentiating between the intravenous effects of cocaine and amphetamines when they are administered in equally potent doses.[1]

At low doses, amphetamine evokes an alerting, arousal, or behavioral-activating response not unlike one's normal reaction to an emergency or to stress—a reaction that is not surprising because, structurally, amphetamine closely resembles both epinephrine (NE) and dopamine (DA), compounds for which most of the criteria for a transmitter substance in the brain have been met (see Appendix II). Indeed, the central stimulant actions of both amphetamine and cocaine appear to result from the ability of both compounds to mimic or potentiate the action of DA and NE in the brain. High doses of these drugs can produce a psychosis that is easily mistaken for schizophrenia, which is thought to be due to their effects on dopamine neurons.

Biological amines appear to be involved in the behavioral activation associated with the fight/flight/fright response (see Appendix II). Thus, one would predict that increased activity of NE synapses within the brain would result in behavioral activation. Similarly, methylphenidate, pemoline, and phenmetrazine appear to elevate mood, relieve depression, depress appetite, and calm hyperkinetic behavior secondary to their ability to augment the action of NE at the synapse. Clinically, these compounds are widely prescribed as amphetamine substitutes both in the treatment of hyperkinetic behavior in children and in the treatment of obesity.

Dopamine neurons have recently been implicated in animals as the sites of action that underlie the self-administration, behavioral reinforcing, and addictive properties of cocaine,[2] and the striatum (limbic system) exhibits a particularly high ability to bind cocaine.[3-4]

Biological Amine Theory of Mania and Depression

Norepinephrine and dopamine play important roles in the body's response to stress and emotion. These two transmitters are released from neurons as part of the fight/flight/fright response; they increase heart rate and blood flow to skeletal muscle and reduce blood flow to the stomach, kidney, liver, and other internal organs. Such reactions generally prepare the body for stress, exertion, or the expression of emotion.

A third biological amine transmitter, serotonin, is also present in large amounts in the CNS. Its possible role in depression has been reviewed recently [*Journal of Clinical Psychiatry* 46 (1986): 4 (Suppl.) 23–35.]

The specific role that NE, dopamine, and serotonin play in the control of emotional disorders is unknown, although researchers believe that such disorders are related to their functional excesses or deficits at the synapses within the brain. Emotional depression, they speculate, is related to a deficiency of these transmitters within the brain and mania is caused by an excessive amount (Figure 5.1). In other words, they are thought to be the synaptic transmitters responsible for maintaining behavior.

According to this hypothesis, drugs that increase the synaptic action of NE, dopamine, and serotonin stimulate behavior relative to the concentration of transmitter at the synapse. Conversely, agents that deplete the store of transmitter in the brain or block receptors at the synapse induce depression. Evidence that amphetamine, cocaine, and the clinical antidepressants (both the MAO inhibitors and the tricyclic compounds) all increase NE activity supports this hypothesis.

For example, studies of amphetamine abuse and withdrawal showed that when the patients were allowed to administer amphetamine to themselves, they became manic and the metabolic byproducts of brain amines were elevated. When the amphetamines were withdrawn abruptly, the metabolites decreased and the patients became depressed. As the depression slowly disappeared and the patients returned to normal, there was a gradual increase in amine metabolites in the urine, indicating that synapses were recovering.

In contrast, the antipsychotic drug, reserpine, depletes NE and

Figure 5.1

Outline of the biological amine hypothesis of mania and depression.

Behavioral state

Depression $\longleftrightarrow$ Normal $\longleftrightarrow$ Behavioral stimulation $\longleftrightarrow$ Mania

Amine levels

Low $\longleftrightarrow$ Normal $\longleftrightarrow$ Slight excess $\longleftrightarrow$ Great excess

Drug	Transmitter levels	Behavior
Amphetamine	Up	Up
Cocaine	Up	Up
MAO inhibitors	Up	Up
Tricyclic compounds	Up	Up
Reserpine	Down	Down
Lithium	Down	Down

serotonin in the brain and produces behavioral depression that can be severe if enough transmitter is lost. Lithium's usefulness in the treatment of mania is due to its ability to block the release of NE from the presynaptic nerve terminal (decreasing the amount available at the receptor). Lithium may also "stabilize" the receptor, decreasing its sensitivity to transmitter. Interestingly, lithium is also used to manage depression. This apparent contradiction of the catecholamine hypothesis of mania and depression is explained by the fact that as lithium slowly relieves manic episodes, brain levels of catecholamine become more stable and the periods of depression decrease. Lithium is discussed at length in Chapter 6.

Neurotransmitters and Mechanisms of Drug Action

It is now clear that drugs interfere with a variety of processes associated with synaptic transmission. Amphetamine and cocaine appear to exert their behavioral effects by increasing the action of NE, serotonin, and dopamine at the synapse. There are at least five ways in which a drug could potentiate the synaptic action of these transmitters. First, it might increase the rate of synthesis of the transmitter substance. Such an action is unlikely, and, indeed, has not been demonstrated because drugs usually depress ongoing processes rather than stimulate reactions.

Second, the compound might potentiate synaptic transmission by blocking the enzymes responsible for the metabolism of the transmitter.

Third, a drug might augment the action of transmitter by inducing its release from the presynaptic nerve terminals, thus increasing the amount of transmitter available to stimulate the postsynaptic receptors. The stimulants amphetamine and methylphenidate do induce such a release of NE and serotonin. Some postulate that this is the primary action responsible for the behavioral effects of these drugs. Release of dopamine by high doses of either drug may produce their psychotomimetic side effects.

Fourth, a drug might prolong the action of transmitter at its postsynaptic receptor by blocking its active uptake from the synaptic cleft back into the presynaptic nerve terminal. The synaptic action of NE, dopamine, and serotonin is apparently terminated by its active uptake from the synaptic cleft back into the presynaptic terminal from which it was originally released. Such a block of active reuptake of dopamine appears to be the primary mechanism of action of cocaine.

Finally, drugs may directly stimulate the postsynaptic NE receptor, mimicking the effect of NE or dopamine. This is thought to be another action of amphetamine, in addition to its ability to induce the release of NE from the presynaptic terminal.

The actions of amphetamine, cocaine, and the clinical antidepressants are summarized in Table 5.2. Despite their varied mechanisms of action, all appear to relieve depression or induce behavioral stimulation in a manner strongly correlated with their ability

Table 5.2

Potentiation of transmission at biological amine synapses by various drugs.

Drug	Action
Amphetamine	Increased release of NE Direct stimulation of postsynaptic NE receptors
Methylphenidate	Increased release of NE Direct stimulation of postsynaptic NE receptors
Cocaine	Blocks reuptake of dopamine by presynaptic nerve terminal
Tricyclic antidepressants*	Blocks reuptake of NE by presynaptic nerve terminal
MAO-inhibiting* antidepressants	Inhibition of enzyme MAO

* See Chapter 6.

to increase the amount of biological amines at the synapse and bearing out the amine hypothesis of mania and depression presented in Figure 5.1.

Amphetamine

Amphetamine is, structurally, closely related to norepinephrine (see Figure 5.2). It mimics and potentiates the synaptic action of NE both in the central nervous system and in the rest of the body. At higher doses, dopamine neurotransmission is also augmented.

Amphetamine was first synthesized in the early 1900s but was not used for medical purposes until the early 1930s, when it was found that it increased blood pressure, stimulated the central nervous system, caused bronchodilatation (useful in treating asthma), and was useful in treating an epileptic seizure disorder called narcolepsy (a disorder in which the patient repeatedly lapses into sleep). Since then, amphetamines have been used for a wide variety of clinical and recreational purposes.

The most common amphetamine derivatives currently available are amphetamine (Benzedrine), dextroamphetamine (Dexedrine), and methamphetamine (Methedrine or Desoxyn). Other chemicals also are available that are structurally related to amphetamine and that share its profile of action. Most are promoted as appetite suppressants. Despite variances in potency (compensated for by an adjustment in dose), the effects of the amphetamine derivatives are similar to those of amphetamine itself; therefore, amphetamine is discussed at length and the other drugs compared with it.

Figure 5.2

Structural formulas of norepinephrine and amphetamine.

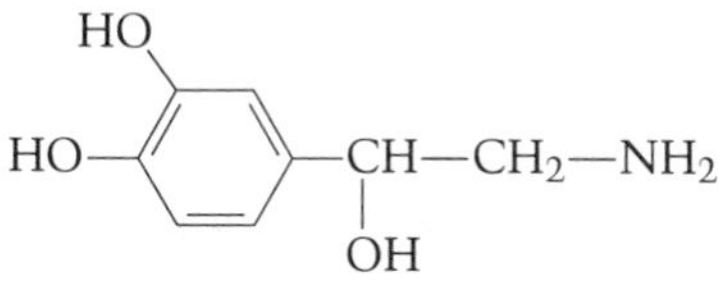

Norepinephrine

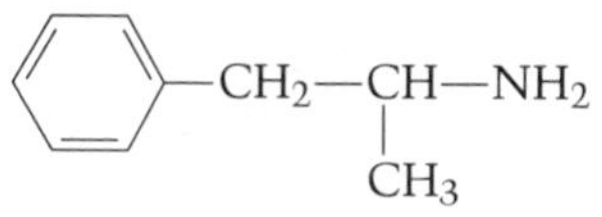

Amphetamine

Therapeutic Uses and Status

The primary *medical* uses of amphetamine are restricted today. Amphetamine was first found useful and specific in the treatment of narcolepsy and is used to treat a form of epilepsy called petit mal epilepsy. It also appears to be useful in treating certain attention deficit (hyperkinetic) disorders in children. Such disorders are characterized by inattentiveness and impulsiveness, usually with impaired learning and behavioral hyperactivity. Amphetamine, and more recently the amphetamine derivatives methylphenidate (Ritalin) and pemoline (Cylert), improve behavior and learning ability in 50–75 percent of children correctly diagnosed. However, indiscriminate use of these behavioral stimulants for "problem children" and *sole dependence* on drug therapy for attention deficit disorders should be discouraged. The family situation of a child diagnosed as hyperkinetic should be investigated to rule out external causes for his or her behavior. Some theorize that a child's hyperkinetic behavior may be a natural defense against his or her own state of depression. Such behavior would be a symptom of a deeper problem, not a disease. Even if the drug does correct the behavioral and learning problems, the home situation should still be explored. Adjunctive treatments such as remedial education, behavioral modification, and counseling with parents and teachers are indicated.

Why stimulants calm hyperactive children is not clear. If one postulates that hyperkinesis is a manifestation of the child's own depression, however, use of an antidepressant drug would serve to alleviate the behavioral symptoms. On the other hand, by increasing attention and learning abilities, a child's anxieties may be relieved and the anxious state replaced by a more pleasant and productive one. Indeed, adults in certain anxiety states (such as studying for final examinations) often find that they become calmer, more alert, and can work more efficiently after taking amphetamine or other stimulants.

These uses of amphetamine are the only ones presently recognized as clinically significant. The amphetamines, however, are strong appetite suppressants and have been sold extensively as "diet pills." Tolerance to the appetite-suppressant action of amphetamines appears within about 2 weeks, however, so the dose must be increased. Once tolerance develops, and unless the dose is increased (usually to the point at which the patient becomes agitated), the patient usually resumes his or her previous eating habits and gains back all the weight lost earlier. As a result, amphetamines are no longer recognized as effective drugs for the long-term control of obesity. Indeed, federal regulations currently require the following labeling information on amphetamine preparations:

Amphetamines have a high potential for abuse. They should thus be tried only in weight reduction programs for patients in whom alternative therapy has been ineffective. Administration of amphetamines for prolonged periods of time in obesity may lead to drug dependence and must be avoided. Particular attention should be paid to the possibility of subjects obtaining amphetamines for nontherapeutic use or distribution to others, and the drugs should be prescribed or dispensed sparingly.

Despite such warnings, pharmacological methods of promoting weight loss continue to be sought by the public. Thus, several drugs chemically related to amphetamines are available for use if such is desired (see the following discussion).

Amphetamines are used nontherapeutically for many and varied reasons, usually because they are euphoriant or because they improve performance.[5] Characteristically, amphetamines produce a state of euphoria—an action that may explain the wide misuse of the drug.

It has been well documented that psychomotor, intellectual, or athletic performance may be improved to a slight but statistically significant degree by amphetamines. It is most likely that such improvements are a result of the increased availability of norepinephrine, which will augment alertness and the fight/flight/fright reactions. The amphetamines also have the ability to produce prolonged periods of wakefulness and induce insomnia, an action that has been postulated to result from an increase in norepinephrine in the reticular formation, especially in the ARAS, which stimulates the centers responsible for maintaining wakefulness.

Amphetamine and many amphetamine derivatives are widely available legally and illegally in a variety of forms, mixtures, and concoctions. In the legal market, there is probably no area of medicine in which one group of drugs has been so misused. The amphetamines are commercially found mixed with barbiturates, other sedatives, atropine, caffeine, vitamins, thyroid, and numerous other drugs, usually in irrational combinations. For example, the Le Dain report of Canada stated that one amphetamine combination was described by its manufacturer as follows: "This is a multicoated tablet of pentobarbital on the outside to induce sleep rapidly, phenobarbital under a delayed dissolving coating to extend the sleep, and under another coating, an amphetamine to awaken a patient in the morning."[6]

Recently, an illegally obtained product, Redotex, became available that contains an amphetamine-like compound (Fenfluramine) plus a diuretic, thyroid, a laxative, atropine, and a sedative such as diazepam (Valium). Weight loss from such a diet cocktail is temporary and places the patient at risk of injury or even death.

Another example of misleading information about amphetamine action occurred during the period of explosive increases in amphetamine use and abuse in the 1950s and 1960s when it was felt by many that children should not be placed on long-term amphetamine therapy for hyperkinetic disorders, even though many physicians prescribed it. Therefore, two "nonamphetamine" stimulants, methylphenidate (Ritalin) and pemoline (Cylert), were introduced for the treatment of these children. As Figure 5.3 shows, methylphenidate and pemoline are structurally so similar to amphetamine that they probably work on the same receptors in the brain as does amphetamine. Thus, despite the fact that methylphenidate and pemoline are *chemically* not amphetamine (which is a chemical term), pharmacologically their effect is virtually identical.

Pharmacological Effects

The physiological responses to amphetamine vary markedly with the dose of the drug.[7] In general, however, they may be categorized as those observed at low-to-moderate doses (5 to 50 milligrams of amphetamine, usually administered orally) and those observed at high doses (doses above approximately 100 milligrams, often administered intravenously). These dose ranges are not the same for all amphetamines. For example, dextroamphetamine is more potent than amphetamine. Low-to-moderate doses of dextroamphetamine

Figure 5.3

Structural formulas of amphetamine, methylphenidate, and pemoline. This shows the close structural similarities among these drugs. Shading indicates the common portions of the molecule.

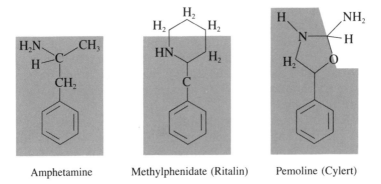

Amphetamine   Methylphenidate (Ritalin)   Pemoline (Cylert)

range from 2.5 to 20 milligrams, while high doses are considered to be 50 milligrams or more. Methamphetamine ("speed") is even more potent, and doses have to be lowered even further.

At *normal, oral* doses, all of the amphetamines induce a significant increase in blood pressure, with a reflex slowing of heart rate, a relaxation of bronchial muscle, and a variety of other responses that are predictable from drugs that mobilize norepinephrine and thus induce the fight/flight/fright response (that is, increased blood sugar, increased blood flow to musculature, decreased blood flow to internal organs, dilation of pupils, increased rate of respiration, and so on). In the central nervous system, the amphetamines are potent stimulants, producing both EEG and behavioral signs of increased alertness and excitement. Characteristically, wakefulness, increased alertness, a reduced sense of fatigue, mood elevation, increased motor and speech activity, euphoria, and an increased feeling of power occur. Task performance is improved, although dexterity may not improve as evidenced by increased errors that can result from the irritability and nervousness that occurs. When short-duration, high-intensity energy output is desired, such as in athletic competition, performance may be enhanced despite the fact that dexterity and fine motor skills may be reduced.[8]

At moderate doses (5 to 50 milligrams), the effects of amphetamine in the brain include stimulation of respiration, production of a slight tremor, restlessness, increased motor activity, insomnia, and agitation. In addition, amphetamine prevents fatigue, suppresses appetite, and promotes wakefulness. The wakefulness is of interest because even with amphetamines the biological need for sleep may not be postponed indefinitely. When the administration of amphetamines is stopped, there is a rebound increase in sleep time. Indeed, such drug-induced sleep deficits, with subsequent rebound, are significant and complete recovery of normal sleeping patterns may take many weeks. Indeed, prolonged use of low doses of amphetamine and single use of high doses of amphetamine are characteristically followed by an intensity of mental depression and fatigue that parallels the behavioral stimulation and euphoria produced by the initial dose of the drug.

During chronic use of amphetamine in high doses (100 milligrams or more), a different pattern of physiological effects is observed, partly because such high doses are usually administered intravenously. Daily doses in the range of 100 milligrams to several grams have been reported. During prolonged, high-dose "sprees," an individual experiences a paranoid mania that is induced by the excessive levels of NE (Figure 5.1), by the chronic lack of sleep and food, and by the drug-induced activation of dopamine neurons. Because dopamine neurons are involved in the pathogenesis of schizophrenia (Chapter 8), it is not surprising that amphetamine produces a schizophrenic-like behavioral response.[9]

The intravenous injection of amphetamine provides a sudden "flash" or "rush," described by users as being extremely pleasurable and very similar to an intense sexual orgasm. These pleasurable effects, however, are offset by the manic paranoia that is induced. Withdrawal of the drug and subsequent termination of the "spree" is followed by fatigue. Deep sleep occurs and may last for several days. Upon awakening, the user is lethargic, emotionally depressed, and intensely hungry. Food and counseling may be helpful in this withdrawal period. Otherwise, the user may try more injections of amphetamine, thus initiating another spree.

The amphetamines have been used widely in the treatment of obesity; however, today such use is considered unwise and has been abandoned.[10] Weight loss following amphetamine use is caused by a depression of appetite that is secondary to the drug's action on feeding and satiety centers in the hypothalamus. Tolerance to this effect develops rapidly and weight loss is usually not maintained. Because the amphetamines were the first drugs widely prescribed to suppress appetite, they remain the standard to which newer drugs are compared (despite the fact that they are no longer recommended because the risk of drug dependence is so great). Newer drugs currently promoted as appetite suppressants include diethylpropion (Tenuate, Tepanil), mazindol (Mazanor, Sanorex), fenfluramine (Pondimin), and phentermine (Ionamin). Formerly, phenmetrazine (Preludin) was used widely, but a high incidence of drug abuse and dependence has rendered it obsolete. All these drugs closely resemble amphetamine both structurally and pharmacologically. Although none of these drugs are superior to the amphetamines as appetite suppressants, few of them are currently associated with significant drug abuse problems. Therefore, they are preferred in those rare instances where drug supplementation may be beneficial in appetite-suppression programs.

Phenylpropanolamine (available in multiple over-the-counter diet aids) is a mild adrenergic stimulant that is promoted as an aid in weight reduction. It has low potency and, as a result, exerts only mild CNS effects. At doses that are equally effective with those of amphetamine, phenylpropanolamine probably would be equally euphoric but, at this point in time, the drug has not been abused widely.

In summary, therefore, despite their continuing availability, nonamphetamine appetite suppressants offer few advantages over the amphetamines, and one must continue to strive for nonpharmacological methods to curb caloric intake. Compulsive overeating will not be solved by drugs, and the CNS stimulation and appetite-suppressant effects of these drugs continue to be inseparable.

Psychological Effects

The psychological effects of amphetamine differ widely, depending upon the dose administered. At low-to-moderate doses, an individual typically experiences increased alertness, wakefulness, elevation of mood, mild euphoria, increased athletic performance, decreased fatigue, possible freedom from boredom, less mental clouding, clearer thinking, improvements in concentration, increased energy, and, in general, increased levels of behavioral activity. All of this corresponds to the role of norepinephrine in behavioral alerting or arousal responses. Some of the effects of these low doses may be bothersome, for they include increased irritability, restlessness and insomnia, blurred vision, increased blood pressure, cardiac palpitations, and anxiety. Occasionally, aggression, hallucinations, and psychosis may occur, but usually only at higher doses.

High-dose intravenous use induces a pattern of psychosis characterized by confused and disorganized behavior, compulsive repetition of meaningless acts, irritability, fear, suspicion of everything and everyone, hallucinations, and delusions. The user may become aggressive and extremely antisocial. Individuals who inject amphetamines either dissolve oral tablets or crystalline methamphetamine ("crystal") that is manufactured illegally. Used intravenously, the amphetamines are known as "speed." Users of injectable amphetamines (or cocaine) often attempt to antagonize high-dose toxic symptoms by adding an opioid analgesic (such as morphine or heroin) to the stimulant. Such a concoction is called a "speedball." Amphetamine abusers also usually consume large amounts of other CNS depressants such as barbiturates, benzodiazepines, or alcohol. Interestingly, the depression and lethargy that follow amphetamine use are markedly accentuated by the presence of depressant drugs, which serve to intensify the fatigue, lethargy, and mental depression. Reinitiation of amphetamine use eliminates this state, but it starts a new cycle.

The majority of amphetamine or methamphetamine in each dose taken is exerted unchanged in the urine. Techniques have been developed to detect in each dose taken these substances in urine up to 24–48 hours after drug use. Positive tests for amphetamines must be confirmed by eliminating the possible presence of such drugs as ephedrine and phenylpropanolamine, which are found in cold remedies and dietary aids.

Side Effects and Toxicity

The side effects induced by low doses of amphetamine are usually extensions of the drug's behavioral actions: restlessness and tremor, anxiety, insomnia, dizziness, irritability, and tenseness. These side effects are usually tolerable and decrease within a few days as tolerance develops. Amphetamines also increase blood pressure and may cause heart palpitations. Sweating, dry mouth, and nausea and vomiting may also occur. Fatalities are rare.

The side effects of prolonged use of high doses are more serious. Psychosis and abnormal mental conditions, weight loss, skin sores, infections resulting from neglected health care, and a variety of other consequences occur because of the drug itself or because of poor eating habits, lack of sleep, and the use of unsterile equipment for intravenous injections.

Most high-dose users show progressive social, personal, and occupational deterioration, and their course is often characterized by intermittent periods of hospitalization for episodes of toxic psychosis.

Fatalities directly attributable to the use of amphetamine, however, are rare. Individuals with no tolerance have survived doses of 400 to 500 milligrams. Even larger doses are tolerated by chronic users. The slogan, "speed kills," does not refer to a direct effect of single doses of amphetamine but, rather, to the deteriorating mental and physical condition and the destructive and aggressive behavior induced by prolonged high-dose amphetamine sprees. Such sprees are detrimental to both the mental and the physical health of the individual and often to those with whom he or she interacts. Only rarely does even high-dose, intravenous use of amphetamine result in lethal rupture of blood vessels as a result of drug-induced increases in arterial pressure.

Dependence

Dependence is twofold: psychological and physiological. Psychological dependence is described as a compulsion to use a drug repeatedly for its enjoyable effects. The euphoric or pleasurable state that follows even moderate doses of amphetamine and the drug-induced "rush" and orgasm that may be induced by intravenous use can lead to a compulsion to misuse the drug.

Physiological dependence to the sedative-hypnotic compounds has been described as a period of rebound hyperexcitability following withdrawal of the drug. Withdrawal of amphetamine produces fatigue, profound and prolonged sleep, EEG changes characteristic of sleep, severe emotional depression, and increased appetite. This certainly is not unexpected; one would predict that if the body and the brain were continually stimulated by amphetamine such stimulation would be followed by depression upon removal of the drug.

Tolerance

Tolerance to the many effects of amphetamine develops at different rates and to different degrees. Tolerance to the appetite-suppressing effect of amphetamine almost invariably develops, accounting for the failure of these compounds to be effective in the long-term treatment of obesity. The mood-elevating action of amphetamine is subject to tolerance but not to quite the same extent as the appetite-suppressant effect. Tolerance to the peripheral effects also develops, so that a habitual user is able to increase the dose considerably in order to attain a desired effect as his or her tolerance to the central effects builds. Yet there are some effects of amphetamine to which only minimal tolerance develops. For instance, in the treatment of behavioral hyperactivity, once an adequate controlling dose is achieved, there may be little need to increase the dose of amphetamine for many years. Tolerance to the psychological effects develops to such a degree that the habitual user may inject up to a gram of amphetamine every few hours.

Cocaine

Cocaine is a naturally occurring alkaloid obtained from the leaves of *Erythroxylon cocca*, trees that are indigenous to Peru, Columbia, and Bolivia. In these countries, the leaves are usually chewed to increase endurance and to promote a sense of well-being.

Pharmacologically, cocaine has two prominent actions: (1) it is a potent local anesthetic, and (2) it is a powerful stimulant of dopamine neurotransmission. Cocaine inhibits the active reuptake of this transmitter into presynaptic nerve terminals in both the brain and the peripheral nervous system[2] (Table 5.2). Such uptake blockade increases the amount of dopamine in the synaptic cleft, thereby stimulating both the central and the peripheral nervous systems. At high doses, cocaine probably augments the synaptic action of NE as well.

In the peripheral nervous system, the potentiation of NE neurotransmission initiates responses characteristic of the fight/flight/fright syndrome: the drug increases heart rate and constricts blood vessels. The net result is an increase in blood pressure. Cocaine also produces bronchodilatation in the lungs, and this action, combined with constriction of blood vessels in the nose, makes breathing easier. When the drug wears off, however, the nasal blood vessels dilate, causing regular users to experience nasal stuffiness and tender, bleeding nasal membranes. As a result, cocaine users often sniff more drug, delaying but intensifying the symptoms. The vasoconstriction after "snorting" can produce ischemia of the nasal tissues with eventual perforation of the nasal septum.

Cocaine is a powerful CNS stimulant and euphoriant, affecting both the cortex and the brainstem.[11] It increases mental awareness and intellectual ability, accompanied by a feeling of well-being and euphoria (identical to that obtained with amphetamine). Although the user's sense of fatigue is decreased and his or her motor activity is increased, coordination decreases rapidly with higher doses because the brainstem centers that coordinate movement are affected. With even higher doses, a progressive loss of coordination is followed by tremors and eventually by seizures. CNS stimulation is followed by depression, and eventually the respiratory control centers in the brainstem are depressed. Death results from respiratory failure.

The syndrome of behavioral and toxic effects (including paranoia) produced by cocaine is generally similar to that produced by amphetamine—a similarity that would be expected, considering the similar sites of action on nerve terminals, resulting in potentiation of norepinephrine and dopamine. As with amphetamine, respiration and heart rate are stimulated and vomiting may be induced. Experienced cocaine users find that the effects of an inhaled dose of about 16 milligrams closely resembles an inhaled dose of about 10 milligrams of amphetamine, except that the effects of amphetamine last longer. The effects of amphetamine may last for several hours. Cocaine, on the other hand, may be active in the body for only a short period of time because it is metabolized by the liver. A dose of cocaine may be metabolized within 60 minutes. Although the average street dose of cocaine is about 20–50 milligrams intranasally,[12] much higher doses are commonly being taken.[13]

Because only about 1 percent of a dose of cocaine is excreted unmetabolized in urine, detection techniques involve urinary detection of metabolites. Such can be detected for up to 2 days after cocaine use; thus, a positive cocaine metabolite test indicates use within this 2-day period. Thus, periodic urinalysis for drug use is less likely to detect cocaine use than that of marijuana or barbiturates, which have a longer detection time.

Oral doses are absorbed well but so slowly that the effects may be missed. Potency is increased several-fold with intravenous administration, though the duration of action is very short (5–15 minutes), and the potential for overdosage is great. Intravenous use of cocaine is extremely dangerous and possibly lethal.[14] Thus, while the euphoric effects are magnified by intravenous use, so is the potential for serious injury.

Undesired side effects are not common for recreational users of low doses of cocaine. When acute anxiety reactions occur they are manifested by increased blood pressure and heart rate, sweating, anxiety, and paranoia. Hallucinations and delusions are rare. More common are the feelings of irritability and lassitude after the effects subside, together with a desire for more drug. Withdrawal after a longer period of using higher doses is followed by profound physical and emotional depression similar to that occasioned by amphetamine withdrawal.

The social misuse of cocaine is not new. In 1884, Sigmund Freud advocated use of cocaine for relief from depression and chronic fatigue, describing it as a "magical drug." He wrote the "Song of Praise" to cocaine, which was published in 1884. In relieving his own depression, Freud described small doses of cocaine as inducing "exhilaration and lasting euphoria, which in no way differs from the normal euphoria of the healthy person."[15] Freud, however, did not immediately perceive the liability of cocaine to produce tolerance, dependency, a state of psychosis, and withdrawal depression.[16]

As amphetamine became available in the 1930s, the use of cocaine diminished, probably because amphetamine cost less and lasted longer. Thus, cocaine was little used until the late 1960s, when tight federal restrictions on amphetamine distribution raised the cost of amphetamine to the point where cocaine was once again attractive. Because their actions at the NE synapse are similar, cocaine and amphetamine can be used almost interchangeably as euphoriants, so their use and popularity in the future will most likely be determined by availability and price. In a 1977 survey,[17] cocaine was ranked first by social-recreational cocaine users as their recreational drug of choice. From their standpoint, the only limitations to its use were its high cost and lack of availability. By 1987, almost 20 percent of young adults reported having used cocaine at least once, with 5 percent indicating use within the preceding month. Cocaine remains widely available, although the quantities ingested and the number of frequent users are decreasing modestly.[18] Unfortunately, increased use of illicit amphetamines (especially methamphetamine) appears to account for this reduced use of cocaine.

In South America, coca paste is made by mashing coca leaves and extracting the drug, which is then treated to produce a hydrochloride salt. It is imported in that form and then diluted with inert substances to increase its bulk and street value. Until recently, this type of preparation was used most frequently. However, with the desire for increased effect and potency, the diluted drug is now commonly either extracted in ether (for "freebasing") or in alkaline water (to make "crack"). Following either method of extraction, the concentrated powder can produce effects of utmost intensity and danger to the user. With such preparations, the low-dose behavioral effects are absent and the high-dose, high-intensity effects predominate. The incidence of acute panic states, toxic psychosis, and paranoid schizophrenia is greatly magnified.

Ephedrine, Metaraminol, Phenylephrine, and Others

There are many drugs structurally related either to amphetamine or to norepinephrine that can alter the synaptic action of NE both in the brain and in the periphery. Some of these agents release NE from presynaptic terminals; others directly stimulate postsynaptic NE receptors. Despite this difference in exact site of action, however, these compounds can induce a pattern of physiological and behavioral responses similar to those induced by amphetamine, even though the central effects of some of these agents are mild and high doses might be required. Although their number is bewildering, many names are likely to be familiar to the reader.

Representative products include ephedrine, tetrahydrazoline (Tyzine), metaraminol (Aramine), phenylephrine (Neo-Synephrine), pseudoephedrine (Sudafed), xylometazoline (Otrivin), nylidrin, (Arlidin) propylhexedrine (Benzedrex), phenmetrazine (Preludin), naphazoline (Privine), and oxymetazoline (Afrin). These compounds differ from one another primarily in the intensity of their effects on the body (heart rate, breathing, and the like) and in the degree to which they stimulate behavior. In general, the responses to these drugs are similar to those observed for amphetamine except that most have very poor CNS effects. Many are used as nasal decongestants and will produce rebound increases in nasal stuffiness when they wear off, a response similar to the stuffy nose induced by cocaine. Ephedrine is found as the active ingredient in approximately 70 percent of illicit preparations alleged to be amphetamine. Ephedrine is also readily available in over-the-counter preparations, especially those available by mail order. It is anticipated, therefore, that the abuse of ephedrine and other amphetamine-like compounds will continue.[19]

Convulsants

Many drugs that exert a generalized stimulation of the central nervous system are capable of inducing convulsions when administered in sufficient quantity. Notable examples are strychnine, picrotoxin, pentylenetetrazol (Metrazol), and bicuculline. These compounds differ from the drugs discussed earlier in this chapter in that they do *not* exert their effects through the NE synapses and therefore do not produce the continuum of behavioral states illustrated in Figure 5.1. They principally stimulate the spinal cord and brainstem and have, in general, less effect on the cerebral cortex. Although seldom useful clinically, the convulsants can stimulate respiration, temporarily counteract the action of depressant drugs, induce hyperactive spinal-cord reflexes, and, in general, increase the excitability of the nervous system without markedly augmenting the higher functions of the cerebral cortex such as creativity or thinking ability.

Each convulsive agent acts by blocking the synaptic actions of certain specific inhibitory neurotransmitters within the brain (Appendix II). The convulsant action of *strychnine* is due to interference with the inhibitory transmitter role of the amino acid glycine, an important inhibitory transmitter in the spinal cord.[20] *Picrotoxin* selectively antagonizes the effects of the inhibitory transmitter gamma-aminobutric acid (GABA) within the CNS. *Bicuculline* and *pentylenetetrazol* (Metrazol) act similarly, although all three of these drugs affect slightly different steps in GABA neurotransmission. These drugs are primarily useful as laboratory tools for investigating the functions of GABA neurons in the brain.

Laboratory studies using these agents to study brain mechanisms are consistent with the general rule that drugs exert both stimulant and depressant effects by blocking ongoing processes. In the case of convulsants, the blockade of inhibitory neurotransmission leads to loss of inhibitory control mechanisms and ultimately to convulsions.

The behavioral stimulation, hyperactivity, and convulsions that they induce occur as a result of their blocking inhibitory synapses in the spinal cord and the brainstem, which has the overall effect of markedly increasing the excitability of the central nervous system. As might be expected, these agents are not considered drugs of any useful therapeutic value. One would also question their recreational value, because they merely increase excitability without producing euphoria or augmenting cortical function. Strychnine and other convulsants are now only rarely encountered in illicit drug preparations.

They are extremely dangerous, especially when injected intravenously. They may induce powerful convulsions that disrupt the brainstem and, consequently, paralyze respiration, leading ultimately to cardiac arrest and death. In addition, because the action of stimulants is followed by behavioral depression, profound CNS depression is observed during recovery from these agents. The drugs are so gross in their action on the nervous system that treatment of overdose is nonspecific and not very effective because there are no specific antidotes. About all one can do is to prevent convulsions and support respiration. Convulsions can be prevented with a sedative-hypnotic drug, but when the convulsant is metabolized and the patient becomes depressed, the sedative-hypnotic deepens the depression, further endangering the patient.

Caffeine

Caffeine, one of the most popular and widely consumed drugs in the world, is found in significant concentrations in coffee, tea, cola drinks, chocolate candy, and cocoa.[21] The average cup of coffee contains between 100 and 150 milligrams of caffeine, and a 12-ounce bottle of a cola drink contains between 35 and 55 milligrams. The caffeine content may be as high as 25 milligrams per ounce in chocolate bars. The annual consumption of caffeine in the United States in the form of coffee alone is estimated at about 15 million pounds.

The main pharmacological actions of caffeine are exerted on the CNS, the heart, the kidneys, the lungs, and the arteries supplying blood to the heart and brain.[22] Most of these actions appear to be the result of caffeine-induced augmentation of cellular metabolism. Current thought holds that this action is exerted through a chemical substance called cyclic adenosine monophosphate (cyclic AMP). Caffeine inhibits an enzyme that ordinarily breaks down cyclic AMP to its inactive end product. The resultant increase in cyclic AMP leads to increased glucose production within cells and thus makes available more energy to allow higher rates of cellular activity.

Absorption, Distribution, Metabolism, and Excretion

Caffeine, existing in the stomach primarily in a water-soluble form, is only slowly and incompletely absorbed into the bloodstream. Thus, absorption is delayed and occurs largely through the intestine. As a result, caffeine is absorbed slowly (only approximately 25 percent in 1 hour), but completely.

Caffeine is freely and equally distributed throughout the total body water and crosses the placenta to the fetus. Thus, caffeine is found in almost equal concentrations in all parts of the body, including the brain. Most of the caffeine is metabolized by the liver before it is excreted by the kidneys. Only approximately 10 percent of the drug is excreted unchanged (that is, without being metabolized). The half-life of caffeine is about 5 hours in most adults; longer in infants, pregnant women, and the elderly; and shorter in smokers. Concentrations in breast milk may exceed that in mothers.

Pharmacological Effects

Caffeine is a powerful stimulant of nerve tissue in the brain. The cortex, being most sensitive, is affected first, followed next by the brainstem. The spinal cord is stimulated last, but only after extremely high doses of the drug. Since the cerebral cortex is affected at doses lower than those necessary to excite the brainstem, the earliest behavioral effects of caffeine are increased mental alertness, a faster and clearer flow of thought, wakefulness, and restlessness. This increased mental awareness may result in sustained intellectual effort for prolonged periods without the disruption of coordinated intellectual or motor activity that usually follows alteration of the function of the medulla (as occurs with amphetamine, cocaine, or the convulsants). The effects on the cerebral cortex may be observed after oral doses of as little as 100 or 200 milligrams, that is, one to two cups of coffee. Heavy consumption (12 or more cups a day, or 1.5 grams of caffeine) can cause more intense effects marked by agitation, anxiety, tremors, rapid breathing, and cardiac arrhythmias.

Only after massive doses (probably 2 to 5 grams) does the spinal cord become stimulated. Increased excitability of spinal reflexes might be observed then and, at even higher doses, convulsions and death may ensue. The convulsive dose, however, is so high (over 10 grams, the equivalent of 100 cups of coffee) that death from caffeine is highly unlikely.

Caffeine has a slight stimulant action on the heart, resulting in increased cardiac contractility and output (an increase in the total amount of blood pumped by the heart per minute). Caffeine also affects the arteries supplying blood to the heart (the *coronary* arteries), causing their dilation. This increases the flow of oxygenated blood to the heart muscle and increases the work capability of the heart. It should be noted, however, that caffeine *decreases* blood flow to the brain by constricting the cerebral blood vessels. Such action affords striking relief from headaches associated with increased blood pressure (hypertensive headaches) and provides some relief of certain types of migraine headaches, conditions for which caffeine is used clinically.

Another action of caffeine is to relax the musculature of the bronchi of the lungs, although a closely related compound, theophylline, is more potent in this regard. Caffeine also exerts a diuretic effect on the kidneys, although therapeutic effectiveness as a useful diuretic might be questioned.

Psychological Effects

In normal doses (100 to 500 milligrams), caffeine potently stimulates the cerebral cortex, promoting wakefulness and improving psychomotor performance. The stimulation, however, is not nearly as great as that induced by amphetamine. It must be remembered that once any stimulant agent is metabolized, there follows a period of behavioral and mental depression. This may be expressed frequently in automobile accidents that occur as a result of people driving for prolonged periods under caffeine stimulation. If people stop drinking coffee, they may become drowsy and fall asleep while driving. Such depression should be considered when any stimulant (such as amphetamine, cocaine, or caffeine) is ingested to maintain wakefulness or performance for prolonged periods.

Side Effects

The side effects associated with caffeine are extensions of its primary effect. One frequently observes periods of wakefulness and insomnia, psychomotor agitation, increases in heart rate with occasional arrhythmias, and either increases or decreases in blood pressure (usually not of great significance). With higher doses, mild delirium may be induced.

Dependence and Tolerance

With the usually administered doses of caffeine, little tolerance of the central stimulant actions develops. Some slight tolerance, however, may develop after prolonged ingestion of larger doses. It is now clear that caffeine does induce physiological dependence. Anyone who drinks five or more cups of coffee daily may experience withdrawal symptoms if he or she abruptly stops drinking coffee. Symptoms include headaches, irritability, lassitude, and sometimes nausea, all of which usually go away in a few days. The etiology of the withdrawal headache is unclear but likely involves dilatation of blood vessels inside the skull, increasing intracranial pressure.

Teratogenesis and Mutagenesis

Certain drugs endanger the fetus when they are ingested during pregnancy. Such toxicities are usually manifested as either mutagenesis (changes in the genetic code) or teratogenesis (abnormal development). Goldstein, Aronow, and Kalman claim that caffeine may induce chromosomal breakage in a variety of nonmammalian species.[23] Indeed, caffeine is used as a laboratory standard for studies of chromosomal breakage. The doses required to induce such breakage, however, are significantly higher than those usually consumed by humans.

It does not appear at this time that ingestion of tea or coffee increases mutation rates in humans, and most researchers have concluded, therefore, that caffeine does not constitute a *significant* toxic hazard to the fetus. One note of caution, however, was expressed by Goldstein et al.: "Caffeine should be regarded as possibly hazardous to the fetus during the first three months of pregnancy."[24] Such caution is warranted whenever *any* drug is ingested, especially a widely used drug that is freely distributed throughout the body and easily crosses the placenta.

Nicotine

Next to caffeine, nicotine, an active ingredient in tobacco, is the most widely used psychoactive agent in our society. Despite the fact that nicotine currently has little therapeutic application in medicine, its extreme potency and widespread use gives it considerable importance. Recent evidence indicates a wide range of toxicity to both nicotine and other ingredients of tobacco. The reader is referred to Brecher for a history of tobacco.[25]

Absorption, Distribution, Metabolism, and Excretion

Nicotine is readily and completely absorbed from the stomach after oral administration and from the lungs upon inhalation. Most cigarettes contain between 0.5 and 2.0 milligrams of nicotine, depending upon the brand. Conservative estimates indicate that approximately 20 percent (between 0.1 and 0.4 milligrams) of this nicotine is actually inhaled and absorbed into the smoker's bloodstream. Indeed, the physiological effects of smoking a single cigarette can be closely duplicated by the intravenous injection of these amounts of nicotine. This is well below the lethal dose of the drug, which is considered to be approximately 60 milligrams.

Like most psychoactive drugs, nicotine is quickly and ubiquitously distributed, rapidly penetrating the brain, all body organs, the fetus, and, in general, all body fluids.

Approximately 80 to 90 percent of the nicotine that is administered to an individual either orally or by smoking must be metabolized by the liver before it is excreted by the kidneys. Nicotine is also excreted in the milk of lactating women who smoke. Indeed, the breast-fed infant may have a blood level of nicotine as high or even higher than that of the mother.

Pharmacological Effects

Nicotine is an extremely potent compound and exerts powerful effects on the brain, the spinal cord, the peripheral nervous system, the heart, and various other body structures. Pharmacologically, nicotine appears to exert this action secondary to a direct stimulation of certain receptors sensitive to the transmitter acetylcholine.[26] This stimulation of acetylcholine receptors is manifested as CNS stimulation, increased blood pressure, increased heart rate, release of epinephrine (adrenalin) from the adrenal glands (including symptoms characteristic of the fight/flight/fright response), and increased tone and activity of the gastrointestinal tract.

Nicotine stimulates the central nervous system at all levels, including the cerebral cortex, producing increased levels of behavioral activity. The drug is capable of inducing tremors and, in large doses, convulsions. As with all stimulant drugs, stimulation of the brain is followed by a period of depression. Nicotine is also capable of stimulating the vomiting and the respiratory centers in the brainstem. It stimulates the hypothalamus to release a hormone called ADH (antidiuretic hormone), which causes an individual to retain fluid because the excretion of urine is reduced. The effect of nicotine on nerve fibers coming from the muscles leads to a marked reduction in muscle tone and may be involved (at least partially) in the relaxation that can accompany smoking.

In addition to its effects on the central nervous system, normal doses of nicotine can increase heart rate and blood pressure and stimulate heart muscle. It also increases blood flow to the heart and to skeletal muscle. Because it also increases the tone and activity of the bowel, nicotine may occasionally induce diarrhea.

Dependency

As many smokers know, nicotine induces both physiological and psychological dependence. It is, in fact, the most widespread example of drug dependence in the country. Over 50 million Americans smoke cigarettes; 60 percent of these persons have tried to quit, and 90 percent state that they would like to quit. Most smokers are physically dependent on nicotine and psychologically dependent on the behavior of smoking. Thus, for most smokers, cigarette smoking is an addiction.[27]

Withdrawal from cigarettes is accompanied by headache, stomach pain, irritability, and insomnia. Withdrawal appears to be quite prolonged, as evidenced by the individual who relapses after successfully completing the early stage of withdrawal. Smoking cigarettes with less nicotine content usually fails to help an individual cut down because he or she merely smokes more cigarettes per day. Attempts to free individuals from nicotine dependence by substituting nicotine-free cigarettes also fail. The newest treatment is the prescription chewing gum (Nicorette), each piece of which contains 2 milligrams of nicotine in a slow-release resin complex.[28] The idea is to substitute the gum for cigarettes, in the hope that the individual will tackle the psychological dependence and social components of smoking by first satisfying his or her physiological dependence on nicotine. Later, gum consumption can be slowly reduced and the individual withdrawn from the physiological dependence. Full withdrawal can take 6 months or longer. Nicotine-containing gum is not intended for nonsmokers because it may induce a physiological dependence on nicotine in them (this is one reason it is restricted to a doctor's prescription). Because it contains a fairly large dose of nicotine, it is not indicated in patients with heart disease, pregnant women, or breast-feeding mothers.

The number of cigarettes one must smoke per day to be considered addicted is unclear, but those who smoke 15 or more are very likely cigarette dependent.

Side Effects and Toxicity

The CNS side effects of nicotine usually consist of cortical stimulation, irritability, and tremors. Peripherally, side effects are usually manifested by intestinal cramps, diarrhea, increased heart rate and blood pressure, possible vomiting, and water retention.

The serious side effects of nicotine are many and alarming when one considers its widespread use. Cigarette smoking induces serious toxicity, which seems to occur secondary to a combination of the nicotine, carbon monoxide, and tars found in cigarette smoke.[29]

It is estimated that 362,000 persons die annually from tobacco use. Of these, 62,000 deaths are caused by lung disease, 130,000 are caused by cancer, and 170,000 result from heart and vascular diseases. One's life is shortened 14 minutes for every cigarette smoked. In other words, a 30- to 40-year-old male cigarette smoker who smokes two packs of cigarettes per day loses an estimated 8 years of his life. Over 50 million people (one of every six Americans alive today) will die from the effects of smoking cigarettes years before they otherwise would. Cigarette smoking, the nation's greatest public health hazard, is, ironically, the nation's most preventable cause of premature death, illness, and disability.[30]

In 1979 and 1981, the Surgeon General released two reports on the health consequences of smoking.[31,32] These and earlier monographs,[33,34] provide extensive discussion of cigarette toxicity. Considering only the *mortality* from cigarettes, increased death rates result from (1) cancers of the lung, voice box, mouth, throat, pancreas, and urinary bladder, (2) heart attacks secondary to coronary artery disease, and (3) chronic lung disease from bronchitis and emphysema.

The effects of the combined action of carbon monoxide and nicotine in cigarette smoke on the heart are as follows: carbon monoxide decreases the amount of oxygen delivered to heart muscle while nicotine increases the amount of work done by the heart (by increasing heart rate and blood pressure). Both carbon monoxide and nicotine serve to increase the incidence of atherosclerosis (narrowing) and thrombosis (clotting) in the coronary arteries. These three actions (and others as well) seem to underlie the five- to nineteenfold increase in the risk of death from coronary heart disease in smokers as compared to nonsmokers. If a smoker also has hypertension (elevated blood pressure) or diabetes, the risk is even further magnified.

In the lungs, chronic smoking results in a smoker's syndrome characterized by difficulty in breathing, wheezing, chest pain, lung congestion, and increased susceptibility to infections of the respiratory tract. Cigarette smoking impairs ventilation and greatly increases the risk of emphysema (a form of irreversible lung damage). About 8 to 10 million Americans suffer from cigarette-induced chronic bronchitis and emphysema.

The relationship between smoking and cancer is now beyond question. Cigarette smoking is the major cause of lung cancer in both men and women, with approximately 92,000 deaths in the United States per year. High incidences of cigarette-induced cancers of the mouth, voice box, and throat are also noted; and, as discussed in Chapter 4, concomitant alcohol ingestion greatly increases their incidence. Finally, cigarette smoking is a primary cause of many, if not most, of the nearly 10,000 deaths per year resulting from bladder cancer. Similar statistics apply to cancer of the pancreas. How cancer is caused by the compounds in cigarette smoke is unclear but the mechanisms probably involve many of the more than 2,000 compounds identified in cigarette "tar."

Historically, society has focused on the adverse effects of smoking in *men*, but some reports also focus on women.[35,36] Data indicate that more women die from cigarette-induced lung cancer than from breast cancer. Female smokers also suffer higher incidences of coronary heart disease and heart attacks than do nonsmoking women.

In addition, the carcinogenic effects of smoking apply to women as well as to men. Despite these data, it is discouraging to note that increasing numbers of females, especially teenagers, are smoking.

In addition to the direct effects of smoking on smokers, data indicate possible adverse consequences on nonsmokers by the environmental pollution caused by smokers.[37]

Effects in Pregnancy

There is now strong evidence that cigarette smoking affects the developing fetus.[32] Cigarettes increase the rates of spontaneous abortion, stillbirth, and early postpartum death. Infants born of smoking mothers are at least twice as likely to be stillborn as infants born of nonsmoking mothers. There even appears to be a relationship between the number of cigarettes smoked per day and the percentage of stillbirths. There is evidence that infants born of nonsmoking mothers may be heavier than those born of smoking mothers, at least during the first year of life.

Thus, as has been so often stressed throughout this book, psychoactive drugs are readily distributed through the placenta and may exert potent effects on the developing fetus. Because nicotine is among the most commonly used psychoactive drugs in our society, the situation is even more serious. Nicotine should be considered deleterious to the fetus and therefore contraindicated during pregnancy. Because a woman often does not realize that she is pregnant until 6, 8, or even more weeks after conception, some suggest the drug is contraindicated for all women who might become pregnant.[23] Further evidence indicates that smoking during the last 6 months of pregnancy results in a statistically significant increase in the numbers of stillbirths.

The evidence is conclusive: if we are interested in the effects of drugs on the fetus, on fetal development, and on the health of the newborn infant, nicotine should be contraindicated throughout the entire 9 months of pregnancy and during breast-feeding thereafter.

As a response to these toxicities, the 1970 warning placed on cigarette packs and advertisements ("Warning: The Surgeon General has determined that cigarette smoking is dangerous to your health") has been replaced by four new statements that are used on a rotating basis. These read as follows:

—Surgeon General's Warning: Smoking causes lung cancer, heart disease, and emphysema.

—Surgeon General's Warning: Quitting smoking now greatly reduces serious health risk.

—Surgeon General's Warning: Smoking by pregnant women may result in fetal injury and premature birth.

—Surgeon General's Warning: Cigarette smoke contains carbon monoxide.

Though these four new statements constitute an improvement on the old warning, they greatly underestimate the toxicities of cigarettes and the health consequences of continued cigarette use.[38,39]

On an encouraging note, during recent years a progression toward intolerance of smoking has occurred, with government and private agencies establishing work spaces that are smoke-free. What continues as a source of discouragement is the continued denial of cigarette-induced toxicity by their manufacturers, the continued smoking of impressionable youth, and the continued political contradictions that lead, on the one hand, to support of the tax-supported growth and production of cigarettes and, on the other hand, to the tax-supported payment of billions of dollars for the social and health consequences that result from cigarette toxicity. More will be said about societal effects of nicotine and cigarettes in Chapter 13.

Notes

1. J. H. Jaffe, "Drug Addiction and Drug Abuse," in A. G. Gilman, L. S. Goodman, T. W. Rall, and F. Murad, eds., *Goodman and Gilman's The Pharmacological Basis of Therapeutics*, 7th ed. (New York: Macmillan, 1985, pp. 550–551.
2. M. C. Ritz, R. J. Lamb, S. R. Goldberg, and M. J. Kuhar, "Cocaine Receptors on Dopamine Transporters Mediate Drug Self-administration," *The Pharmacologist* 29 (1987): 126.
3. J. Sharkey and M. J. Kuhar, "H-6BR 12935 Labels the Cocaine Binding Site Associated with Dopamine Uptake Inhibition," *The Pharmacologist* 29 (1987): 126.
4. D. O. Calligaro and M. E. Eldefrawl, "Putative Cocaine Receptors in Rat Brain Striatum Associated with Dopamine Transporter," *The Pharmacologist* 29 (1987): 126.
5. U. G. Laties and P. Weiss, "The Amphetamine Margin in Sports," *Federation Proceedings* 40 (1981): 2689–2692.
6. *Interim Report of the Commission of Inquiry into the Non-medical Use of Drugs.* Gerald Le Dain, chairman (Ottawa: Information Canada, 1970), p. 52.
7. N. Weiner, "Norepinephrine, Epinephrine, and the Sympathomimetic Amines," in A. G. Gilman, L. S. Goodman, T. W. Rall, and F. Murad, eds., *Goodman and Gilman's The Pharmacological Basis of Therapeutics*, 7th ed. (New York: Macmillan, 1985), pp. 166–168.
8. G. Smith and H. K. Beecher, "Amphetamine Sulfate and Athletic Performance," *Journal of the American Medical Association* 170 (1959): 542–547.

9. M. E. Lickey and B. Gordon, *Drugs for Mental Illness* (New York: W. H. Freeman and Co., 1983).

10. American Medical Association, "Drugs Used in Obesity," in *Drug Evaluations*, 6th ed. (Chicago: American Medical Association, 1986), pp. 927–936.

11. J. M. Ritchie and N. M. Greene, "Local Anesthetics," in A. G. Gilman, L. S. Goodman, T. W. Rall, and F. Murad, eds., *Goodman and Gilman's The Pharmacological Basis of Therapeutics*, 7th ed. (New York: Macmillan, 1985), p. 309.

12. L. Grinspoon and J. B. Bakalar, "Adverse Effects of Cocaine: Selected Issues," in *Research Developments in Drug and Alcohol Use, Annals of the New York Academy of Science* 362 (1981): 125–131.

13. J. Grabowski, ed., "Cocaine: Pharmacology, Effects and Treatment of Abuse," *National Institute on Drug Abuse, Research, Monograph No. 50*, Department of Health and Human Services, Publication No. (ADM) 84–1326. Washington, D.C.: U.S. Government Printing Office, 1984.

14. R. E. Mittleman and C. V. Wetli, "Death Caused by Recreational Cocaine Use," *Journal of the American Medical Association* 252 (1984): 1889–1893.

15. E. Jones, *Life and Work of Sigmund Freud*, vol. I (New York: Basic Books, 1961), pp. 82–83.

16. S. Freud, *Cocaine Papers* (New York: Stonehill, 1974).

17. R. C. Petersen and R. C. Stillman, eds., *Cocaine: 1977*. National Institute on Drug Abuse, Research Monograph No. 13 (Washington, D.C.: U.S. Government Printing Office, 1977).

18. N. J. Kozel and E. H. Adams, eds., "Cocaine Use in America: Epidemiologic and Clinical Perspectives," *National Institute on Drug Abuse, Research Monograph No. 61*, Department of Health and Human Services (Washington, D.C.: U.S. Government Printing Office, 1985).

19. P. Pentel, "Toxicity of Over-the-Counter Stimulants," *Journal of the American Medical Association* 252 (1984): 1898–1903.

20. D. N. Franz, "Central Nervous System Stimulants: Strychnine, Picrotoxin, Pentylenetetrazol, and Miscellaneous Agents," in A. G. Gilman, L. S. Goodman, T. W. Rall, and F. Murad, eds., *Goodman and Gilman's The Pharmacological Basis of Therapeutics*, 7th ed. (New York: Macmillan, 1985), pp. 582–588.

21. D. Grady, "Don't Get Jittery over Caffeine," *Discover* 7(7) (1986): 73–79.

22. T. W. Rall, "Central Nervous System Stimulants: The Methylxanthines," in A. G. Gilman, L. S. Goodman, T. W. Rall, and F. Murad, eds., *Goodman and Gilman's The Pharmacological Basis of Therapeutics*, 7th ed. (New York: Macmillan, 1985), pp. 589–603.

23. A. Goldstein, L. Aronow, and S. M. Kalman, *Principles of Drug Action* (New York: Harper & Row, 1968), pp. 647–653 and 663–668.

24. A. Goldstein, L. Aronow, and S. M. Kalman, *Principles of Drug Action* (New York: Harper & Row, 1968), pp. 733.

25. E. M. Brecher, and *Consumer Reports* editors. *Licit and Illicit Drugs: The Consumers Union Report on Narcotics, Stimulants, Depressants, Inhalants, Hallucinogens, and Marihuana—Including Caffeine, Nicotine, and Alcohol*. Mount Vernon, N.Y.: Consumers Union, 1972, pp. 272–277 and 302–307.

26. P. Taylor, "Ganglionic Stimulating and Blocking Agents," in A. G. Gilman, L. S. Goodman, T. W. Rall, and F. Murad, eds., *Goodman and*

Gilman's *The Pharmacological Basis of Therapeutics*, 7th ed. (New York: Macmillan, 1985), pp. 215–218.

27. American Medical Association, "Drugs Used in Other Mental Disorders," in *Drug Evaluations*, 6th ed. (Chicago: American Medical Association, 1986), p. 157.

28. J. Grabowski and S. M. Hall, ed., "Pharmacological Adjuncts in Smoking Cessation," *National Institute on Drug Abuse, Research Monograph No. 53*, Department of Health and Human Services Publication No. (ADH) 85–1333 (Washington, D.C.: U.S. Government Printing Office, 1985).

29. M. E. Jarvik, "Biological Factors Underlying the Smoking Habit," in M. E. Jarvik, J. W. Cullen, E. R. Gritz, T. M. Vogt, and L. J. West, eds., *Research on Smoking Behavior*, National Institute on Drug Abuse, Research Monograph 17 (Washington, D.C.: U.S. Government Printing Office, 1977), pp. 122–146.

30. W. Pollin, in M. E. Jarvik, J. W. Cullen, E. R. Gritz, T. M. Vogt, and L. J. West, eds. *Research on Smoking Behavior*, (Washington, D.C.: U.S. Government Printing Office, 1977), pp. v–vi.

31. *Smoking and Health: A Report of the Surgeon General*, U.S. Department of Health, Education and Welfare (Washington, D.C.:U.S. Government Printing Office, 1979).

32. *The Changing Cigarette: Health Consequences of Smoking. A Report of the Surgeon General.* U.S. Department of Health and Human Services (Washington, D.C.: U.S. Government Printing Office, 1981).

33. M. E. Jarvik, J. W. Cullen, E. R. Gritz, T. M. Vogt, and L. J. West, eds., *Research on Smoking Behavior*, National Institute on Drug Abuse, Research Monograph 17 (Washington, D.C.: U.S. Government Printing Office, 1977).

34. N. A. Krasnegor, ed., *Cigarette Smoking as a Dependence Process*, National Institute on Drug Abuse, Research Monograph 23 (Washington, D.C.: U.S. Government Printing Office, 1979).

35. *The Health Consequences of Smoking for Women: A Report of the Surgeon General*, U.S. Department of Health, Education and Welfare (Washington, D.C.: U.S. Government Printing Office, 1980).

36. *Voices for Women: 1980 Report of the President's Advisory Committee for Women* (Washington, D.C.: U.S. Government Printing Office, Dec. 1980).

37. J. R. White and H. F. Froeb, "Small-Airways Dysfunction in Non-Smokers Chronically Exposed to Tobacco Smoke," *New England Journal of Medicine*, 27 March 1980, pp. 720–723.

38. American Cancer Society, *Dangers of Smoking: Benefits of Quitting* (New York: American Cancer Society, 1980).

39. H. Ashton and R. Stepney, *Smoking: Psychology and Pharmacology* (London: Tavistock Publications, 1982).

CHAPTER 6

Antidepressants and Lithium

Drugs Used in Affective Disorders

Depressive illness, manic illness, and manic-depressive illness are mood, or affect, disorders in contrast to schizophrenia, which is a thought disorder. A depressive episode is characterized by dysphoria or loss of interest or pleasure in all, or almost all, of an individual's usual activities or pastimes. Depression that is clinically significant is characterized by feelings of intense sadness and dispair, inability to experience joy or pleasure in usual activities, decreased sexual drive, mental slowing and loss of concentration, pessimism, feelings of helplessness, worthlessness or self-reproach, inappropriate guilt, agitation, self-depreciation, recurrent thoughts of death and hopelessness, blunted affect, tearfulness, anorexia with weight loss, fatigue, insomnia, decreased energy, and so on. Anxiety almost invariably occurs in depressed individuals, which can lead to misdiagnosis and inappropriate or improper treatment. About 15 percent of depressed individuals may display suicidal thoughts or acts at some point during their lives.[1]

Individuals who experience major depressions respond to tricyclic or other antidepressant drugs, to monoamine oxidase inhibitors, and, in severe or drug-resistant individuals, to electroconvulsive shock therapy (ECT) and psychotherapy.

Attempts to identify the underlying causes of major depressive orders have led to elusive results.[2] Most investigators agree that a neurochemical imbalance is probably involved and, in some cases, may be genetically transmitted. Pharmacological evidence has pointed to an involvement of norepinephrine and perhaps serotonin (discussed in Chapter 5 and Appendix II). First, reserpine has been shown both to induce severe depression and, concomitantly, to deplete norephinephrine and serotonin transmitter neurons. Second, the antidepressant drugs exert important actions on these transmitters to potentiate their role in transmission. Third, strong evidence for genetic predisposition has led to speculation that the underlying biological ideology of major depressive episodes may include an abnormal hypoactive function of norepinephrine and serotonin neurotransmission or of their receptors. Antidepressant drugs do not potentiate dopamine neurotransmission very effectively—a situation that is different from that of the behavioral stimulants cocaine and amphetamine, which potentiate transmission at both norepinephrine and dopamine synapses. Indeed, cocaine and the amphetamines are poor antidepressants despite the fact that they are behavioral stimulants and euphoriants. Thus, although the stimulant action of drugs such as cocaine and the amphetamines may be caused by intensifying dopamine neurotransmission, relief of major depression can result from increased norephenephrine and serotonin neurotransmission.

One difficulty with the biologicalamine hypothesis of depression is that the time course of action of these drugs is delayed. Although neurotransmission of norepinephrine and serotonin is activated soon after drug administration, the antidepressant effect may not appear for 2 weeks or longer. Thus, altering the rate of neurotransmission may be only an initial step in a more complex series of events that eventually results in clinical antidepressant activity. Also, some newer antidepressant agents (see the following discussion) do not appear to exert the same degree of catecholamine alteration as that seen with the earlier antidepressants. Thus, for the present discussion, the biological amine hypothesis is still the most pharmacologically consistent explanation of drug action.[3–5]

More recently, however, investigations into this delay in therapeutic effectiveness have given rise to the *catecholamine receptor hypothesis*. This hypothesis postulates that the receptors for catecholamines, serotonin, or both mediate the clinical effects of antidepressant drugs. Thus, by blocking the uptake or inhibiting the action of monoamine oxidase, longer-term biochemical changes might occur (such as reductions in the numbers of catecholamine or serotonin receptors). Conversely, depression might be caused by an abnormality (genetically or otherwise induced) in the regulation of these receptors, which may be corrected by the administration of an antidepressant drug (that "down-regulates the receptors").[6] Such receptor pathology in depression remains to be demonstrated.

Mania and alternate periods of mania and depression (so-called *bipolar affective disorder*) are less common than major depression (a *unipolar disorder*). Mania (and its milder form, hypomania) are treated with lithium for both short-term treatment and long-term prevention of recurrence of manic episodes. Mania is characterized by emotional euphoria, insomnia, flight of ideas, excessive speech, hyperactivity, excessive sociability, extreme self-confidence, impaired judgment, and delusions of grandeur.

Lithium, at therapeutic blood levels (see the following discussion), appears to inhibit the release of norepinephrine and dopamine (but not serotonin) from nerve terminals. This finding is consistent with the biolgical amine hypothesis of mania and depression (Chapter 5). In addition, lithium inhibits the breakdown of certain chemical intermediates that serve to modulate the action of several CNS transmitters. This occurrence may lead to a decreased neuronal responsiveness, especially in hyperactive neurons, thus modulating the function of those neurons that might contribute to states of mania. Again, much remains to be learned about the biological and neurochemical basis of mania and the pharmacological action of lithium in ameliorating this disorder.

Therapy for Major Depressive Illness

Therapy for treatment of major depression involves the use of (1) the tricyclic antidepressants, (2) the newer "second-generation" antidepressants, (3) monoamine oxidase (MAO) inhibitors, and (4) electroconvulsive therapy. Inhibitors of serotonin reuptake will be added to this list shortly. One such drug, fluoxetine (Prozac), has recently become available for use in treating depression.

Tricyclic Antidepressants

The term *tricyclic antidepressant* is derived from the fact that these drugs all have a three-ring molecular core (Figure 6.1) and produce relief from depression in individuals who experience major depressive illness.[7] In general, these drugs also share the ability to inhibit, or block, the neuronal uptake of norepinephrine and serotonin into the presynaptic nerve terminals from which they were originally released. Because of these neuronal effects, these drugs should be used with caution in manic-depressive individuals because they may unmask the mania. These drugs do not produce euphoria or other pleasurable effects, and they have few discernible psychological effects in normal patients. Thus, they have no recreational value and their abuse and psychological dependency are not of concern. The choice of drug is determined by effectiveness, tolerance of side effects, and duration of action (Table 6.1).

The tricyclic antidepressants are the drugs most widely used for the treatment of major depression. This use is well established and their therapeutic effectiveness is well delineated. They elevate

Figure 6.1

Tricyclic and second-generation antidepressants.

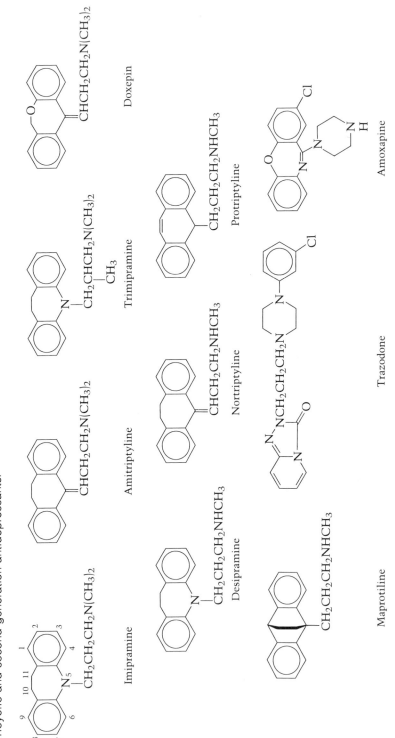

Table 6.1

Drugs used in affective disorders

Classification	Drug name Generic (trade)	Sedative activity	Anticholinergic* activity	Elimination half-life (hours)
Antidepressants				
1. Tricyclic compounds	Imipramine (Tofranil)	Moderate	Moderate	4–17
	Desipramine (Norpramin)	Low	Low	12–25
	Trimipramine (Surmontil)	High	High	Unknown
	Protriptyline (Vivactil)	Low	Moderate	55–125
	Nortriptyline (Pamelor, Aventyl)	Moderate	Low	12–48
	Amitriptyline (Elavil)	High	High	10–25
	Doxepin (Adapin, Sinequan)	High	High	8–24
2. Second-generation compounds	Amoxapine (Asendin)†	Low	Low	8–10
	Maprotiline (Ludiomil)	Moderate	Moderate	27–58
	Trazodone (Desyrel)	Moderate	Low	6–13
3. MAO inhibitors	Phenelzine (Nardil)	NA‡	NA	Unknown
	Isocarboxazid (Marplan)	NA	NA	Unknown
	Tranylcypromine (Parnate)	NA	NA	Unknown
Antimanic Drug	Lithium carbonate (Eskalith)	NA	NA	17–36

* Anticholinergic side effects include dry mouth, blurred vision, tachycardia, urinary retention, and constipation.
† Also has antipsychotic effects due to dopamine receptor blockade (Chapter 7).
‡ NA—Data not applicable.

mood, increase physical activity, increase mental alertness, improve appetite and sleep patterns, and reduce morbid preoccupation in 60 to 70 percent of individuals experiencing major depression. They are most useful in treating acute episodes of depression, although they are effective in preventing relapses, serving as maintenance therapy for individuals who are prone to major depressive episodes.

Pharmacological Effects

As stated previously, the tricyclic antidepressants do not have a stimulating or mood-elevating effect in normal individuals. In such persons, drowsiness, hypotension, dry mouth, and blurred vision commonly occur. These effects are often interpreted as unpleasant and may resemble those seen in individuals using phenothiazines.

In contrast to the effects in normal individuals, when tricyclic antidepressants are administered over a 2-to-3-week period to depressed patients, an elevation of mood occurs. Although this slow onset of effectiveness is well documented, its explanation remains elusive. The antidepressant effect may represent a dulling of depressive ideation rather than euphoric stimulation.[7]

The tricyclic antidepressants markedly alter sleep patterns. Indeed, they are among the most effective depressants of REM sleep known. They also increase stage 4 sleep and decrease the number of nocturnal awakenings. The depression of REM sleep can be used as a predicator of drug effectiveness for some individuals.

Mechanism of Neuronal Action

These drugs augment neurotransmission in norepinephrine and serotonin neurons (discussed previously). They do this by blocking the major mechanism by which these transmitters are inactivated physiologically: their reuptake from the synaptic cleft back into the presynaptic nerve terminal.[4–5] The limitations of this action prevent it from being considered a definitive mechanism that is responsible for antidepressant effects (discussed previously).

The tricyclic antidepressants exert a variety of effects on the peripheral nervous system. These effects result primarily from blockade of acetylcholine receptors, which results in blurred vision, dry mouth, constipation, and urinary retention (Table 6.1). However, the potentiation of catecholamine neurotransmission results in a complex picture of cardiac depression that is combined with increased electrical irritability of the heart. Cardiac depression becomes most prominent and even life-threatening when an overdose of one of these drugs is taken (as in a suicide attempt).

Drug Administration

The tricyclic antidepressants are quite well absorbed when administered orally. Since most of them have relatively long half-lives, single daily administration at bedtime tends to minimize many of their untoward side effects. The drugs most likely to produce sedation (Table 6.1) are most ideally administered in this fashion. Although it is possible to administer tricyclic antidepressants intramuscularly, it is rarely done.

The initial treatment period is considered to be in a range of 4 to 8 weeks, a time period necessary for reasonable evaluation. Excessive sedation can occur in the first few weeks of therapy and this occurrence can reduce patient compliance; this is a critical point at which drug failures should be evaluated (that is, to determine whether the drug was ineffective or was not taken). For long-term therapy, continuous administration of lower doses is usually preferred. Therapy is usually continued long enough to encompass a period of time that is equivalent to several equal cycle lengths. Following this initial phase, dosage can be reduced gradually; however, if signs of relapse are observed, the initial dosage can be reinstituted. In the elderly, dosages should be markedly reduced and close medical supervision maintained. Elderly patients with cardiac disease are especially susceptible to serious side effects.

Second-Generation Antidepressants

The slow onset of action and the relative severity of real and potential side effects of the tricyclic antidepressants has led to a continued search for more effective, more rapid onset, and less toxic antidepressant agents. Drugs that have a different chemical structure have been the goal of research in the hope that an alteration in structure would produce less toxic and more effective drugs. However, those drugs that have been developed that are structurally different are not necessarily more effective than the tricyclic antidepressants. They are termed *second-generation* (or atypical) *antidepressants* to distinguish them from the older tricyclic antidepressants.

The effectiveness of *amoxapine* (Figure 6.1) is equivalent to that of imipramine and amitriptyline (both tricyclic antidepressants), although amoxapine may be slightly more effective in relieving anxiety and agitation than is imipramine. Also, amoxapine is claimed to have a more rapid onset of action than the older agents (for example, 2 weeks instead of 3 to 4 weeks), but this claim is poorly substantiated.

Maprotiline is also similar to imipramine in its spectrum of action. However, it may be more selective for blocking uptake of norepinephrine than that of serotonin. It is occasionally effective after 1 to 2 weeks of therapy, but 2 to 3 weeks are most commonly needed. Differences between maprotiline and the older agents are not remarkable.

Trazodone is chemically the most unique of the antidepressants (Figure 6.1). Trazodone primarily blocks the reuptake of serotonin and leaves the norepinephrine neurons relatively unaffected. Of all the antidepressants, it has perhaps the shortest onset ($\frac{1}{2}$ to 1 week), but it still takes 2 to 5 weeks for its optimal effect to occur. Since the drug does not affect norepinephrine neurons, behavioral agitation is unusual, cardiac toxicity is less severe, and other side effects are either less frequent or less severe. Drowsiness is the most common side effect, occurring in about 20 percent of patients. The biological half-life of trazodone is shorter than that of most of the other antidepressants, frequently necessitating divided daily dosages rather than a single bedtime dose. Other inhibitors of serotonin uptake are being evaluated,[5] and one, fluoxetine, is available clinically.

Monoamine Oxidase Inhibitors

The monoamine oxidase (MAO) inhibitors are a small group of drugs that have long been considered alternative drugs for the treatment of major depressive illness; they all have in common the ability to block the enzyme monoamine oxidase.[8] Monoamine oxidase is an enzyme located within the nerve terminals of norepinephrine, dopamine, and serotonin neurons. Blockade of this enzyme (which normally modulates the amount of transmitter present) allows transmitters to accumulate in the nerve terminals. As a result, larger amounts of the transmitter are released when neuronal stimulation occurs. Today, the use of MAO inhibitors is quite limited because the predominant treatment of depression is use of the tricyclic antidepressants. MAO inhibitors are used when other therapy has been proved inadequate or incomplete. However, these drugs are effective and they exhibit periodic increases in clinical use. Severe and often unpredictable side effects limit their widespread use. The most severe problems involve drug interactions between MAO inhibitors and (1) other drugs that the patient might be taking or (2) numerous foods that patients might occasionally eat (see the following discussion). Use of these agents is, therefore, potentially hazardous, and extensive patient education combined with close supervision by a physician is necessary.

Three MAO inhibitors are currently available for clinical use (Table 6.1). All three are irreversible inhibitors of this enzyme. Although this action occurs quite rapidly (just as with the tricyclic antidepressants), the onset of therapeutic response is delayed. Thus, the association between enzyme inhibition, increased transmitter activity, and antidepressant effectiveness is still elusive. Because these drugs inhibit MAO irreversibly, drug action is quite prolonged, and recovery depends on the body's synthesis of new enzyme.

Besides localization of MAO to brain tissue, it is also found in the liver where it is required for the metabolism of circulating transmitters and transmitter-like substances such as *tyramine*. Tyramine is a substance that is widely found in foods such as aged cheese, red wine, kippered and pickled herring, chicken livers, figs, yeast, and numerous other foods. A buildup of tyramine in the body can precipitate a hypertensive crisis that is characterized by increased blood pressure, headache, increased heart rate, palpitations, and other effects that follow severe increases in blood pressure. Complete lists of tyramine-containing foods can be obtained from physicians familiar with the use of these drugs.

Electroconvulsive Therapy

Electroconvulsive therapy (ECT) is effective in the treatment of individuals with major depression, but such therapy is reserved for those who are either unresponsive to drug therapy or considered to be at risk for suicide.[9] Although ECT is frequently considered a controversial treatment, its use is currently on an upswing. In England, about 200,000 treatments are administered every year compared to the United States, where approximately 100,000 treatments are administered every year.

The history of inducing seizures to treat depressive illness dates back to 1934, and it has involved insulin overdose, pentylene-tetrazol-induced seizures (Chapter 5), and electrically induced seizures. Currently, electroconvulsive therapy is the only modality used. The safety of ECT has been greatly increased by modern anesthesia techniques, which include administration of low doses of barbiturates to produce unconsciousness and muscle relaxants to prevent body injury.[10] Indeed, ECT combined with short-acting intravenous barbiturates and muscle relaxants results in a technically simple, safe regimen to produce brain seizures that can effectively ameliorate depression.

Individuals who exhibit "endogenous" depression are most susceptable to ECT therapy, and those with a history of failed drug therapy and recurrent bouts of depression or with suicidal tendencies are prime candidates.

Physiological effects are characterized by increases in heart rate and blood pressure and occasionally by cardiac arrythmias. Cardiac arrythmias usually resolve spontaneously or can be treated relatively easily by the anesthesiologist who is invariably present when therapy is administered. CNS effects include seizures (which are not usually accompanied by muscle contractions because the patient is paralyzed for the procedure) and the resultant increases in oxygen consumption and multiple transmitter release.

Memory loss is the most troublesome side effect of ECT; however, only a small minority of patients claim or exhibit long-term major impairments of memory. Following the induction of seizures, tremendous alterations occur in multiple aspects of brain activity; thus, it is very difficult to determine which alterations in transmitter function contribute to antidepressant effectiveness. However, it is known that ECT activates norepinephrine transmission, reduces serotonin reuptake, and increases the sensitivity of dopamine receptors. Thus, improved transmitter function may correlate with clinical effectiveness.

Current estimates of complications average about 1 in 1700 treatments, and the risk generally correlates with the risk of the short-acting barbiturate anesthesia. The memory losses are difficult to substantiate, and most arguments concerning ECT therapy now focus on that unknown factor.

At present, the number of yearly ECT treatments is increasing, perhaps because the limitations of pharmacological treatment of depression are being recognized. Although correlation of clinical effectiveness with neurotransmitter alterations is incomplete, several lines of evidence are consistent with the biological amine hypothesis of mania and depression.

Lithium

Lithium carbonate is effective in treating 60 to 80 percent of persons with manic-depressive ("bipolar depression") illness. It calms manic patients and functions as a mood-stabilizing drug when used chronically to prevent recurrent manic episodes. Lithium is an alkali metal, like sodium and potassium. It was used in the 1920s as a sedative-hypnotic compound, and in 1940 lithium chloride was available as a salt substitute. This latter use produced disastrous consequences, including deaths. In the late 1940s, after an Australian scientist noted that lithium administered to guinea pigs made these animals lethargic, lithium was administered to manic patients with somewhat spectacular effects. However, it took longer than 20 years for this agent to be accepted by the medical community as an effective treatment for mania.

In therapeutic doses, lithium has almost no discernible psychotropic effect in normal persons. It does not induce sedation and exhibits few effects on the brain aside from its specific action on mania. The drug is not a euphoriant. The mechanism through which lithium exerts its antimania effect is still a matter of speculation, but it does decrease the release of both NE and serotonin and increase their reuptake into nerve terminals—actions in agreement with the biological amine hypothesis.[4] These effects on amines, on the other hand, occur very rapidly, while the antimania effect often takes 1 or 2 weeks. Alternative hypotheses for the slow onset of lithium's clinical effectiveness are that it invokes abnormal NE and serotonin receptors and that it "stabilizes" the receptor membrane, reducing excessive receptor stimulation that would ordinarily lead to an episode of mania.[11]

Lithium is rapidly absorbed when administered orally.[12] Peak blood levels are reached within 1 to 3 hours and correlations exist between the levels of lithium in the blood and therapeutic efficacy. Because lithium closely resembles normal salt (sodium chloride), when salt intake is lowered or when excessive salt is lost (as through sweating), lithium blood levels rise and intoxication may follow. Therefore, in patients on low-salt diets or in all patients exposed to warm weather, lithium blood levels must be closely monitored. Toxic reactions consist primarily of fatigue, muscle weakness, slurred speech, and tremor. At high concentrations, more serious toxic effects consisting of muscle rigidity and coma may be observed. Thus, lithium therapy should only be prescribed by a physician familiar with its side effects. Despite these risks, lithium's effectiveness and relative safety make it irreplaceable in the treatment and prevention of mania, a disorder that was previously quite resistant to treatment.

Notes

1. American Medical Association, "Drugs Used in Affective Disorders," in *Drug Evaluations*, 6th ed. (Chicago: American Medical Association, 1986), pp. 131–152.
2. H. M. Van Praag, "Depression," *Lancet* 2 (1982): 1259–1264.
3. R. J. Baldessarini, *Biomedical Aspects of Depression* (Washington, D.C.: American Psychiatric Press, Inc., 1983).
4. F. E. Bloom, G. Baetge, S. Deyo, et al., "Chemical and Physiological Aspects of the Actions of Lithium and Antidepressant Drugs," *Neuropharmacology* 22 (1983): 359–365.

5. M. Asberg, B. Eriksson, B. Martensson, L. Traskman-Bendz, and A. Wagner, "Therapeutic Effects of Serotonin Uptake Inhibitors in Depression," *Journal of Clinical Psychiatry* 47 (1986): 4 (Suppl.): 23–35.

6. S. M. Stahl and L. Palazidou, "The Pharmacology of Depression," *Trends in Pharmacological Sciences* 7 (1986): 349–354.

7. R. J. Baldessarini, "Drugs and the Treatment of Psychiatric Disorders," in A. G. Gilman, L. S. Goodman, T. W. Rall, and F. Murad, eds., *Goodman and Gilman's The Pharmacological Basis of Therapeutics*, 7th ed. (New York: Macmillan, 1985), pp. 412–445.

8. G. D. Tollefson, "Monoamine Oxidase Inhibitors: Review," *Journal of Clinical Psychiatry* 44 (1983): 280–288.

9. R. R. Crowe, "Electroconvulsive Therapy: Current Perspectives," *New England Journal of Medicine* 311 (1984): 163–166.

10. B. L. Selvin, "Electroconvulsive Therapy—1987." *Anesthesiology* 367–385, 1987.

11. M. E. Lickey and B. Gordon, "Drugs for Mental illness" (New York: W. H. Freeman & Co., 1983), pp. 195–200.

12. R. J. Baldessarini, "Drugs and the Treatment of Psychiatric Disorders," in A. G. Gilman, L. S. Goodman, T. W. Rall, and F. Murad, eds., *Goodman and Gilman's The Pharmacological Basis of Therapeutics*, 7th ed. (New York: Macmillan, 1985), pp. 426–431.

CHAPTER 7

The Opiates

Morphine and Other Narcotics

In this chapter, we discuss the pharmacological, physiological, psychological, and behavioral effects induced by a group of compounds referred to as *opiates, narcotic analgesics,* or *strongly addictive analgesics.* The term *opiate* refers to any natural or synthetic drug that exerts actions upon the body similar to those induced by morphine, the major pain-relieving agent obtained from the opium poppy. The term *narcotic* has numerous meanings and usually is defined in widely varying terms by law-enforcement officers, lawyers, physicians, scientists, and laymen. Here, the term narcotic is considered obsolete, and the term opiate refers to all drugs, natural and synthetic, that possess morphinelike actions.

The major medical uses of the opiates are for the relief of pain, the treatment of diarrhea, and the relief of coughing. Because the opiates are addictive (that is, are capable of inducing tolerance and physiological and psychological dependence), many drugs that are like morphine in action have been synthesized in attempts to duplicate its usefulness and avoid its addictive qualities. With only one or two exceptions, these attempts to separate the analgesic effects from the euphoria-producing effects, which are those associated with compulsive abuse, have been unsuccessful.

Historical Background

Opium occurs naturally and is obtained from the opium poppy, *Papaver somniferum.* The earliest descriptions of the psychological and physiological effects of opium were written in about 300 B.C., although references to opiates have been found dating to about 3000 B.C. Opium appears to have been used in early Egyptian, Greek, and Arabian cultures primarily for its constipating effect in the treatment of diarrhea. Later, opium's sleep-inducing properties were noted by Greek and Roman writers such as Homer, Virgil, and Ovid. Opium was frequently used by the Greeks to treat a variety of medical problems, including snake bite, asthma, cough, epilepsy, colic, urinary complaints, headache, and deafness. The Greeks also appeared to use the drug recreationally, and opium cakes and candies were commonly available on the streets. Addiction to opium was common, even among high-standing military and political figures of Rome.

From the early Greek and Roman days through the sixteenth and seventeenth centuries, the medicinal and recreational uses of opium were well established throughout Europe. Because much of the opium came from the Near East and the Orient, a bustling trade in opium existed between East and West. Indeed, control of opium was a central issue in the opium wars in China in 1839.

Through the centuries, from 3000 B.C. to A.D. 1800, the opiates used medicinally and recreationally consisted of the crude opium obtained from the opium poppy. Opium, however, is a resinous material that contains at least 20 different substances. It was not until the early 1800s that a chemist named Serturner isolated the primary active drug in opium, *morphine.* The development of morphine revolutionized the use of the opiates, and since then morphine (rather than crude opium) has been used throughout the world for the medical treatment of pain and diarrhea.

In the United States, morphine and opium are both widely used and have been since the nineteenth century. Until 1914, both drugs, for prescription and nonprescription use, were as accessible as aspirin is today, being freely available from physicians, drug stores, and general stores, by mail order, and in patent medicines sold through a variety of channels. It was not until after the Civil War (when opiate addiction was referred to as "soldier's disease") and the invention of the hypodermic needle in 1856 that a new type of drug user appeared in the United States: one who administered opiates to himself by injection. At about this time, there was a large influx of Chinese laborers who freely smoked opium.

By the early part of the twentieth century, opium use was widespread and it was estimated that one out of every 400 Americans was addicted to opium or one of its derivatives. Concern began to mount over the possible dangers of opiates and the dependence that they might induce. By 1914, the Harrison Narcotic Act was passed and the use of most opiate products was placed under strict controls. Nonmedical uses of opiates were banned.

The use of opiates is deeply entrenched in society, widespread, attractive, difficult to treat, and impossible to stop. The pharmacology of the opiates should be discussed in the same manner as that of any other class of psychoactive drugs whose effects can be pleasurable to the user, affect behavior, produce a pattern of tolerance and physiological dependence, and potentially can be compulsively misused. Emotional reactions and extensive legal efforts have failed and will probably continue to fail to eradicate the recreational use of these drugs. The opiates will continue to be used in medicine because, as pain-relieving agents, they are irreplaceable by other compounds. In addition, the profound effects of the opiates on the central nervous system induce an enormous liability for compulsive abuse, a liability that is likely to resist any efforts at total control.

Chemistry

The term *opium* refers to the crude resinous exudate obtained from the opium poppy. Crude opium contains a wide variety of ingredients, including *morphine* and *codeine,* both of which are widely used in medicine. The bulk of the ingredients of opium, however, consists of such organic substances as resins, oils, sugars, and proteins that account for more than 75 percent of the weight of the opium but exert little pharmacological activity. Morphine is the major pain-relieving drug found in opium, being approximately 10 percent of the crude exudate. Codeine is structurally closely related to morphine, although it is much less potent and amounts to only 0.5 percent of the opium extract. *Heroin* does not occur naturally but is a semisynthetic derivative produced by a chemical modification of morphine that increases the potency. It takes only 3 milligrams of heroin to produce the same analgesic effect as 10 milligrams of morphine (heroin being three times as potent as morphine). However, at equally effective doses (3 milligrams of heroin compared with 10 milligrams of morphine), it may be difficult to distinguish between the effects of the two compounds.

Several totally synthetic opiates are available. These are drugs that exert effects like those of morphine but are synthetically produced in a laboratory. Meperidine (Demerol) and methadone (Dolophine) are both synthetic opiate narcotics. Meperidine is between 10 and 20 percent as potent as morphine (100 milligrams of meperidine is approximately equal in potency to between 10 and 20 milligrams of morphine). Methadone has approximately the same analgesic potency as morphine but induces less euphoria. Currently, methadone is being used in the treatment of opiate dependence.

Medical Uses

The primary medical uses of the opiates are for the relief of pain, the treatment of diarrhea, and the relief of cough, all disorders for which the opiates have been used since well before the sixteenth century.[1] Despite intensive research, few other drugs have come even close to the opiate narcotics for use in the treatment of either pain or diarrhea. Although codeine is an extremely effective drug for the relief of cough, several newer synthetic compounds have been shown to be effective. In most nonprescription cough preparations, the codeine has been replaced by newer drugs such as dextromethorphan, a synthetic, nonnarcotic, nonanalgesic cough depressant with a very low potential for compulsive abuse. Nevertheless, morphine and related opiates will retain a vital and special place in the armamentarium of the physician as essential agents in the struggle against pain.

As the name *narcotic* implies, the opiates are capable of inducing sleep, but because of the euphoria they induce and because they are likely to be misused, they are seldom used medically for inducing sleep. However, when pain is present and sleep is necessary, the use of an opiate narcotic to supplement the sleep-inducing properties of a barbiturate is indicated. The barbiturates and other sedative-hypnotic compounds are not analgesic—that is, they do *not* relieve pain—and if pain is present, barbiturates may have little sedative or hypnotic effect.

Classification

The classification of opiates is changing rapidly.[2] Early classification was based on either the drug's potency (compared to morphine) or its natural or synthetic origin. A subsequent concept (Table 7.1) resulted from a search for potent analgesics that would not have the potential to produce addiction. Although generally unsuccessful, such a search led to the identification of a class of drugs that possesses varying degrees of analgesic effectiveness as well as the ability to antagonize certain actions of morphine. These compounds were referred to as *mixed agonist-antagonists,* a classification that distinguished them from the strongly addicting opiates (such as morphine), which were called *pure agonists,* and, at the other extreme, compounds that were devoid of analgesic effect but could antagonize the effects of morphine. These latter compounds were referred to as *pure narcotic antagonists.*

About 1970, it was recognized that this means of distinguishing between opiates was inadequate and that a new classification was

Table 7.1

Classification of opioid analgesics by their ability to produce analgesia (agonists) or block the actions of morphine (antagonists).

Pure agonists	Mixed agonist–antagonists	Pure antagonists
Morphine	Nalbuphine (Nubain)	Naloxone (Narcan)
Codeine	Butorphanol (Stadol)	Naltrexone (Trexan)
Heroin	Pentazocine (Talwin)	
Meperidine (Demerol)	Buprenorphine (Buprenex)	
Methadone (Dolophine)		
Oxymorphone (Numorphan)		
Hydromorphone (Dilaudid)		
Fentanyl (Sublimaze)		

needed to explain the physiological interaction of drugs with specific opiate receptors. Since 1970, binding sites for opiate drugs have been meticulously researched, located, and are now being studied intensively. At the same time, naturally occurring substances in the brain that interact with these opiate receptors have been identified. These naturally occurring substances (especially the enkephalins) and the receptors upon which they may act are discussed in Appendix II.

Although the receptor classification of opiates is still incomplete, at least four major categories of receptors are known to exist, and three of them are reasonably well characterized pharmacologically. These three receptors are designated as *mu, kappa*, and *sigma* (Table 7.2). The mu receptors are associated with analgesia, respiratory depression, euphoria, and physical dependence. The kappa receptors are associated with spinal analgesia, miosis (pinpoint pupils), and sedation. The sigma receptors (located primarily in the limbic system of the brain) are associated with dysphoria, hallucinations, and other psychotomimetic effects that are occasionally encountered in persons who use opiates. Drugs that stimulate any of these receptors are termed *agonists* while drugs that block the receptors are termed *antagonists*. Drugs that stimulate one receptor but block another are termed mixed agonists-antagonists. Of note is the observation that the pure narcotic antagonist naloxone (Narcan) binds to (and blocks) all opiate receptors, but its affinity for mu receptors is at least tenfold higher than its affinity for kappa receptors. This characteristic explains naloxone-induced reversal of respiratory depression, which occurs with only minimal reversal of the analgesia that results from stimulation of kappa receptors in the spinal cord.

Table 7.2

Classification of opioid agonists and antagonists by actions at opioid receptors.

Compound	Receptor types*		
	Mu	Kappa	Sigma
Morphine	Ag†	Ag	0
Naloxone‡	Ant	Ant	§
Pentazocine	Ant	Ag	Ag
Butorphanol	0	Ag	Ag
Nalbuphine	Ant	pAg	Ag§
Buprenorphine	pAg		0

* The mu receptor is thought to mediate supraspinal analgesia, respiratory depression, euphoria, and physical dependence; the kappa receptor, spinal analgesia, miosis, and sedation; the sigma receptor, dysphoria, hallucinations, and respiratory and vasomotor stimulation. Categorizations are based on best inferences about actions in humans. See text for further explanation.

† Ag = agonist; Ant = competitive antagonist; pAg = partial agonist; the absence of an entry means that the compound has not yet been fully studied; 0 = no significant action.

‡ Naloxone is more potent in antagonizing the effects of mu agonists than kappa or sigma agonists and is thus thought to have the highest affinity for the mu receptor.

§ Some effects of sigma agonists are antagonized by naloxone; others are not. The reason for this is not understood but may indicate that there are several subtypes of sigma receptors. With nalbuphine, sigma-like effects are minimal.

Adapted with permission from J. H. Jaffe and W. R. Martin, "Opioid Analgesics and Antagonists," in A. G. Gilman, L. S. Goodman, T. W. Rall, and F. Murad, eds. *The Pharmacologic Basis of Therapeutics,* 7th ed. (New York: Macmillan, 1985), p. 494.

Thus, the unfolding classification of opiates depends on the actions of all these drugs in terms of their interactions with mu, kappa, or sigma receptors.[3]

Absorption, Distribution, Metabolism, and Excretion

The opiates (morphine and codeine) and their synthetic or semi-synthetic equivalents (meperidine, heroin, and methadone) may be given by different routes. They may be administered orally, parenterally, or by inhalation. In general, absorption from the gastrointestinal route is slower and considerably less complete than absorption from either parenteral or inhalation routes. The opiate narcotics, when given orally, exist in the stomach in a fat-insoluble form that is only poorly absorbed into the bloodstream. Absorption is delayed, incomplete, and occurs largely from the intestine. The blood levels of drug that are reached after a given oral dose are usually only half or less than that achieved when the drug is injected. One of the few advantages of giving an opiate by mouth rather than by injection is that, because of this slow rate of absorption, the drug reaches the bloodstream slowly and is therefore metabolized at a slower rate, which may result in a somewhat longer duration of action in the body. In general, oral administration of an opiate results in erratic and unpredictable absorption when compared with administration by injection or by inhalation.

The opiates may be administered by intramuscular, subcutaneous, or intravenous injection; in nonmedical situations, the subcutaneous ("skin-popping") and intravenous ("main-lining") techniques are commonly used. The problems and limitations of the injection of drugs, delineated in Chapter 1, include accidental overdose, rapid onset of adverse drug reaction, necessity of sterile technique, and inability to recall the drug if too much is administered. The latter point may sometimes be circumvented, however, by a specific pharmacological antagonist, naloxone (Narcan), which is discussed later in this chapter.

As is well known from the history of opium smoking among Eastern cultures, the opiates may be administered by inhalation and absorbed through the lungs, either by sniffing the powdered drug or, more commonly, by inhalation of the smoke from burning crude opium. In either case, the opiates are rapidly and completely absorbed. In fact, the rapidity of onset of drug action rivals that of intravenous injection. (Refer to Chapter 1 for a more complete discussion of the absorption of drugs from the lungs following inhalation.)

Opiates achieve significant levels in the brain within seconds to minutes of intravenous injection. More water-soluble (fat-insoluble) opiates such as morphine penetrate the blood-brain barrier somewhat slower than do fat-soluble opiates such as fentanyl. Fentanyl is a very short-acting opiate used in anesthesia and, when available on the street, is referred to as "china white." Its extreme potency has led to multiple fatalities following its intravenous use in illicit situations.

Morphine exists in the bloodstream in a relatively fat-insoluble form and, because the blood-brain barrier is fairly impermeable to such compounds, only small amounts (20 percent) ever penetrate the brain. In contrast, fentanyl and heroin cross the blood-brain barrier easily. Perhaps this may explain why the "flash" or "rush" with intravenous heroin is so much more intense than that perceived after injection of morphine. The opiates also reach all body tissues, including the fetus, and infants born of addicted mothers are physically dependent on opiates and may exhibit withdrawal symptoms unless they are given the drug.

Numerous papers have been published on the metabolism and excretion of morphine and the other opiates. In general, these studies demonstrate that the opiates are largely metabolized by the liver before they are excreted by the kidneys. Small amounts of both codeine and heroin are metabolized by the body into morphine, which is further metabolized into inactive products that are finally excreted by the kidneys. Metabolism of most opiates is rapid. The durations of action of these drugs average 4 to 5 hours, a factor of considerable importance to the addict who must continually seek and administer the drug at intervals as short as 3 to 5 hours.

Urine screening tests for opiates detect codeine and morphine (either free or metabolized) as well as dihydrocodeine, dihydromorphine, and hydromorphone. Because heroin (diacetylmorphine) is metabolized to morphine and, further, street heroin also contains acetylcodeine, which is metabolized to codeine, heroin use is suspected by the presence of both morphine and codeine in urine. Thus, assays cannot be used to determine whether heroin, codeine, or morphine has been used. Furthermore, codeine is widely available in cough and analgesic preparations, and poppy seeds contain small amounts of morphine. Thus, poppy seed ingestion can yield positive screens for morphine. Morphine and codeine can be detected in the urine for 2 to 4 days after use.

Pharmacological Effects

Morphine and the other natural and synthetic opiates exert their major effects primarily on opiate receptors located in the central nervous system and the gastrointestinal tract. In chronic morphine use or in acute morphine poisoning, a syndrome consisting of sedation, chronic constipation, decreased respiratory rate, and pinpoint pupils is observed.

One of the prime medical uses of morphine and the other opiates is for the relief of pain; the drugs raise the pain threshold and alter an individual's reaction to the painful experience. Recent evidence indicates that their pharmacological effects result from interaction with both mu and kappa receptors that are located in areas within the brain and spinal cord where pain is felt or appreciated. Recent studies have implicated these receptors in the analgesic effects of acupuncture, electrical stimulation, and the analgesia induced by opiates and anesthetics.

The Central Nervous System
Analgesia   Morphine exerts a narcotic action manifested by analgesia, drowsiness, changes in mood, and mental clouding. The major medical action of morphine sought in the CNS is analgesia,

which may usually be induced by doses below those that cause other effects on the CNS, such as sedation or respiratory depression. Morphine seems to relieve pain without simultaneously depressing vision, hearing, touch, or pressure sense. In fact, its analgesic action appears to result not from a decrease of pain impulses into the CNS but from an altered perception of the painful stimulus; the pain is still present and felt, but it is not appreciated as being painful. Thus, it would appear that, rather than decreasing the stimulus of pain, opiates decrease the suffering associated with the pain by altering the patient's awareness of it.

Respiration   A second major action of morphine and the other opiates on the CNS is to depress respiration through interaction with mu receptors located in the brainstem. The result of this action is a marked decrease in the rate of respiration. At high doses, respiration may become so slow and irregular that life is threatened. The cardinal acute toxic effect of opiate narcotics, respiratory depression, far outweighs all other adverse effects of this class of drugs. Death, when induced by opiates, is almost always secondary to respiratory failure.

Cough   Opiates suppress the "cough center," which is also located in the brainstem. Such an action is thought to underlie the use of opiate narcotics as cough suppressants. Codeine appears to be particularly effective in this action and is widely used for this purpose.

EEG   Morphine exerts EEG effects similar in many respects to those produced by the barbiturates. The EEG may appear to be characteristic of alertness and then shift to being characteristic of sleep or drowsiness. Also, like the barbiturates, morphine suppresses REM (dream) sleep and, with repeated administration, the EEG patterns once again become characteristic of alertness. The EEG patterns observed in a tolerant individual differ from the EEG patterns seen in an individual who has no tolerance.

Pupil   Morphine as well as other mu and kappa agonists cause pupillary constriction (miosis), which follows from a stimulant action on an ophthalmic control center in the brainstem. Such pupillary constriction in the presence of analgesia is characteristic of narcotic ingestion.

Nauseant Effects   Opiate narcotics stimulate receptors in an area of the brainstem called the *chemoreceptor trigger zone* (CTZ). Such stimulation of the CTZ produces nausea and vomiting, the most characteristic and unpleasant side effect of narcotics.

The Gastrointestinal Tract

The opiates have been used for centuries for the relief of diarrhea and for the treatment of dysentery, uses developed long before these agents were used as analgesics or euphoriants. Opiates appear to exert their effects on the gastrointestinal tract primarily in the intestine, where peristaltic movements (or waves), which normally propel food down the intestine, are markedly diminished. Also, the tone of the intestine is greatly increased to the point where almost complete spastic paralysis of movement occurs. This combination of decreased propulsion and increased tone leads to a marked decrease in the movement of food through the intestine. This stasis is followed by a dehydration of the feces, which hardens the stool and further retards the advance of material. All these effects contribute to the constipating properties of opiates. Indeed, nothing more effective has yet been developed for treating severe diarrhea.

Psychological Effects

Morphine produces analgesia, drowsiness, mood changes, and mental clouding. In most people, opiates induce an extremely pleasant euphoric state, but such a reaction is not universal. On first use of an opiate, some individuals experience a dysphoria, consisting of anxiety and fear, lethargy, apathy, sedation, mental clouding, lack of concern, inability to concentrate, nausea, and vomiting. The effects of the opiate narcotics therefore vary considerably from person to person and may be influenced by the set and setting in which the drug is administered. Even if the first exposure to opiates results in dysphoria, repeated exposures usually result in a state of euphoria, consisting of warmth, a feeling of well-being, peacefulness, and contentment, accompanied by feelings of boundless energy and strength or, conversely, a pleasant dreamlike state, a turning inward, and sleep.

These psychological alterations appear to follow the interaction of opiates with sigma receptors located in those areas of the brain that are largely responsible for emotional activity (that is, the limbic system). Although there is still no consensus in the literature, drugs that displace either opiates or naturally occurring enkephalins decrease both auditory hallucinations in chronic schizophrenic patients and self-mutilation in autistic children. This finding suggests that opiate receptors located in the limbic system may be involved in some aspect of complex behavior. In addition, some studies suggest that these enkephalins are involved in the mediation of stress. Patients with chronic pain, whether of psychogenic or physiological origin, have altered levels of enkephalins. Thus, the profound effects of opiates on behavior, mood, emotions, and pain may be explained eventually by the interactions of drugs with specific opiate receptors.

Regular users and those who are psychologically attracted to these drugs describe the effects of intravenous injection in ecstatic and often in sexual terms. This euphoria induces a powerful compulsion to continue to use the drug. The euphoric effect becomes progressively *less* intense, however, and users then inject the drug for one or more of several possible reasons: in an attempt to reexperience the extreme euphoria of the first few injections, to maintain a state of pleasantness and well-being, to prevent mental discomfort associated with reality, or to prevent withdrawal.

Perhaps part of the psychological attraction to the opiates is related to their ability to alter the perception of pain by inducing a lack of concern for or indifference to it. Medical practitioners and researchers often tend to describe pain in physical terms: a person who has cancer or breaks a leg is in pain. However, we cannot discount the possibility of emotional or psychological pain to which no organic cause may be ascribed. Thus, in certain individuals who are attracted to the opiates, it is perhaps their ability to dull an indeterminable psychological pain that may be partly responsible for the profound psychological effects and the feeling of well-being that the drug induces.

Tolerance and Dependence

Tolerance to morphine and to the other opiate narcotics varies with the particular physiological response, the dose, and the frequency of administration. With all opiates, tolerance to the respiratory depressant, analgesic, euphoric, and sedative effects develops, but it does not usually occur with the pupil-constricting and constipating effects.

The rate at which tolerance develops varies widely. With intermittent use, little if any tolerance develops. When "sprees" of drug use are separated by prolonged drug-free periods, the opiates retain their initial efficacy. For example, if a person uses opiates for recreational purposes only on weekends, low doses may continue to be effective and not have to be markedly increased (unless, of course, a greater or more intense effect is desired). However, usually within a year, Saturday and Sunday "sprees" tend to begin on Friday night and go through Monday morning. Soon the drug is also used on Tuesday, Wednesday, and Thursday, and the "spree" is now a seven-day-a-week addiction.

As soon as this pattern of repeated administration occurs, tolerance develops and may become so marked that phenomenal doses have to be administered in order to maintain a state of euphoria or prevent discomfort. This tolerance appears to be due to both the induction of drug-metabolizing enzymes in the liver and the adaptation of neurons in the brain to the presence of the drug, the latter being the more important mechanism.

In addition to the development of tolerance to one opiate, *cross-tolerance* develops, so that an individual who becomes tolerant to one opiate will also exhibit a tolerance to all other natural or synthetic opiates, even if they are chemically dissimilar. This cross-tolerance is similar to that exhibited with various sedative-hypnotics (see Chapter 3). Cross-tolerance, however, does *not* develop between the opiate narcotics and the sedative-hypnotics. An individual who has developed a tolerance to morphine will also be tolerant to heroin but not to alcohol or barbiturates. This latter point is extremely important, because accidental death may result from the additive effects of a sedative and an opiate. For example, if an individual takes moderate doses of opiates and then drinks alcohol or takes a sedative, additive depression of respiration will occur and could lead ultimately to coma and death. Deaths from the combined effects of opiates and general depressants are not at all uncommon.

In Chapter 1, we described *physical dependence* as a state in which a person does not function properly without a drug. Physical dependence is characterized by a withdrawal syndrome when the drug is not administered. Physical dependence on the sedative-hypnotic compounds is characterized by hyperexcitability when the drug is withheld. Withdrawal of the central stimulants such as amphetamine is followed by profound physical and emotional depression. Symptoms of withdrawal from the opiate narcotics are characterized by restlessness and craving for the drug, sweating, extreme anxiety, fever, chills, violent retching and vomiting, increased respiratory rate (panting), cramping, insomnia, explosive diarrhea, and nearly unbearable aches and pains. The magnitude of these withdrawal symptoms depends upon the dose and frequency of drug administration, the duration of drug dependence, and the opiate used. For example, withdrawal signs following the removal of methadone are usually less severe than those observed following the removal of heroin.

Withdrawal from the opiates also differs from barbiturate withdrawal in that the effects are seldom life-threatening, although they are uncomfortable and seemingly unbearable. Convulsions leading to respiratory paralysis and death are not observed during opiate withdrawal.

Too often, extremely vivid accounts of the withdrawal symptoms are presented as part of an attempt to discourage the recreational use of heroin, opium, morphine, or other opiate narcotics. The dependence and withdrawal syndrome should not be held as the *only* reason that these drugs should not be used for recreational purposes. The opiates are extremely potent, valuable, and irreplaceable drugs for the treatment of pain. But they also have the capability of inducing a state of euphoria and relief from psychological pain, which may lead to a powerful compulsion to misuse them. In addition, intravenous injection of these drugs is capable of inducing a "rush" that can be described only in ecstatic or sexual terms.

The opiates induce profound tolerance and physiological dependence, the consequences of which are important both medically and sociologically because the dependent and tolerant opiate user is difficult to treat and must frequently resort to crime to support the habit and reach a source of supply. Tolerance leads to the need for massive doses of drugs in order to prevent withdrawal, alleviate pain (physical or psychological), and attempt to maintain a state of euphoria. Drugs are extremely expensive when it becomes necessary to purchase them illegally, even though they may be inexpensive when purchased legitimately. It may not be the tolerance and dependence that are so harmful as the lengths to which the individual is forced to go in order to procure adequate supplies of drugs. A person who has access to inexpensive, medical-quality narcotics and sterile needles and syringes supplied through legitimate sources may be capable of leading a fairly normal life despite his or her tolerance to and physical dependence upon an opiate. The same may be said for patients on chronic methadone maintenance (see the following discussion).

Synthetic Narcotic Analgesics

There are several other narcotics that are structurally related to morphine but which differ primarily in their potency. Examples include oxymorphone (Numorphan) and hydromorphone (Dilaudid), both of which are six to ten times more potent than morphine, meaning that only one-sixth to one-tenth of each is needed to achieve the same intensity of analgesia or respiratory depression that a higher dose of morphine would induce. Aside from this difference in potency there is little to distinguish these drugs from morphine.

Figure 7.1 presents the structural formulas of morphine, heroin, and four synthetic agents. These agents are structurally unrelated to either morphine or heroin, though they have about the same qualitative pharmacological actions as morphine and differ from it only quantitatively. We will discuss these synthetic analgesics with reference to morphine and emphasize the differences.

Figure 7.1

Structural formulas of morphine, heroin, and four synthetic narcotic analgesics.

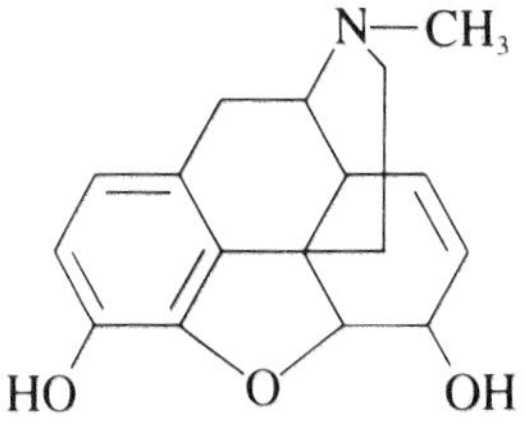

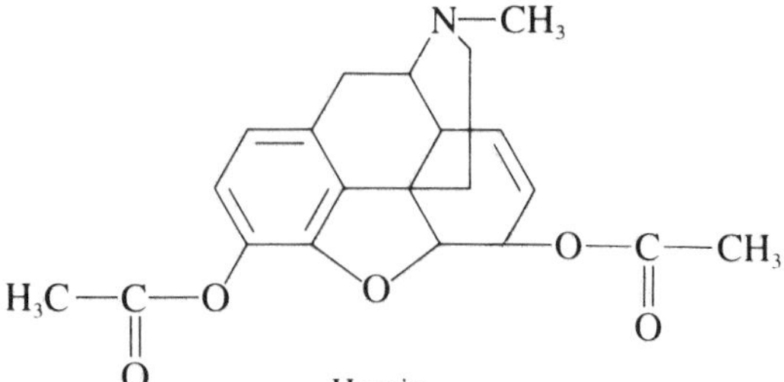

Heroin

Morphine

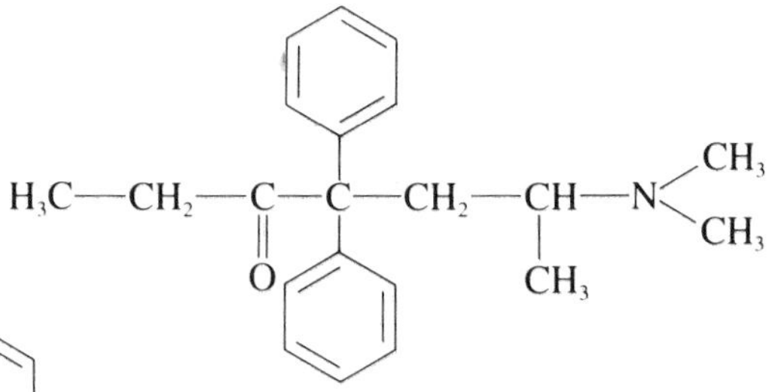

Methadone (Dolophine)

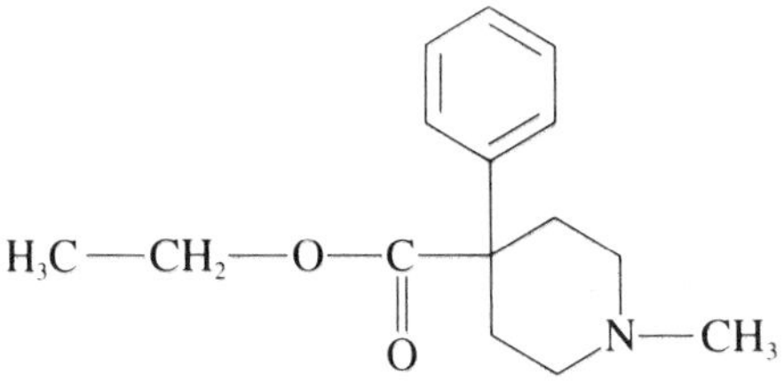

Meperidine (Demerol)

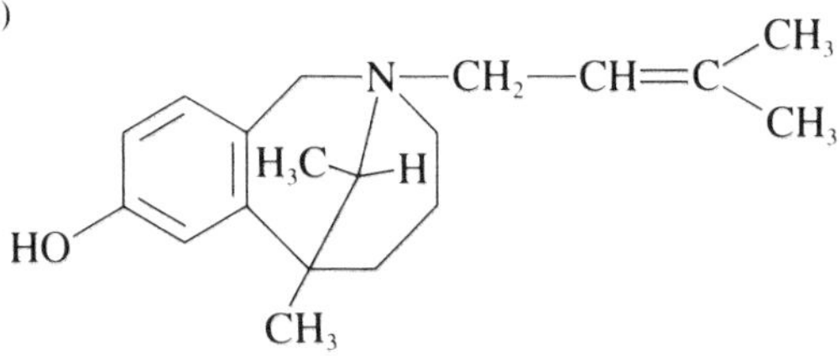

Pentazocine (Talwin)

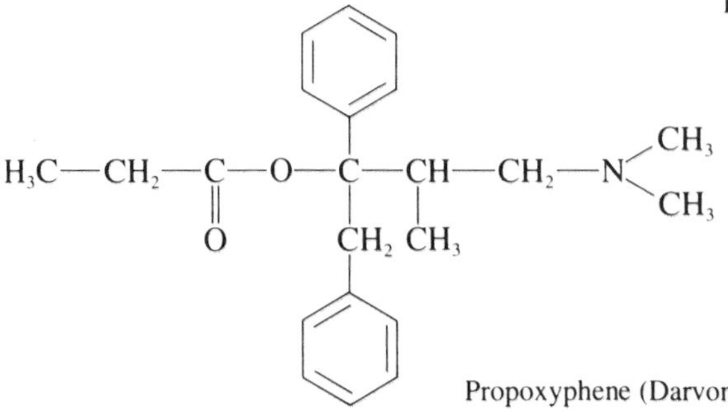

Propoxyphene (Darvon)

Meperidine

Meperidine (Demerol) is a synthetic compound that was introduced into medicine in 1939. Although not originally studied as an analgesic, meperidine was soon discovered to have considerable analgesic activity. As Figure 7.1 shows, it is chemically quite dissimilar to morphine, and for many years it was thought to be free of many of the undesirable properties associated with the use of opium alkaloids. It is now recognized that meperidine is addictive and will substitute for morphine or heroin in addicts. Meperidine is widely available commercially and is probably the narcotic most frequently abused by physicians and others in the medical profession. Because it is the narcotic analgesic most widely prescribed for pain relief in hospitalized patients, it is therefore a very commonly encountered agent in physician-induced addiction of patients.

Like morphine, its pharmacological effects are characterized by analgesia, sedation, euphoria, and respiratory depression. One interesting difference is that meperidine does not cause pinpoint pupils but causes the pupils to dilate. Unlike morphine, meperidine is quite well absorbed when taken orally and is therefore frequently prescribed when an orally administered, potent analgesic is needed.

Given by injection (subcutaneous or intramuscular), meperidine has a rapid onset of action (within 10 minutes) but a duration of action (2 to 4 hours) that is considerably shorter than that of morphine (4 to 6 hours). This short duration necessitates frequent reinjections for the relief of continuing pain. Unlike morphine, meperidine is not clinically useful for the treatment of cough or diarrhea.

Methadone

Methadone (Dolophine) is a synthetic opiate first synthesized by German chemists during World War II. Its pharmacological activity is very similar to that of morphine. As stated by Jaffe and Martin, "The outstanding properties of methadone are its effective analgesic activity, its efficacy by the oral route, its extended duration of action in suppressing withdrawal symptoms in physically dependent individuals, and its tendency to show persistent effects with repeated administration."[4]

One of the most important uses of methadone today is in the controlled withdrawal of opiate addicts. In this situation, orally administered methadone is substituted for the injected opiate of addiction and the patient is later slowly withdrawn from methadone. The withdrawal is milder and less acute than that from morphine. Another important use is in methadone maintenance programs for opiate dependence. Methadone is an effective agent when administered orally and it has an extended duration of action; thus it is used as a substitute for other opiate narcotics. These uses of methadone are further discussed on pages 143–144.

Propoxyphene

Propoxyphene (Darvon) is an analgesic compound that is structurally very similar to methadone (Figure 7.1). As an analgesic its potency is considerably less than that of codeine but greater than therapeutic doses of aspirin. In large doses, opiate-like effects are seen, and when used intravenously, propoxyphene is recognized by addicts as a narcotic. Used orally, however, the abuse liability of propoxyphene is relatively low. Some cases of drug dependence have been reported but to date they have not been of major concern. Abuse difficulties arise primarily when the drug is administered intravenously. Because commercial intravenous preparations are not available, such abuse is encountered only when individuals attempt to inject solutions of the powder taken from the capsules intended for oral use.

Opiates with Mixed Actions

Four drugs that all bind in varying degrees to the three types of opiate receptors are pentazocine, butorphanol, buprenorphine, and nalbuphine. These drugs are either unable to exert any actions at all on the receptor (and thus act as competitive *antagonists* of more potent opiates) or their actions are limited, whereupon they are termed *partial agonists* at their receptors. Their characterization (as far as it is known for each agent) is presented in Table 7.2.

Pentazocine (Talwin) and butorphanol (Stadol) are sigma agonists. Their actions are often characterized by prominent behavioral alterations, including, at high doses, psychotomimetic effects. Both are agonists of spinal kappa receptors, whereas neither has much stimulant effect, and they even seem to have some antagonistic effect at mu receptors. Therefore, neither of these drugs has much potential for producing respiratory depression or physical dependence. Obviously, this characteristic also limits their analgesic effectiveness. Administered to morphine- or heroin-dependent persons, these drugs only poorly substitute for more potent agents and, indeed, the drug-dependent individual may experience withdrawal symptoms.

In recent years, however, abuse of pentazocine has been on the increase—especially popular has been the combination of pentazocine with tripelennamine, an antihistamine. The combination is called "T's and blues," and it has caused serious medical compli-

Figure 7.2

Structural formulas of two morphine antagonists. Naloxone (right) is a *pure* antagonist while nalbuphine has *mixed* agonistic-antagonistic properties.

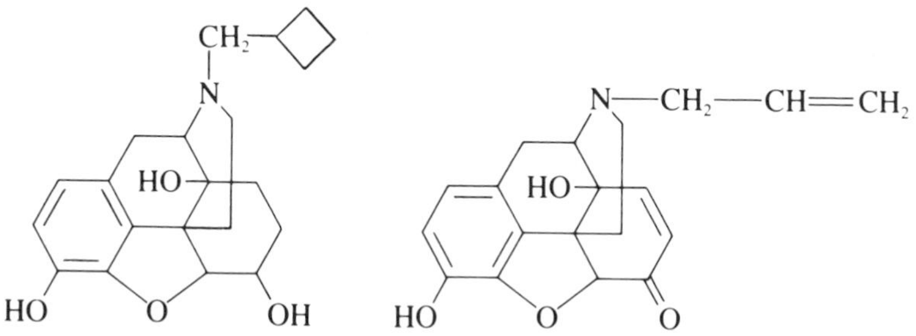

Nalbuphine

Naloxone

cations, including seizures, psychotic episodes, skin ulcerations, abscesses, and muscle wasting. (The latter three resulting from repeated injection of the drugs.)

Buprenorphine (Buprenex) is a newer agent whose action is characterized by a limited stimulation (partial agonist) of mu receptors; this action is responsible for its analgesic effectiveness. It has a very long duration of action, presumably because of its strong binding to mu receptors. Such binding, however, occasionally limits its reversibility by naloxone when such reversal is thought necessary.

Nalbuphine (Nubain) is primarily a kappa agonist, which accounts for its limited analgesic effects. Because it is a mu antagonist, it is not likely to produce analgesia, respiratory depression, or patterns of abuse. It is relatively devoid of sigma effects, and psychotomimetic alterations are rarely observed. Structurally (Figure 7.2), nalbuphene is closely related to naloxone (Narcan), which is a pure narcotic antagonist (discussed in the following section).

All four of these agents are poor substitutes for these potent mu agonists. When they are administered to morphine- or heroin-dependent individuals, withdrawal symptoms will occur.

Anesthetic Narcotics

Three potent, short-acting narcotics have been introduced for use during surgery: fentanyl (Sublimaze), sufentanil (Sufenta), and, more recently, alfentanyl (Alfenta). Occasionally, these drugs, which are obtained from legitimate manufacturers, appear on the illicit market. More commonly, however, illicitly manufactured derivatives appear, usually as a "designer drug" under such names as "China white."

All are extremely potent (about 200 to 1000 times as potent as morphine) and produce immediate and intense analgesia. Unfortunately, they also produce severe respiratory depression and, occasionally, spasm of the muscles of the chest wall. These two effects can lead to a paralysis of respiration that necessitates an injection of a curare-like muscle relaxant followed by artificial ventilation. Because time does not often permit this, deaths from illicitly manufactured derivatives are common when they are self-administered or otherwise abused. Over 100 deaths from "China white" have occurred in California alone.

In attempts to control the manufacture and distribution of illicit fentanyl derivatives ("designer drugs"), the Federal Drug Enforcement Agency (DEA) responded by adding an emergency provision to the Comprehensive Crime Control Act of 1984. This provision authorized the DEA to temporarily declare any drug a Schedule I narcotic substance if it poses an immediate public health hazard. Since 1985, dozens of analog drugs have been placed under Schedule I control, including the fairly widespread hallucinogenic amphetamine MMDA (methoxy-methylene dioxyamphetamine) popularly known as "ecstasy;" certain meperidine (Demerol) derivatives, especially MPPP (1-methyl-4-phenyl-4-propionoxy-piperidine) and MPTP (1-methyl-4-phenyl-1, 2, 5, 6-tetrahydropyridine), both of which are neurotoxin by-products of meperidine, which induce a severe, irreversible, and progressive parkinsonian disease state; and numerous fentanyl analogs.

The Emergency Scheduling Provision of the Comprehensive Crime Control Act was first invoked for the fentanyl analog 3-methylfentanyl in 1985. Since then, nine other fentanyl analogs have been controlled under the Emergency Scheduling Provision: acetyl-alphamethyl fentanyl, alpha-methylthiofentanyl, benzylfentanyl, beta-hydroxyfentanyl, beta-hydroxy-3-methylfentanyl, 3-methyl-thiofentanyl, para-fluorofentanyl, thiofentanyl, and thenylfentanyl.

New legislation has been proposed that would make it illegal to engage in any drug activities using illicit analogs regardless of whether the "designer drug" in question has been duly scheduled under the DEA's Controlled Substance Act. The language of the proposed law would make it "unlawful to manufacture, distribute, or possess, with the intent to distribute, a controlled substance analog intended for human consumption unless the action is in conformance with section 505 of the Federal Food, Drug, and Cosmetic Act."

Antagonists of Opiate Narcotics

In the previous discussion, we noted that when opiates with mixed actions were administered to nonaddicts, a morphine-like action was observed but when administered to morphine- or heroin-dependent individuals, they would not substitute and a withdrawal syndrome might be precipitated. This apparent contradiction in action can be explained this way: when the drugs are administered to nonaddicted individuals, they attach to kappa or mu receptors in the brain and produce the characteristic (although mild) narcotic actions of analgesia, sedation, euphoria, and respiratory depression. However, when they are administered to a person who is physically dependent on morphine, heroin, or another narcotic analgesic, they block the access of the more potent drug to the mu receptor.

In contrast, two drugs (naloxone and naltrexone) have no agonist effects of their own but antagonize the effects of opiates at all of their receptors. These two drugs are called *pure narcotic antagonists.*

Naloxone

Naloxone (Narcan), when administered to normal individuals, produces no analgesia, euphoria, or respiratory depression. However, it rapidly precipitates withdrawal in narcotic-dependent individuals. It is devoid of agonist (morphine-like) effects and therefore is not subject to abuse. It antagonizes the actions of morphine at all its receptors, with mu receptors being most sensitive.

The uses of naloxone include the reversal of the respiratory depression that follows acute narcotic intoxication (overdoses) and the reversal of narcotic-induced respiratory depression in newborns of mothers who have received narcotics. The use of naloxone is limited by a short duration of action and the necessity of a parenteral route of administration (the drug is poorly absorbed orally).

Naltrexone

Naltrexone (Trexan) became clinically available in 1985 as a new narcotic antagonist. Its actions resemble those of naloxone, but naltrexone is well absorbed orally and is long acting, necessitating only a single dose of 50 to 100 milligrams. Therefore, it is useful in narcotic treatment programs where it is desired to maintain an individual on chronic therapy with a narcotic antagonist. In individuals taking naltrexone, subsequent injection of an opiate will produce little or no effect. Naltrexone appears to be particularly effective for the treatment of narcotic dependence in addicts who have more to gain by being drug-free rather than drug-dependent.

Opiate Narcotics and Crime

The relationship between the use of opiates and the occurrence of crime is complex and emotionally charged. Blum and his associates state that "no known drug, by itself, can be shown to 'cause' crime, although when the use of a drug is illegal, the 'crime' clearly rests upon the person's decision to acquire, possess, or use the drug illicitly."[5] If the use of a drug is defined as a crime, drug use *must* lead to crime. Laws have been passed to control the manufacture, distribution, and sale of opiates and many other psychoactive drugs so that in the mere possession, use, or selling of any drug illegally a crime is necessarily committed.

Other factors in the relationship between opiates and crime are perhaps more serious. For example, the illegal procurement of opiates is extremely expensive. A well-developed heroin habit may cost from $100 to $500 a day. The same quantity of drug obtained legally would cost only a few dollars. Obviously, there are very few legitimate ways in which most people can earn this amount of extra money. The individual has one of two choices: either stop taking the drug, lose the euphoria, and go through withdrawal, or else attempt to meet the necessary expenditure by turning to illegal, usually nonviolent, activities. The present laws seem to encourage crime. By making these drugs illegal, by making the addict a criminal, and by restricting trade by incarcerating the small-volume dealer (which forces prices upward), the laws encourage the addict to commit crimes in order to obtain his or her drug supply.

There is little evidence to indicate that crimes of violence are a direct consequence of the use of opiate narcotics. Individuals on opiates are usually quiet, passive, and seldom prone to violence. This is in contrast to the cocaine abuser, since cocaine is a stimulant and can cause a manic paranoia (Chapter 5). Still, while there is no evidence that opiates are a *cause* of violent crime, there is little doubt that among those addicts with a background of delinquency, the use of opiates is part of their total social activity, which includes crime. The use of opiates by these individuals may encourage or perpetuate associations in social or antisocial groups that may pose problems for the community and for society.

An important footnote must be added: Within the last few years there has been a drastic change in the pattern of illicit drug use in our society. Whereas most opiate use was formerly confined to antisocial elements in our society, the use of opiates and other psychoactive drugs has spread into the suburbs and permeated all facets of community life. This tends to weaken even further the causal relationship between drugs and crime. This new generation of drug users often does not use them continuously and thus may not develop tolerance or physical dependence. They use opiates, at least initially, only on "sprees" and do not need to buy large quantities. An addict is not necessarily a degenerate criminal or shabby, ill-shod, or malnourished. An individual tolerant to and dependent upon an opiate who is socially or financially capable of obtaining an adequate supply of good quality drug, sterile syringes and needles, and other paraphernalia may maintain his or her proper social and occupational functions, remain in fairly good health, and suffer little serious incapacitation as a result of the dependence.

Treatment of the Opiate User

The precise motivations for a person's becoming dependent upon opiate narcotics are far from clear. In the United States, there are three basic patterns of opiate use and dependence, as described by Jaffe:

One involves individuals whose drug use begins in the context of medical treatment and who obtain the initial supplies through medical channels. This group constitutes a very small percentage of the addicted population. Another pattern begins with experimental or recreational drug use, progresses to more intensive use, and involves adolescents and young adults, with males far outnumbering females. Most of these users are introduced to the drug by other users. This is true both of the initial contact and of those subsequent contacts which lead to relapse after periods of withdrawal. The way in which drug use spreads from one friend to another in epidemic fashion has been well documented. A third pattern involves users who begin in one or another of the preceding ways but later switch to oral opiates (methadone) obtained from organized treatment programs.[6]

The analgesia and euphoria induced by opiate narcotics are attractions to their use. However, additional contributions to the incidence of opiate dependence appear to be sociological or psychological, rather than necessarily the result of a physiological or organic deficit in the individual. For example, in 1971, with the wide availability of opium and heroin in the Far East, about 45 percent of U.S. Army enlisted men in Vietnam had used opiates at least once.[7] About half of these users reported that at some time during their tour of duty in Vietnam they were physically dependent. It is unlikely that in this large number of young men there was a consistent organic deficit. Rather, the ready availability of opiates and the traumatic situation in which the soldiers were involved predisposed them to the use of these agents. It can therefore be seen that before any attempt is made to withdraw an addict permanently from opiate use, his or her underlying motivation for seeking the drug's positive reinforcement or reward (the euphoria, sedation, and analgesia) must be determined. In recent years, it has become clear that treatment and rehabilitation of opiate users cannot reside *solely* in attempts to withdraw them from the drug but must include withdrawal from the positive reinforcements or life situations that were associated with opiate use. As Jaffe states:

The indications for treatment vary with the drugs being used as well as with the social and cultural factors determining the particular pattern of drug use. Some patterns of drug use, such as the "recreational" use of marijuana, do not require treatment any more than does the occasional smoking of tobacco or the social use of alcohol. Such casual use is not without hazard, but this does not imply a treatable disorder. It is likely that changing views about drug use will continue to create grey areas where the indications for treatment are unclear. However, there is general agreement that treatment is appropriate for the adverse consequences of drug use and for the compulsive drug user who voluntarily seeks help.[8]

Until recently, few thought a heroin addict could ever be satisfactorily rehabilitated and maintained in a functional, drug-free state, and addicts were routinely sentenced to imprisonment. Statistics indicate that such periods of imprisonment were not an effective treatment or sufficient rehabilitation for the addict. At least 90 percent of those incarcerated for opiate use relapsed within 6 months of their release.

We have recently entered a more enlightened time and recognize that an addict is ill and not necessarily criminal (recall the discussion of alcoholism). We handle the treatment and rehabilitation of the narcotic addict with a more positive, medically oriented approach. No longer do all physicians adhere to the concept that drug withdrawal must be the first step in treatment or that effective rehabilitation requires a carefully controlled, drug-free environment. The latter concept of rehabilitation started with the development of residential communities such as the Synanon Foundation in California, which are comprised of social programs of group living and community involvement to assist former addicts in facing their problems, learning to understand themselves, and altering their behavior and life-styles. Such programs are effective. One frequently raised objection, however, is that addicts do not adjust to living in the "real world," because they are so completely involved in the small communal group. In addition, these programs are expensive and not capable of handling large numbers of drug-dependent individuals—an important point, since more and more persons within our society are using opiates.

Such considerations have led to the development of new programs designed to withdraw addicts, while they remain functioning members of their own communities, on oral doses of narcotic so that they need not purchase drugs on the street. By so doing, the dependence on the needle, the subcultural involvement, and criminal orientation are decreased. It would be possible, of course, to continue to give patients the drugs they were using (heroin, morphine, and so on) and either maintain them on that dose (provided by a legitimate source) or else simply reduce the dose over a period of several days. However, as mentioned previously, methadone is an effective drug administered orally for suppressing withdrawal symptoms. Methadone can be substituted for any of the opiate analgesics currently available.

With *methadone substitution*, the opiate originally used (usually injected) is replaced by an orally administered agent. The dose of methadone is then slowly reduced over a period of 10 to 14 days. The withdrawal symptoms are rarely worse than those of a moderate "flu-like" syndrome. The dose of methadone employed varies with the patient's health and the amount of drug formerly used. Unfortunately, the relapse rate following methadone substitution is high, approaching 60 to 70 percent.

With *methadone maintenance*, addicts are stabilized on methadone and, it is postulated, remain productive members of their communities so that it may not be necessary to withdraw the methadone. More recently, however, it has been found that after 1 to 2 years, many former heroin addicts maintained on methadone can be gradually withdrawn from this drug over a period of several weeks. The withdrawal discomforts are relatively minor and some patients are able to complete the withdrawal processes and not relapse to the use of heroin, morphine, or other opiate. Others have completed the withdrawal but have later returned to heroin. Still other patients have discontinued withdrawal and have remained on methadone maintenance.[9]

Methadone-substitution and methadone-maintenance programs have been in operation for several years, and studies conclude that methadone is an effective aid in the treatment of heroin addiction. It is also clear that methadone must be combined with intensive psychological counseling and adoption of a productive life-style. It is not enough merely to switch addicts from heroin to methadone and return them to the street. This has happened in some programs and the result is often either compulsive abuse of methadone or return to the use of heroin. Alternatives must be provided to the addict's life-style and positive reinforcements introduced to replace the use of opiates before they will be successfully adjusted. Once these reinforcements are found, consideration can be given to discontinuing the methadone. Too rapid removal of methadone should be avoided, however, since it may be more socially acceptable to maintain an individual on methadone than to return him or her to the street and to former habits of drug acquisition and use.

Several nonnarcotic drugs have been tried to aid in opiate withdrawal, and one agent has been found to be moderately successful. Clonidine (Catapres) is an antihypertensive drug, used clinically to lower blood pressure in patients with hypertension. Pharmacologically, it stimulates certain specialized catecholamine receptors in the brain and spinal cord (alpha-2 receptors). It effectively suppresses withdrawal symptoms in addicts withdrawing from low-to-moderate doses of methadone.[11–12] Its mechanism of action is speculative, but it probably involves activation of certain inhibitory pathways that are suppressed during periods of opiate dependency.

In treatment, methadone is abruptly discontinued and clonidine is administered for 7 to 10 days to suppress symptoms. The clonidine is then withdrawn gradually over 3 to 4 days. The drug is more effective in suppressing the physical signs and symptoms of withdrawal (nausea, vomiting, and diarrhea) than it is in treating the psychological discomforts and drug craving.

In addicts who desire more rapid withdrawal, methadone doses can be lowered gradually until the patient becomes uncomfortable, at which time either naloxone or naltrexone are administered to precipitate complete withdrawal. Clonidine is then administered to ameliorate the symptoms of the precipitated withdrawal. Such therapy, however, is seldom used.

At present, the pharmacologically optimal method of withdrawing an addict is to place him or her on oral methadone and, after prolonged methadone maintenance and gradual dosage reduction, the patient is withdrawn with the assistance of clonidine. This is followed with long-term maintenance with the antagonist naltrexone. Such a scheme appears to provide the safest and the most effective method of withdrawal in those patients who desire to remain drug-free.

Notes

1. American Medical Association, "Drug Evaluations," 6th ed. (Chicago: American Medical Association, 1986), pp. 53–79.
2. J. H. Jaffe and W. R. Martin, "Opioid Analgesics and Antagonists," in A. G. Gilman, L. S. Goodman, T. W. Rall, and F. Murad, eds., *The Pharmacological Basis of Therapeutics*, 7th ed. (New York: Macmillan, 1985), pp. 493–499.

3. R. M. Brown, D. H. Clouet, and D. Friedman, eds., "Opiate Receptor Subtypes and Brain Function," National Institute on Drug Abuse, Monograph No. 71, Department of Health and Human Services Publication No. ADM. 86-1462 (Washington, D.C.: U.S. Government Printing Office, 1986).

4. J. H. Jaffe and W. R. Martin, "Opioid Analgesics and Antagonists," in A. G. Gilman, L. S. Goodman, T. W. Rall, and F. Murad, eds., The Pharmacological Basis of Therapeutics, 7th ed. (New York: Macmillan, 1985), pp. 517–518.

5. R. H. Blum and Associates, Society and Drugs, vol. 1 (San Francisco: Jossey-Bass, 1969), p. 290.

6. J. H. Jaffe, "Drug Addiction and Drug Abuse," in A. G. Gilman, L. S. Goodman, T. W. Rall, and F. Murad, eds., The Pharmacological Basis of Therapeutics, 7th ed. (New York: Macmillan, 1985), p. 541.

7. L. Robins, The Vietnam Drug User Returns: Final Report, September 1973. Special Action Office Monograph, Series A, No. 2 (Washington, D.C.: U.S. Government Printing Office, 1974).

8. J. H. Jaffe, "Drug Addiction and Drug Abuse," in A. G. Gilman, L. S. Goodman, T. W. Rall, and F. Murad, eds., The Pharmacological Basis of Therapeutics, 7th ed. (New York: Macmillan, 1985), pp. 567–568.

9. J. H. Jaffe, "Drug Addiction and Drug Abuse," in A. G. Gilman, L. S. Goodman, T. W. Rall, and F. Murad, eds., The Pharmacological Basis of Therapeutics, 7th ed. (New York: Macmillan, 1985), pp. 568–569.

10. G. E. Woody, C. P. O'Brien, and R. Greenstein, "Multimodality Treatment of Narcotic Addiction: An Overview," in R. C. Petersen, ed., The International Challenge of Drug Abuse. National Institute on Drug Abuse, Research Monograph 19, Washington, D.C.: U.S. Government Printing Office, 1978), pp. 226–240.

11. J. H. Jaffe, "Drug Addiction and Drug Abuse," in A. G. Gilman, L. S. Goodman, T. W. Rall, and F. Murad, eds., The Pharmacological Basis of Therapeutics, 7th ed. (New York: Macmillan, 1985), p. 569.

12. D. S. Charney et al., "Clonidine and Naltrexone," Archives of General Psychiatry 39 (1982): 1327–1332.

CHAPTER 8

Antipsychotic Tranquilizers

Drugs for Treating Schizophrenia and Other Psychoses

No one class of psychoactive drugs is effective in all mental disorders. Therefore, such mental states as anxiety, neurosis, psychosis, schizophrenia, mania, and depression must be carefully differentiated.

Anxiety is a commonly used term referring to an unpleasant state of tension and uneasiness not usually associated with any specific stimulus.

Neurosis is similar and involves some degree of emotional disability, usually accompanied by anxiety. Neurotics have difficulty dealing with the common frustrations of life and with accepting themselves, and they are frequently troubled by chronic feelings of guilt.

Mania in its broadest sense refers to abnormal, uncontrollable, and possibly dangerous behavior. More commonly, mania is considered to be the excited phase of a mental disorder referred to as *manic-depressive psychosis.*

Depression refers to a state of sadness, hopelessness, pessimism, and uselessness that can be so severe as to lead to impairment of function. Depression often occurs cyclically with mania, so that prolonged periods of manic behavior alternate with prolonged periods of depression.

Schizophrenia literally means "splitting of the mind" and refers to an inappropriateness or imbalance between the emotional reactions and the thought content associated with the emotions (that is, a split in the mind between emotions and mentation).

Schizophrenia represents a group of ill-defined, chronic, idiopathic, psychotic disorders characterized primarily by distinctive changes in concept formation and reality relationships.[1] Symptoms typically become evident during adolescence or early adulthood. Schizophrenia probably has some degree of genetic transmission or involvement, but the exact etiology remains unknown. Exacerbations of schizophrenia are common and signify the presence of a state of chronic schizophrenia. Patients with chronic schizophrenia often experience progressive impairment of insight, judgment, and affect. Chronic schizophrenia is particularly important from a pharmacological point of view because antipsychotic drugs are most effective in acute exacerbations of schizophrenia, whereas they are less effective in sustained or progressive impairments. Indeed, the principal benefit of antipsychotic drugs may lie in their ability to prevent acute exacerbations; in such instances, they reduce the exacerbation rate in chronic schizophrenia by about one-half to two-thirds that seen in nontreated patients.

Thought disturbances include a distortion of reality, delusions, and hallucinations (usually auditory). Mood and behavioral disorders consist of ambivalence, apathy, withdrawal, and bizarre activity. The incidence of schizophrenia is estimated as 0.5 to 1 percent of the general population. Indeed, schizophrenics occupy approximately two-thirds of beds in mental hospitals and more than one-quarter of all hospital beds.

Psychosis is a general term referring to any mental disorder in which a person's mental capacity to recognize reality, communicate, and associate with others is impaired enough to interfere with his or her ability to deal with the ordinary demands of life. The psychoses are severe psychiatric disorders in which there is not only a marked impairment of behavior but also a serious inability to think coherently, to comprehend reality, or to gain insight into the abnormality. These conditions often include delusions and hallucinations.

The psychoses are often subdivided into two major subclassifications according to their origin: (1) psychoses associated with a "brain syndrome" (a loss of nerve-cell function) such as would occur in drug intoxication or dementia (see Chapter 3), and (2) those for which no organic cause has yet been found (such as schizophrenia). Schizophrenic persons retain their sense of orientation and memory, but they exhibit severely disordered emotions, thoughts, and behaviors.

Minor versus Major Tranquilizers

Many of the sedative-hypnotic drugs discussed in Chapter 3 are helpful in treating anxiety states and neurotic behavior. They are not clinically useful in the management of schizophrenia or manic-depressive psychosis, nor can they be relied upon to calm a psychotic patient without inducing pronounced depression of behavior or even deep sleep or anesthesia. The clinical antidepressants (Chapter 6) are useful in the treatment of some forms of depression but have little value in the treatment of psychosis. In contrast, the antipsychotic tranquilizers can calm persons who are suffering from acute psychotic states and reduce their frequency of relapses, making these patients more manageable.

The "minor tranquilizers" discussed in Chapter 3 as being low-potency, sedative-hypnotic compounds—chlordiazepoxide (Librium), diazepam (Valium), and meprobamate (Equanil)—differ from the drugs classified as "major tranquilizers" or, more correctly, "antipsychotic tranquilizers." A minor tranquilizer is useful in the treatment of anxiety and neurosis. A major or antipsychotic tranquilizer is capable of relieving symptoms of psychosis (usually schizophrenia) and inducing a behavioral state characterized by psychomotor slowing, emotional quieting, and an indifference to external stimuli.

It is also important to note that the word *tranquilizer* implies the induction of a tranquil, calm, or pleasant state. This may indeed be true in the case of the minor tranquilizers because sedative-hypnotic compounds can induce a state of disinhibition, euphoria, and relief from anxiety. In contrast, the psychological effects induced by the antipsychotic (or major) tranquilizers are seldom pleasant, seldom euphoric, and may be unpleasant or dysphoric when administered to individuals who are not psychotic. Hence, these agents are seldom encountered as drugs of abuse. Their importance in medicine, however, is well established. In addition, these agents have contributed in the laboratory to our knowledge of the physiological and biochemical bases of behavior and of mental disease.

Historical Background

Clinical descriptions of psychotic patients (especially schizophrenics) date back to at least 1400 B.C. However, the isolation of these patients was the only known therapy until the early twentieth century. The concept of caring for individuals with mental disorders, rather than simply keeping them, did not become entrenched until the eighteenth century. Shock treatment in the eighteenth and nineteenth centuries consisted of twirling patients on a stool until they lost consciousness or dropping them through a trap door into an icy lake.

The only alternative to such drastic therapy was moral treatment, consisting of individualized attention, which today would resemble group and social therapy. Such treatment was probably an effective therapeutic approach to schizophrenic patients. However, with the introduction of huge mental hospitals, in which the personal approach disappeared, moral treatment and the therapeutic gains by such individualized attention were lost.

This therapeutic vacuum persisted until the mid-1930s, when Sakel introduced insulin coma as a therapeutic treatment. In this method, insulin was injected until the patient became hypoglycemic enough to lose consciousness and lapse into coma. Several such treatments were reported to aid schizophrenic patients. Shortly thereafter, electroconvulsive therapy was introduced. In this technique, electrodes were placed on the patient's head and a current was applied until the patient had a seizure. A series of such seizure treatments was frequently effective in relieving an acute psychotic episode.

Prior to 1950, effective drugs for the treatment of psychotic patients were virtually nonexistent, and such patients were usually permanently hospitalized. Between the end of World War II and the mid-fifties, more and more patients were residing in mental hospitals because more facilities were available, funds for the support and care of psychotic patients were increased, and there was more concern for the protection of other members of the community from psychotic patients. By 1955, there were over half a million people in the United States residing in the state and local mental hospitals.

As can be seen from Figure 8.1, however, in 1955 there began a dramatic and steady reversal in this trend. By 1970, there were fewer than 340,000 institutionalized patients, and this number has remained rather stable over the past 20 years. This decline in the number of residents in mental hospitals has occurred despite dramatic *increases* in the numbers of *admissions* to state hospitals. Indeed, between 1955 and 1965, the yearly rate of admissions almost doubled. The crucial factor has been that psychotic patients are now spending only one-quarter to one-third as long in hospitals as they were in 1955. Much of the change has been brought about by the introduction of new drugs effective in the management of psychotic behavior. Since these drugs have played such an important role within our society, a brief look at their historical development may be in order.

Although the prototype of the largest class of antipsychotic drugs (the phenothiazines) was synthesized in the late 1800s, it was not until approximately 1950 in France that a derivative of phenothiazine called promethazine (Phenergan) was found to have a strong sedative effect. In 1952, the French surgeon Laborit introduced the drug as an agent to deepen anesthesia induced by barbi-

Figure 8.1

Numbers of resident patients in state and local government mental hospitals in the United States from 1946 through 1970. Note the dramatic change in the total population of mental hospitals that began in 1956 with the introduction into therapy of psychoactive drugs. [From V. C. Longo, *Neuropharmacology and Behavior* (San Francisco: W. H. Freeman and Company, Copyright © 1972), fig. 1.3, p. 11. Modified from D. H. Efron, ed., *Psychopharmacology: A Review of Progress* (Washington, D.C.: U.S. Department of Health, Education, and Welfare, 1968).]

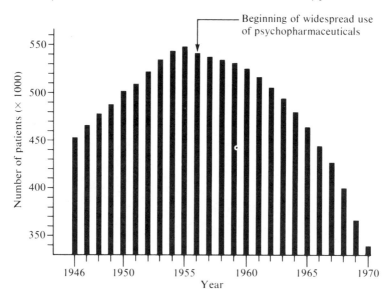

turates. Later in 1952, researchers in a French pharmaceutical company developed another phenothiazine derivative, chlorpromazine (Thorazine), and included it in a "cocktail" administered to patients the night before surgery to allay their fears and anxieties. Chlorpromazine was then found to lower the amount of anesthetic drugs needed without itself inducing loss of consciousness, for it appeared to alter profoundly the patient's mental awareness. Thus, chlorpromazine appeared to be distinct from the barbiturates and the other sedative-hypnotic drugs. Patients who had received chlorpromazine were quiet, conscious, sedated, and quite uninterested in and unconcerned about what was going on about them. Because of these effects, chlorpromazine was tried in the treatment of mental illness and was found to ameliorate psychotic episodes. Thus, for the first time, a drug had been found that specifically altered the manifestations of the psychotic process itself.

Chlorpromazine was introduced into the United States in 1954 and released for marketing in 1955. Its rapid success in the treatment of institutionalized psychotic patients is clearly seen in Figure 8.1.

At approximately the same time that chlorpromazine was introduced into the United States, another antipsychotic agent, unrelated to phenothiazine, was discovered and introduced into therapy. This compound was a drug called reserpine (Serpasil). If reserpine had been introduced and the phenothiazines not discovered, reserpine itself would have been the drug of choice for the treatment of psychotic patients, despite the fact that reserpine produces a number of bothersome side effects. Thus, because both drugs were introduced almost simultaneously and both were effective, the drug that produced fewer side effects was the one more widely used.

More recently, there have been attempts to develop antipsychotic drugs that might be superior to chlorpromazine and the other phenothiazines. One such class of drugs is the butyrophenones developed in Belgium in the mid-sixties. These compounds are structurally unrelated to the phenothiazines, but their pharmacological actions are similar. At the present time, two butyrophenones are available in the United States: haloperidol (Haldol) and droperidol (Inapsine). These compounds seem to have few significant advantages over the phenothiazines but they are used occasionally for patients intolerant of phenothiazines.

In recent years, emphasis has been placed on the understanding of a drug's mechanism and site of action in the brain as well as its possible involvement with certain neurotransmitters in mentally ill patients rather than on the development of new drugs. Attention has also focused on the limitations of treatment with antipsychotic drugs, especially their limited effectiveness in patients with chronic illness, as well as the production and prevention of serious toxic effects. Although these are not the curative "wonder drugs" they promised to be in the 1950s, antipsychotic drugs have had a remarkable impact on psychiatry—an impact that can legitimately be called revolutionary.

Three Biological Theories of Schizophrenia

As mentioned, two broad categories of psychotic states exist—those that can be explained by a loss of neurons in the brain and those for which no organic basis has been identified. Of the latter psychoses, two subcategories have been described: (1) manic-depressive psychoses and (2) schizophrenia. The biological amine theory of mania and depression was discussed in Chapter 5. Here we focus on current theories of the biological basis of schizophrenia. Several reviews of this topic are recommended.[1-7]

The Altered Amine Theory

The altered amine hypothesis of schizophrenia is an older theory based upon evidence that some schizophrenics excrete in their urine abnormal products of amine metabolism that are not found in the urine of normal patients. These altered substances are presumed to be methylated metabolites of dopamine, a normal transmitter within the central nervous system (see Appendix II). The relationship of these methylated metabolites of dopamine to schizophrenia is based in part on the fact that some methylated products of normally occurring amines are hallucinogenic (see Chapter 9, the section on Psychedelics Acting on Norepinephrine Neurons). For example, mescaline and dimethyltryptamine are methylated derivates of dopamine and norepinephrine and can induce a state resembling psychosis. It is not yet clear, however, whether drug-induced psychosis is related to schizophrenia or, indeed, if schizophrenics produce a common methylated amine that underlies the disorder.

The Inherited Gene Theory

A second theory of schizophrenia is that this disease is a specific *inherited* disease resulting from a single mutant inherited gene. It has been hypothesized that there is as yet an undiscovered metabolic error that leads to schizophrenic illness. Evidence in favor of this theory is based upon the fact that while the incidence of schizophrenia in the general population is approximately 1 percent, this increases to 7 to 16 percent in children with one schizophrenic parent and 40 to 68 percent if both parents are schizophrenic. Though no specific genetic deficit has yet been identified, a predisposition to schizophrenia almost certainly is inherited. However, genetic studies have provided evidence that inheritance can account for only a *portion* of the cause of mental illnesses, necessitating other explanations. Thus, early hopes for the identification of genetically determined causes of psychiatric disease have not been realized.

The Dopamine Theory

The leading hypothesis concerning the biological basis of schizophrenia, the dopamine theory, is based on the fact that antipsychotic agents antagonize the actions of dopamine (as a neurotransmitter) in the limbic system; thus, a state of functional overactivity of dopamine may occur in the limbic system of schizophrenic patients.[8] This theory is based on pharmacological evidence that drugs that block dopamine receptors (see Appendix II) are clinically useful in the treatment of schizophrenia. Indeed, because antipsychotic drugs block the action of dopamine in the brain, both their clinical action (in ameliorating schizophrenia) and their side effects (see the following discussion) are mediated by the antagonism of dopaminergic neurotransmission in the brain. What is missing, however, is clear evidence that dopamine antagonism is *necessary* for an antipsychotic effect or that schizophrenia directly results from hyperactivity of dopamine neurotransmission.

Dopamine receptors are located in several sites within the brain (see Appendix II). It is known that antipsychotic drugs antagonize dopamine (1) in the limbic and frontal cortical areas of the brain, which correlates with the therapeutic action of antipsychotic agents, (2) in the extrapyramidal system, which correlates with many of the motor dysfunctions produced by these drugs, (3) in the hypothalamic-pituitary axis, which correlates with the hormonal alterations induced by these agents, and (4) at certain centers of the brainstem (especially the chemoreceptor trigger zone of the medulla), which correlates with the antivomiting effect of these antipsychotic agents. Thus, antagonism of dopamine neurotransmission appears to underlie the therapeutic effects and most of the side effects of these drugs.

The phenothiazines are a class of drugs that block these dopamine receptors. Conversely, drugs that stimulate these dopamine receptors produce a state that closely resembles schizophrenia. Amphetamine (Chapter 5) stimulates dopamine (and NE) receptors, and amphetamine-induced psychosis is at the present time the best available model of acute schizophrenia. Klawans et al. have proposed that the physiological basis of schizophrenia is an increased sensitivity of dopamine receptors within the brain to the normal amounts of dopamine present;[8] others note increased numbers of dopamine receptors in the brains of schizophrenic patients and believe this is the physiological mechanism responsible.[9] Thus, schizophrenia is associated with excessive or hyperactive neurotransmission at dopamine synapses, possibly at a specific subdivision.[10] Causative correlations have not yet been demonstrated.

Classification of Antipsychotic Drugs

The drugs with antipsychotic activity are classified as the phenothiazines, the thioxanthenes (closely related to phenothiazines), and the butyrophenones. Available preparations are listed in Table 8.1 along with two drugs structurally unrelated to the above three classes. The table also lists the therapeutic dose equivalents and relative extent of major side effects for each drug. Because all the drugs have similar properties, emphasis is placed primarily on the phenothiazines.

Table 8.1

Antipsychotic drugs.

Chemical classification	Drug name Generic (trade)	Dose equivalent (mg)	Sedation	Autonomic side effects*	Involuntary movement
Phenothiazine	Chlorpromazine (Thorazine)	100	High	High	Moderate
	Prochlorperazine (Compazine)	15	Moderate	Low	High
	Fluphenazine (Prolixin)	2	Low	Low	High
	Trifluoperazine (Stelazine)	5	Moderate	Low	High
	Perphenazine (Trilafon)	8	Low	Low	High
	Acetophenazine (Tindal)	20	Moderate	Low	High
	Carphenazine (Proketazine)	25	Moderate	Low	High
	Triflupromazine (Vesprin)	25	High	Moderate	Moderate
	Mesoridazine (Serentil)	50	High	Moderate	Low
	Thioridazine (Mellaril)	100	High	Moderate	Low
Thioxanthene	Thiothixene (Navane)	4	Low	Low	High
	Chlorprothixene (Taractan)	100	High	High	Moderate
Butyrophenone	Haloperidol (Haldol)	2	Low	Low	High
	Droperidol (Inapsine)	NA	Low	Low	High
Miscellaneous	Loxapine (Loxitane)	10	Moderate	Low	Moderate
	Molindone (Moban)	10	Moderate	Moderate	Moderate

* Autonomic side effects include dry mouth, blurred vision, constipation, urinary retention, and reduced blood pressure.

Reserpine and promazine (Sparine), two drugs formerly used to treat schizophrenia, are absent from Table 8.1. Reserpine is an effective antipsychotic drug but is rarely used today because of a high incidence of drug interactions, emotional depression, and reduced blood pressure. Promazine is now considered obsolete because of poor effectiveness and a significant incidence of bone marrow depression.

Phenothiazine Derivatives

The phenothiazine derivatives are the most widely used antipsychotics. They are also used extensively in the treatment of nausea and vomiting, for preanesthetic sedation, to delay ejaculation, and for relief of severe itching. Other, less frequent uses include the treatment of alcoholic hallucinosis, hallucinations induced by psychedelic agents (see Chapter 9), certain movement disorders (such as Huntington's chorea), and intractable hiccups.

Table 8.1 lists 10 phenothiazine derivatives available for clinical use. Our present discussion focuses on the prototype agent of this class, chlorpromazine (Thorazine). Chlorpromazine is the most widely known and the most studied of the phenothiazine derivatives. Figure 8.2 shows its chemical structure together with the structures of reserpine and haloperidol. The mechanism underlying the antipsychotic action of chlorpromazine and other phenothiazines involves antagonism of dopamine receptors in various locations within the brain. Of the various subdivisions of the brain (see Appendix III), dopamine receptors occur most prominently in the reticular formation of the brainstem, the hypothalamus, the limbic system, and the basal ganglia. Examination of the consequences of blocking dopamine receptors in each of these structures will serve to explain the physiological and psychological effects of these drugs.

Absorption, Distribution, Metabolism, and Excretion

Although the phenothiazines are effectively absorbed from the gastrointestinal tract, such absorption is slow and incomplete. However, since a patient usually takes these drugs for long periods of time (even for a lifetime), the oral route of administration is still effective and is commonly used. Intramuscular injection of phenothiazines is quite effective, increasing the effectiveness of the drug by about four to ten times that achieved with oral administration. Once in the bloodstream, the phenothiazines are rapidly distributed throughout the body. The phenothiazine levels in the brain are low compared with those found in other body tissues, the highest con-

Figure 8.2

Structural formulas of three representative antipsychotic tranquilizers. Chlorpromazine is a representative of the group of phenothiazine tranquilizers; nine other phenothiazine derivatives are available.

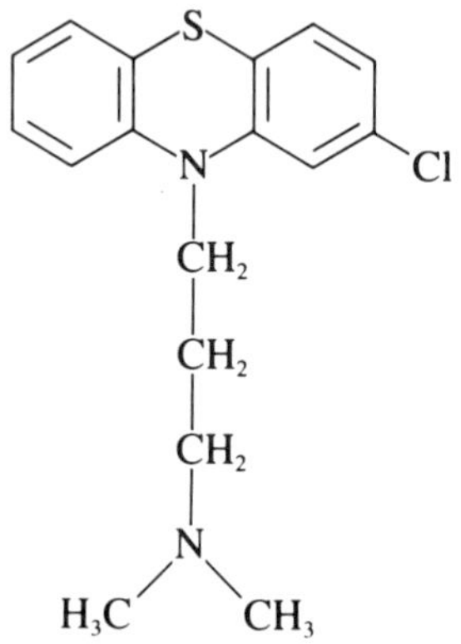

Chlorpromazine (Thorazine)

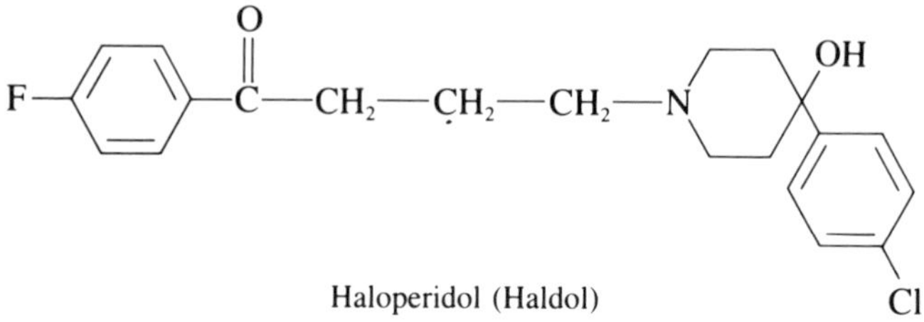

Haloperidol (Haldol)

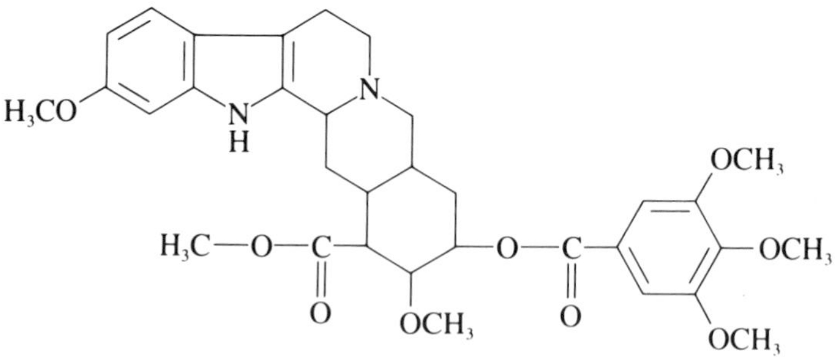

Reserpine (Serpasil)

centrations being found in the lungs, liver, adrenal glands, and spleen.

The metabolism and excretion of the phenothiazines are complicated and their half-lives are quite long—in a range of 1 to 2 days. Thus, clinical effects of single doses persist for at least 24 hours, allowing the entire daily dose to be given at bedtime, minimizing certain side effects (such as excess sedation). The phenothiazines are extensively bound to body tissues, which further delays drug elimination. Indeed, metabolites of some of the phenothiazines can be detected for as long as several months after the drug has been discontinued. Such slow elimination may contribute to the slow rate of rebound of psychotic episodes following cessation of drug therapy.

Pharmacological Effects

The phenothiazines produce dry mouth, dilated pupils, and blurred vision. Constipation, retention of urine, and increased heart rate may also be observed. These effects result from a partial blockade of acetylcholine receptors (Appendix II) that occurs in addition to the drug-induced blockade of dopamine neurons. There may be dilatation of blood vessels, with resulting decreases in blood pressure, especially when an individual rises from a reclining position. The phenothiazines also affect certain hormones; they may disturb the menstrual cycle or block menstruation completely. They may induce lactation in women who are not pregnant.

In the central nervous system, which is the primary site of antipsychotic action, phenothiazines induce a syndrome characterized by psychomotor slowing, indifference to sensory stimuli, emotional quieting, and reduction of initiative. They tend to decrease paranoia, fear, hostility, and agitation and reduce the intensity of schizophrenic delusions and hallucinations. In normal individuals, phenothiazines produce dysphoria and impair intellectual functioning.

These effects are thought to be caused by drug-induced blockade of dopamine receptors in the limbic system. As is discussed in Appendix III, the limbic system is involved in the regulation of emotion and emotional expression. Such suppression of limbic system activity appears to account for the emotional quieting and the calming effects induced by these drugs.

Through actions on the brainstem, the phenothiazines suppress certain centers involved both in behavioral arousal and in vomiting. By suppressing activity in the reticular formation, the phenothiazines induce an indifference to external stimuli such that greater levels of sensory input are necessary in order to alert or arouse an individual. In another area of the brainstem (the vomiting center), the phenothiazines block additional dopamine receptors and thereby inhibit vomiting. Indeed, these drugs are among the best antivomiting agents available.

It is also important to note that the phenothiazines exert prominent effects on an area of the brain referred to as the basal ganglia. Dopamine is an important neurotransmitter in this area, and, when absent, the result is expressed as Parkinson's disease. Replacing the absent dopamine (through the use of l-dopa) is an accepted treatment for this disease (Chapter 11). Since the phenothiazines are dopamine blockers, they have the same effect as depriving the individual of the transmitter itself and produce a parkinsonian syndrome. Parkinsonian movements, including dulled expressions of the face, rigidity and tremor of the limbs, and slow movements are prominent side effects frequently associated with the use of antipsychotic drugs (Table 8.1). In addition, it is now becoming increasingly evident that some of these drug-induced movement disorders may persist for prolonged periods after the drug is discontinued.

As discussed in Appendix III, the *hypothalamus* is intimately involved in emotional, eating and drinking, and sexual behavior and in control over the secretion of some hormones. By suppressing the function of the hypothalamus (again, by blocking dopamine receptors), phenothiazines interrupt these functions. By suppressing the appetite, food intake may be reduced. Sexually, the individual is difficult to arouse. In the male, ejaculation may be blocked. In the female, libido may be decreased, ovulation blocked, and normal menstrual cycles suppressed, resulting in infertility. Breast enlargement may occur in the male, and females may begin lactating. Temperature-regulating centers of the hypothalamus are suppressed, and body temperature will fall in a cold room and rise in a hot room. Occasionally, large doses of phenothiazines may precipitate convulsions, and epileptic patients may have to increase their doses of antiepileptic drug in order to counteract this action. The frequency and severity of the side effects induced by the different phenothiazine derivatives vary, but, in general, all must be tolerated to some extent by the patient.

Psychological Effects

In general, chlorpromazine improves the mood and behavior of psychotic patients by producing an indifference to external stimuli and a reduction of initiative and anxiety without inducing excessive sedation or causing dependence or tolerance. The sedation induced by phenothiazines differs markedly from that induced by the sedative-hypnotic compounds (see Figure 3.1). The patient who is in a state of phenothiazine-induced indifference can easily be aroused with only mild external stimulation. The phenothiazines do not produce euphoria, and the psychological syndrome induced by these drugs is not usually considered particularly pleasant. The agitation, restlessness, and hyperactivity of the acute szhizophrenic attack are often dramatically relieved by treatment. The delusions and hallucinations associated with an acute paranoid attack are particularly sensitive to such treatment. Slightly less susceptible to phenothiazine treatment are the apathy and withdrawal states seen in certain psychotic persons.

The behavioral effects of the phenothiazines may be demonstrated in an animal trained to make a conditioned response. For instance, a rat may be placed in a cage on a wire grid and, immediately after a buzzer is sounded, subjected to a small electric shock. The rat will quickly climb a pole to escape the shock. Within very few trials, the animal will learn to associate the buzzer with the electric shock and will climb the pole whenever it hears the buzzer (a *conditioned-avoidance* response). After very small doses of chlorpromazine, the rat will take no notice of the buzzer but will still be able to escape the shock by climbing the pole.

Chlorpromazine is said to block conditioned-avoidance behavior. Other drugs able to block conditioned-avoidance responses are also useful antipsychotic agents, and still others are being tested. Traditional sedative-hypnotic drugs such as the barbiturates, chlordiazepoxide (Librium), or meprobamate (Equanil) do not block conditioned-avoidance responses; instead, they depress the response to the buzzer and the response to the shock to approximately the same extent.

Side Effects and Toxicity

The phenothiazines differ from the barbiturates not only in their medical uses and behavioral actions but also in their toxicities. In contrast to the barbiturates and other sedative-hypnotics, the phenothiazines are not likely to cause death by respiratory depression. Massive doses may be ingested without producing significant depression of respiration. The compounds are frequently used in large doses for prolonged periods of time. The side effects associated with the use of these compounds, however, are many, and some invariably accompany the therapeutic use of these drugs (Table 8.1).

Phenothiazines produce a variety of disturbances of movement, including tremors, muscle rigidity, walking disorders, and involuntary movements. Other side effects include increased heart rate, dry mouth, blurred vision, and constipation. More serious side effects are altered pigmentation of the skin, pigment deposits in the retina, permanently impaired vision, decreased pituitary function, menstrual disorders, allergic reactions, and possible liver dysfunction (jaundice). These adverse effects cause significant clinical problems, since nonhospitalized patients tend to stop taking their medicine in order to avoid them and inevitably suffer a return of psychotic behavior.

Tolerance and Dependence

One of the positive attributes of the phenothiazines is that they are not addicting. Tolerance does not develop, nor does physical or psychological dependence. Psychotic patients may take phenothiazines for years without necessarily having to increase their dose because of tolerance; if a dose is increased, it is usually to obtain better control of the psychotic episodes. Cessation of these drugs is not followed by symptoms of withdrawal, possibly because it may take up to a year for the compounds to be excreted completely. Because phenothiazines do not induce a state of euphoria, there is little psychological dependence or compulsion to misuse them.

Haloperidol and Droperidol

In 1967, haloperidol (see Figure 8.2) was introduced for sale in the United States as the first of a series of compounds referred to as butyrophenone derivatives. A second compound, droperidol, has subsequently been introduced. Pharmacologically, both compounds are similar to the phenothiazines. They inhibit motor activity in animals and block conditioned-avoidance behavior. In humans, they produce sedation, indifference to external stimuli, and reduce initiative, anxiety, and activity. Both compounds, however, are metabolized and excreted at a much faster rate than the phenothiazines, and the drugs are almost totally excreted within several days after administration is discontinued.

The mechanism of the antipsychotic action of these drugs is like that of the phenothiazines, which is thought to involve antagonism of dopamine neurotransmission. Haloperidol and droperidol do not exhibit most of the serious toxicities occasionally seen with the phenothiazines (jaundice, blood abnormalities, and so on), but the involuntary movements are even more pronounced than those induced by the phenothiazines. In general, however, haloperidol and droperidol are interesting, effective drugs for the treatment of psychoses, and they offer alternatives for patients who may be unresponsive to the phenothiazines. Haloperidol and droperidol are also extremely effective antivomiting agents.

Reserpine

As stated earlier, reserpine (Serpasil) is effective in the treatment of psychoses, but its significant side effects make the phenothiazines preferable. Its most bothersome side effects include mental depression, significant depression of blood pressure, and severe diarrhea. Reserpine, however, is of interest because its mechanism of action is well understood, making it useful in the delineation of chemical pathways in the brain and mechanisms that may possibly underlie mental disorders.

Reserpine's antipsychotic effect correlates with a drug-induced depletion of norepinephrine, serotonin, and dopamine from the central nervous system. It blocks the uptake of these biological amines from inside the presynaptic nerve terminal into the storage granules, thus exposing the intraneuronal amines to the enzyme MAO, by which they are rapidly metabolized. The depletion of amines is so effective that severe mental depression may be induced. Since the phenothiazines do not deplete the brain of amines, their sedative and antipsychotic actions are not accompanied by such intense mental depression. This depleting action of reserpine, however, was important in establishing the initial correlation between biological amines and the continuum of behavioral states from depression to mania (Chapters 5 and 6).

Notes

1. American Medical Association, "Drug Evaluations," 6th ed. (Chicago: American Medical Association, 1986), pp. 111–130.
2. S. H. Snyder, S. P. Banerjee, H. T. Yamamura, and D. Greenberg, "Drugs, Neurotransmitters, and Schizophrenia," *Science* 184 (1974): 1243–1253.
3. S. S. Kety, "Recent Genetic and Biochemical Approaches to Schizophrenia," in L. L. Simpson, ed., *Drug Treatment of Mental Disorders* (New York: Raven Press, 1976), pp. 1–11.
4. M. E. Lickey and B. Gordon, *Drugs for Mental Illness* (New York: W. H. Freeman and Co., 1983), pp. 63–74 and 105–120.
5. T. C. Manschreck, "Schizophrenic Disorders," *New England Journal of Medicine* 305 (1981): 1628–1632.
6. R. J. Baldessarini, *Chemotherapy in Psychiatry*, 2nd ed. (Cambridge: Harvard University Press, 1985).
7. R. J. Baldessarini, "Drugs and the Treatment of Psychiatric Disorders,"

in A. G. Gilman, L. S. Goodman, T. W. Rall, and F. Murad, eds., *The Pharmacological Basis of Therapeutics*, 7th ed. (New York: Macmillan, 1985), pp. 387–412.

8. H. L. Klawans, C. Goetz, and R. Westheimer, "The Pharmacology of Schizophrenia," in H. L. Klawans, ed., *Clinical Neuropharmacology*, vol. 1 (New York: Raven Press, 1976), pp. 1–26.

9. M. E. Lickey and B. Gordon, *Drugs for Mental Illness* (New York: W. H. Freeman and Co., 1983), p. 119.

10. S. H. Snyder, "Dopamine Receptors, Neuroleptics, and Schizophrenia," *American Journal of Psychiatry* 138 (1981): 460–463.

CHAPTER 9

Psychedelic Drugs

Mescaline, LSD, and Other "Mind-Expanding" Agents

Psychedelic drugs are a group of heterogeneous compounds, all with the ability to induce visual, auditory, or other hallucinations and to separate the individual from reality. These agents may induce disturbances in cognition and perception and, in some instances, may produce behavioral patterns that are similar to components seen in psychotic behavior. Because of this wide range of psychological effects, it is difficult to assign a single term that adequately classifies these agents.

The term *hallucinogen* has been widely used because most of these agents can induce hallucinations if the dose is high enough. Hallucinogen, however, appears to be a somewhat inappropriate term because it does not adequately describe the range of pharmacological actions of such a diverse group of substances. The term *psychotomimetic* has been assigned to these compounds because of their alleged mimicking of psychoses or inducement of a psychotic state. However, careful analysis of the action of these drugs indicates that their effects are unlike the behavioral patterns observed during psychotic episodes. It appears that the behavioral responses to high doses of amphetamines (Chapter 5) more closely resemble a true psychotic episode.

Because no term comprehensively yet briefly characterizes the pharmacology of these drugs, we must rely on a descriptive term such as *phantasticum* (proposed by Lewin in 1924) or *psychedelic* (proposed by Osmond in 1957) to imply that these agents all have the ability to alter sensory perception and thus may be considered "mind expanding."

The psychedelic agents have a long and colorful history. Indeed, many are natural in origin, being derived from plants. Today, however, more are synthetically produced in the laboratory (such as LSD and derivatives of tryptamine and amphetamine). Psychedelics have been used for thousands of years. Because of the effects of these naturally occurring drugs on sensory perception, they were frequently ascribed magical, religious, or mystical properties and were used as sacraments in religious rites. For many years, the compounds were primarily restricted to local religious rituals and people in the larger world were barely aware of their existence. In the late 1960s and 1970s, however, the psychedelic agents were "discovered" and advocated by members of modern society as agents that "enhance perception, expand reality, promote personal awareness, and stimulate or induce comprehension of the spiritual or supernatural."

As stated by Jaffe:

There is heightened awareness of sensory input, often accompanied by an enhanced sense of clarity, but a diminished control over what is experienced. Frequently there is a feeling that one part of the self seems to be a passive observer (a "spectator ego") rather than an active organizing and directing force, while another part of the self participates and receives the vivid and unusual sensory experiences. The environment may be perceived as novel, often beautiful, and harmonious. The attention of the user is turned inward, preempted by the seeming clarity and portentous quality of his own thinking processes. In this state the slightest sensation may take on profound meaning. Indeed, "meaningfulness" seems more important than what is meant, and the "sense of truth" more significant than what is true. Commonly, there is a diminished capacity to differentiate the boundaries of one object from another and of the self from the environment. Associated with the loss of boundaries there may be a sense of union with "mankind" or the "cosmos." The drug-induced sensation that the mind is capable of seeing more than it can tell and of experiencing more than it can explain has led some to apply the term *mind expanding* to these agents.[1]

Classification

Since the psychedelics differ widely in chemical structure, they produce a wide range of behavioral alterations. Thus, their classification by chemical structure is difficult. However, because they are thought to produce behavioral changes as a result of alterations in the synaptic transmission processes, it is possible to classify them by the transmitter upon which they are thought to act or that they most closely resemble.

As discussed in Appendix II, several chemical substances are commonly thought to serve as synaptic transmitters within the brain. These substances include acetylcholine (ACh), norepinephrine (NE), dopamine, and 5-hydroxytryptamine (serotonin). Such compounds as physostigmine and diisopropyl fluorophosphate (DFP) increase the amounts of acetylcholine available at its synapses within the brain and induce nightmares, confusion, delirium, agitation, and slowing of intellectual and motor functions. Thus, physostigmine and DFP may be considered as *acetylcholine psychedelics* (see Table 9.1) because they affect ACh transmission. Besides physostigmine and DFP (both of which increase levels of ACh), there are other psychedelic agents that block ACh neurotransmission, thereby decreasing the activity of ACh. Such drugs include atropine and scopolamine.

The action of amphetamine and cocaine on NE neurons in the brain was discussed in Chapter 5. The behavioral stimulation induced by these drugs appears to be related to the potentiation of NE. At high doses, mania and a paranoid psychosis are induced and are accompanied by delusions, hallucinations, and disturbances in sensory perception. Thus, amphetamine and cocaine might well have been discussed as psychedelic agents as well as behavioral stimulants and should be classified, with the wide variety of compounds structurally similar to NE, as *norepinephrine psychedelics*. As Table 9.1 shows, this classification includes mescaline, DOM (also called STP), TMA, MDA, MMDA, DMA, and certain drugs obtained from

Table 9.1

Classification of psychedelic drugs.

1. Acetylcholine psychedelics
   Physostigmine
   DFP, sarin, soman, malathion, parathion
   Atropine
   Scopolamine
   Muscarine

2. Norepinephrine psychedelics
   Mescaline
   DOM (STP), MDA, MMDA, TMA, DMA
   Myristin, elemicin

3. Serotonin psychedelics
   Lysergic acid diethylamide (LSD)
   Dimethyltryptamine (DMT)
   Psilocybin, psilocin, bufotenin
   Ololiuqui (morning glory seeds)
   Harmine

4. Psychedelic anesthetics
   Phencyclidine (Sernyl)
   Ketamine (Ketalar)

nutmeg (myristin and elemicin). All of these compounds differ from one another and from amphetamine and cocaine in their relative intensities of psychedelic action and behavioral stimulation. Amphetamine and cocaine produce more behavioral stimulation than psychedelic action, whereas the reverse is true for the NE psychedelics listed in the table.

Serotonin, as discussed in Appendix II, appears to be involved in (among other things) sensory perception. The synthesis of lysergic acid diethylamide (LSD) and the discovery of its hallucinogenic prop-

Figure 9.1

Structural formulas of acetylcholine (a chemical transmitter), muscarine, atropine, and scopolamine. The latter are three psychedelic drugs thought to act on acetylcholine neurons.

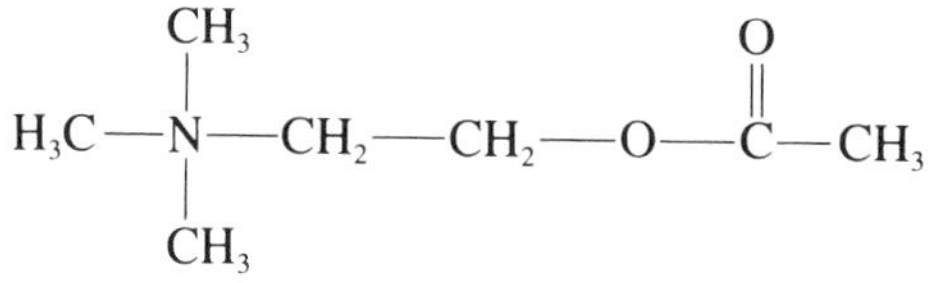

Acetylcholine

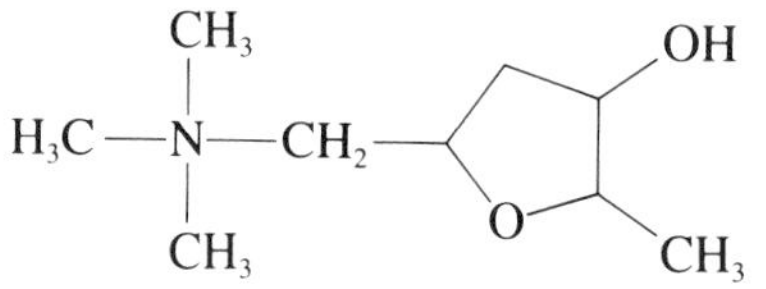

Muscarine

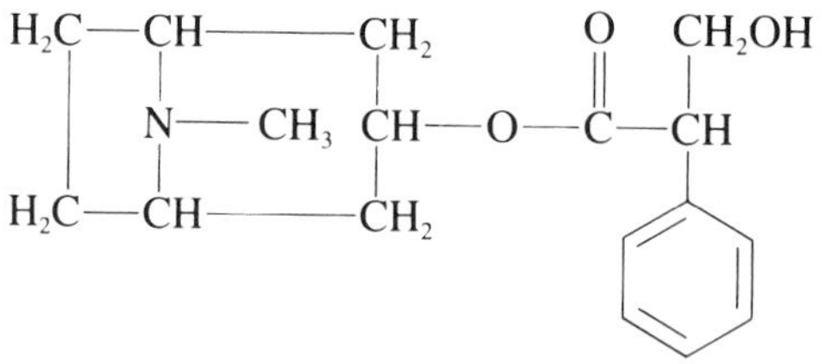

Atropine

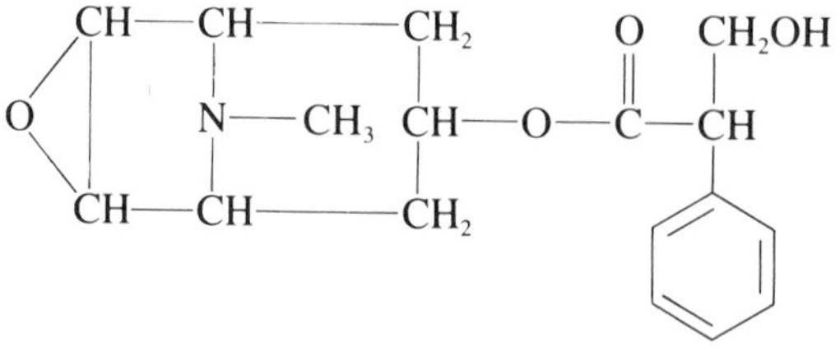

Scopolamine

erty and its structural resemblance to serotonin initiated a class of psychedelics that is presented in Table 9.1 as *serotonin psychedelics*. This group includes psilocybin and psilocin (both from the magic mushroom, *Psilocybe mexicana*), dimethyltryptamine (DMT), bufotenin, muscimol, and ibotinic acid (the latter two isolated from the poisonous mushroom known as fly agaric, or *Amanita muscaria*).

Finally, there is a fourth classification of psychedelic drugs referred to as the *psychedelic anesthetics*. These agents, phencyclidine and ketamine, are structurally unrelated to the other psychedelic compounds and, to date, the neurotransmitters upon which they exert their activity have yet to be identified. The structural relationships among these three transmitters and the various psychedelic drugs are presented in Figures 9.1, 9.2, 9.3, and 9.4.

Psychedelics Acting on Acetylcholine Neurons

The activity of acetylcholine (ACh) in the body can be altered through at least three mechanisms. First, ACh levels can be *increased* by drugs that inhibit the enzyme that normally destroys the transmitter. Second, ACh activity can be *decreased* by drugs that block the ACh receptors, limiting the access of ACh to its receptors. Third, some drugs will directly stimulate ACh receptors, mimicking the action of the transmitter. Specific drugs that produce these effects are discussed in the following section. (More extensive discussion of ACh neurotransmission may be found in Appendix II.)

Acetylcholinesterase (AChE) Inhibitors

Acetylcholinesterase (AChE) is the enzyme responsible for terminating the transmitter action of ACh both within the brain and in the peripheral nervous system. Drugs that have the ability to inhibit or inactivate AChE are called *anticholinesterases*, or AChE inhibitors. As a result of AChE inhibition, ACh accumulates in the synaptic cleft and exerts a stronger or more prolonged action. Because these ACh synapses are widely distributed in the brain and peripheral nervous system, it is not surprising that AChE inhibitors produce a wide variety of effects on both the brain and the body.

Historical Background   The prototype AChE inhibitor is a drug called physostigmine, which occurs naturally and was originally obtained from the Calabar, or ordeal, bean *Physostigma venenosum*) of the Calabar region of Nigeria. This bean was once used by natives of West Africa as an ordeal poison. As a test of guilt, a suspect was forced to swallow the beans. If he died, his guilt was proved. If he were confident of his innocence and ate the beans rapidly, he would promptly vomit and survive the ordeal. (It is rumored, however, that proof of innocence or guilt was not always left to chance. Apparently, a placebo was given to those judged to be innocent by the tribal elders in order that justice might not miscarry.)

In the mid-1800s, the Calabar bean was taken to England and studied by several English pharmacologists. Physostigmine was isolated as the active ingredient in the bean and introduced into medicine for the treatment of glaucoma (a disease resulting from increased pressure inside the eye). Subsequently, synthetic AChE inhibitors were produced. It was found that they increased the strength of muscular contraction, so they were used in the treatment of myasthenia gravis (a disease characterized by weakness of the skeletal muscles).

More recently, a new type of AChE inhibitor has been synthesized. The newer agents produce extremely long-lasting inhibition of AChE, to the extent of being irreversible in their action. These substances are compounds such as diisopropyl fluorophosphate (DFP), malathion, parathion, sarin, and soman. Because of their toxicity, some of these irreversible AChE inhibitors are widely used as agricultural insecticides. Because these compounds are toxic not only to insects but also to humans, their use as insecticides has been responsible for an increasing number of accidental poisonings and deaths, especially among field workers. Sarin and soman, among the most potent synthetic toxic and lethal agents known, have been stockpiled for use as nerve gases in chemical warfare.

Pharmacological Effects   The effects of AChE inhibitors in the body are predictable if one knows the location and function of ACh synapses throughout the body. However, because we have very little information about either the location or function of the brain's ACh synapses, we cannot predict the effects of AChE inhibitors on the brain. In the body, AChE inhibitors increase the levels of ACh and cause any or all of the following effects: constriction of the pupil, constriction of the bronchi, contraction of the bladder and intestinal muscle, profuse salivation and sweating, decreased blood pressure with a slowing of the heart rate, and increased muscle tone followed by paralysis of respiratory muscles, which leads to failure of respiration and eventually death. In the brain, behavioral alterations induced by AChE inhibition consist of anxiety, restlessness, dreaming, nightmares, delirium, and insomnia.

With higher doses, toxic effects include depression, drowsiness, confusion, incoordination, ataxia, slurring of speech, convulsions, coma, and paralysis of the medulla, which leads to failure of respiration and death. The respiratory failure that can result in death can therefore be produced by either of two means: by direct paralysis of the respiratory muscles or by paralysis of the respiratory control center in the brainstem.

Since these agents block the enzyme that destroys ACh, ACh accumulates at the synapse. A true antidote would remove the AChE inhibitor from the enzyme AChE, thus restoring the enzyme's ability to metabolize the transmitter. Such antidotes are available for certain AChE inhibitors, although usually only in hospital emergency rooms. An incomplete antidote might block the action of ACh at the receptor, although it could not regenerate the enzyme. ACh would still be available in excess (owing to AChE inhibition), but it would be prevented from reaching its receptor. One such incomplete antidote is atropine, a drug that blocks many of the ACh receptors both in the brain and in the body.

The wide range of behavioral effects of AChE inhibitors (including their ability to induce delirium, nightmares, vivid dreaming, and so on) dictates their inclusion as psychoactive drugs. However, because of their extreme toxicity and numerous side effects, these agents are seldom encountered as drugs of abuse, because the compulsion to misuse them is low and the risk associated with their use outweighs the benefits received.

Blockers of ACh Receptors (Anticholinergic Drugs)

AChE inhibitors exert their effects by increasing ACh activity as a result of increasing the concentration of ACh at the ACh receptors. The drugs to be discussed now (atropine and scopolamine) decrease ACh activity by blocking ACh receptors and consequently preventing transmission across these synapses.

Historical Background   The history of atropine and scopolamine is long and colorful. These two drugs are widely distributed in nature. They are found in especially high concentrations in the plant known as belladonna, or deadly nightshade (*Atropa belladonna*). These drugs are also found in *Datura stramonium* (Jamestownweed, Jimson-weed, stink-weed, thorn-apple, or devil's-apple), and in *Mandragora officinarum* (mandrake). Scopolamine is found in the shrub *Hyoscyamus niger* (henbane). Preparations of these plants containing atropine and scopolamine have been used for centuries. Both professional and amateur poisoners of the Middle Ages frequently used the deadly nightshade as a prime source of poison. In fact, the name *Atropa belladonna* is derived from Atropos, the Greek goddess who supposedly cuts the thread of life. *Belladonna* means "beautiful woman."

If an extract of the plant is applied to the eyelids or, more usually, in the conjunctival sac, the pupils will dilate. To the Romans and Egyptians, dilated pupils were considered beautiful. Even today a woman with dilated pupils is sometimes thought to be more beautiful than a woman with constricted pupils, simply because her eyes look larger. These drugs were often used recreationally for their psychological and behavioral effects. The use of atropine and scopolamine may have persuaded certain individuals that they had the ability to fly—that they were witches.

Plants containing atropine and scopolamine have been used and misused for centuries. Even today, cigarettes made from the leaves of *Datura stramonium* and *Atropa belladonna* are frequently smoked to induce intoxication. Such cigarettes were, until recently, widely sold in drug stores for use in the treatment of asthma, but because they have been misused, they are not now generally available. Throughout the world, leaves of plants containing atropine or scopolamine are still used to prepare intoxicating beverages, and marijuana and opium preparations from the Far East are quite frequently fortified with atropine obtained from *Datura stramonium*.

Pharmacological Effects   In general, the actions of atropine and scopolamine on body function are the opposite of those of the AChE inhibitors. Atropine and scopolamine depress salivation, reduce sweating, dilate the pupils, increase heart rate, and cause loss of tone in the urinary bladder and the gastrointestinal tract. Because these drugs also inhibit the secretion of acid into the stomach, they are frequently used in the medical treatment of ulcers, although their effectiveness is limited by rather significant side effects.

Low doses of scopolamine depress the arousal centers in the ascending reticular activating system (ARAS) of the brain, induce a cortical brain-wave pattern characteristic of sleep, and produce drowsiness, euphoria, amnesia, fatigue, delirium, mental confusion, dreamless sleep, and loss of attention. Low doses of atropine, however, do not seem to affect EEG or behavior. Although atropine and scopolamine can produce delirium and euphoria, they cloud consciousness, produce amnesia, and do not expand sensory perception. Therefore, they differ from the norepinephrine and serotonin psychedelics to be discussed later in this chapter. Physostigmine will antagonize their effects, but such antagonism is limited by physostigmine's short duration of action.

As psychedelic agents, atropine and scopolamine would seem to be less attractive than those to be discussed later in this chapter because they cloud rather than expand consciousness and impair the memory rather than increase awareness, so that the user cannot remember much of the experience. In addition, the side effects of these compounds tend to limit their recreational use.

Activator of ACh Receptors (Muscarine)

Apart from the Mexican mushroom, *Psilocybe mexicana*, which yields psilocybin and psilocin, there are other mushrooms from which psychoactive drugs may be extracted. One such is fly agaric (*Amanita muscaria*), a mushroom found throughout Europe, especially in Scandinavia (where it is thought to have been used by the Vikings) and northern Siberia.

Amanita muscaria and its close relative *Amanita pantherina* are also found in the United States. Both of these mushrooms contain as their major psychoactive ingredients ibotenic acid and muscimol. A third drug, muscarine, is also found in *Amanita*, although usually in much lower quantities. The name *fly agaric* for *Amanita muscaria* is derived, apparently, from the insecticidal properties of the drug. The compound is not lethal to the fly but, apparently, when a fly ingests the extract of *Amanita muscaria* it goes into a prolonged stupor and thus may be easily killed.

The extract of *Amanita muscaria* is intoxicating and results in a depressed state (a stupor), with concomitant sleep, hallucinations, delirium, and muscle spasms. Stupor may be followed by behavioral excitement accompanied by visual and auditory hallucinations and distortions of sensory input. The active drugs are well absorbed orally and appear to be excreted without being metabolized by the liver to inactive products. Thus, the compounds remain in an active form in urine; this property led to the Siberian practice of many centuries of sharing the intoxication by ingesting the urine of those who had previously eaten the mushroom. It has been reported that the active agents remain effective to the fourth or fifth individual.

While the pharmacological properties of ibotenic acid and muscimol have not been clearly evaluated (they may resemble serotonin psychedelics, discussed in the following section), muscarine itself directly stimulates ACh receptors both in the brain and in the body, causing profound sweating, increased salivation, pupillary constriction, increased bladder tone, decreased heart rate, increased blood pressure, and other effects similar to those produced by the AChE inhibitors. This similarity is not unexpected because both muscarine and the AChE inhibitors increase the activity of ACh neurons.

Interestingly, these same effects are reported by those who use *Amanita muscaria* and *Amanita pantherina* for recreational purposes. Apparently, one man's meat is another man's poison. When medical aid has been sought, atropine has frequently been administered as an antidote. Several reports of prolonged periods of suffering with an intensification of symptoms may make it prudent to withhold the use of atropine as an antidote for mushroom poisoning until the mushrooms involved are identified and the ingredients known.

These mushrooms exert profound effects on the body in addition to their effects on the brain. These peripheral effects would seem to limit the recreational usefulness of *Amanita* except for those willing to tolerate rather profound and unpleasant symptoms in order to achieve sensory distortion.

Psychedelics Acting on Norepinephrine Neurons

In Appendix II, the norepinephrine synapse is discussed as the site of action of several psychoactive drugs and, in Chapters 5 and 8, as the site of action of cocaine, amphetamine, the antidepressants, and lithium. The norepinephrine synapses are also important sites of action for a large group of psychedelic drugs. As may be seen in Figure 9.2, several psychedelic drugs are structurally similar to both norepinephrine and amphetamine. Such psychedelic agents include mescaline, DOM (also called STP), TMA, MDA, MMDA, DMA, myristin, and elemicin. Each of these agents is discussed, with particular attention payed to those actions that differentiate them from amphetamine and cocaine, which were classified in Chapter 5 as behavioral stimulants rather than as psychedelics.

Figure 9.2

Structural formulas of norepinephrine (a chemical transmitter) and eight psychedelic drugs. These eight drugs are structurally related to norepinephrine and are thought to exert their psychedelic actions through alterations of transmission at norepinephrine synapses in the brain.

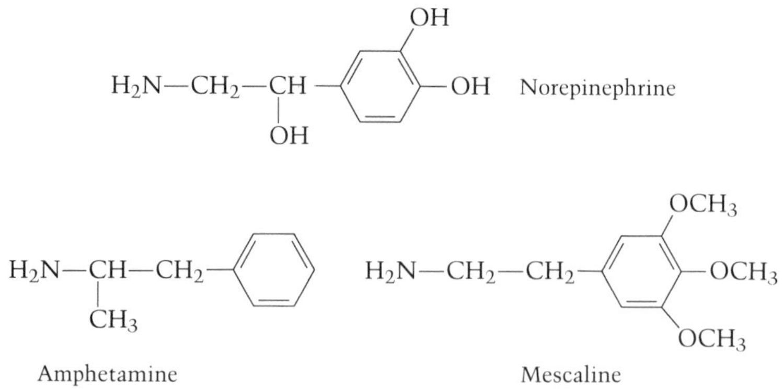

Figure 9.2 (*continued*)

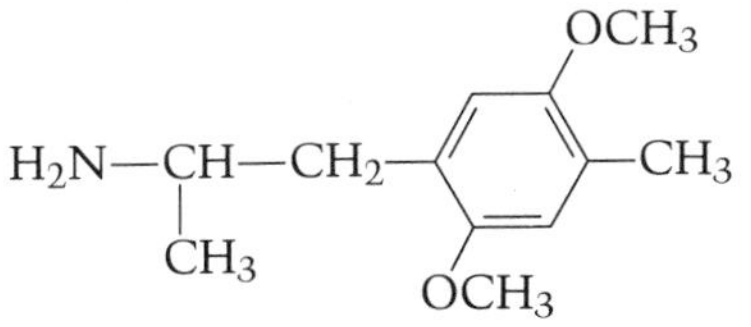

H_2N—CH—CH_2— [ring with OCH_3, CH_3, OCH_3] DOM (STP)
|
CH_3

H_2N—CH—CH_2— [ring with O—CH_2—O] MDA
|
CH_3

H_2N—CH—CH_2— [ring with OCH_3, OCH_3, OCH_3] TMA
|
CH_3

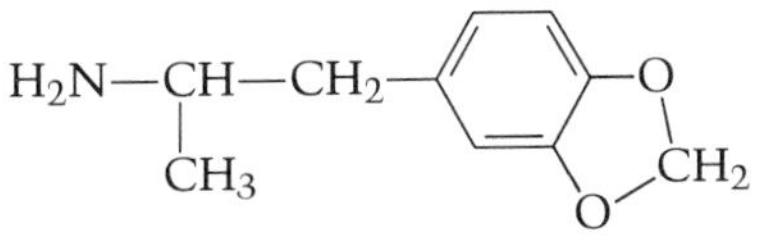

H_2N—CH—CH_2— [ring with OCH_3, O—CH_2—O] MMDA
|
CH_3

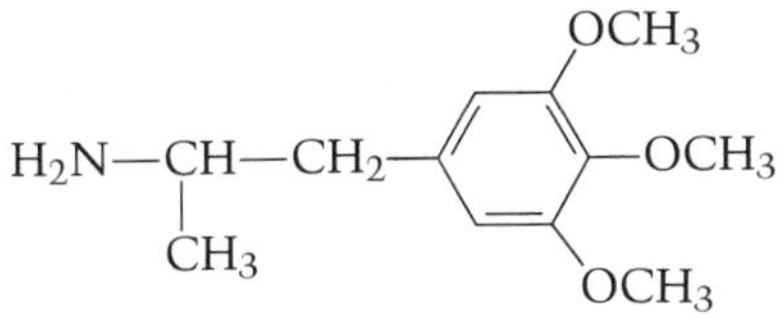

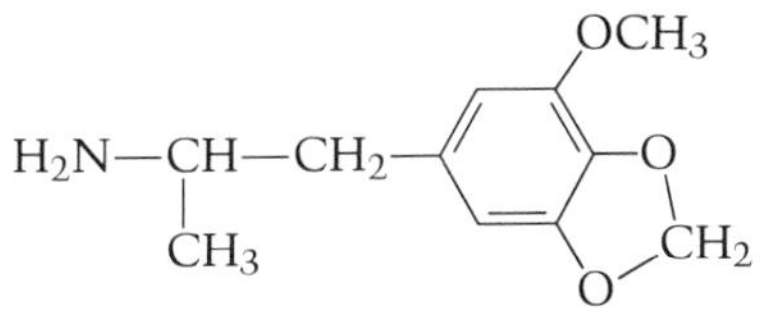

H_2C=CH—CH_2— [ring with OCH_3, O—CH_2—O] Myristin

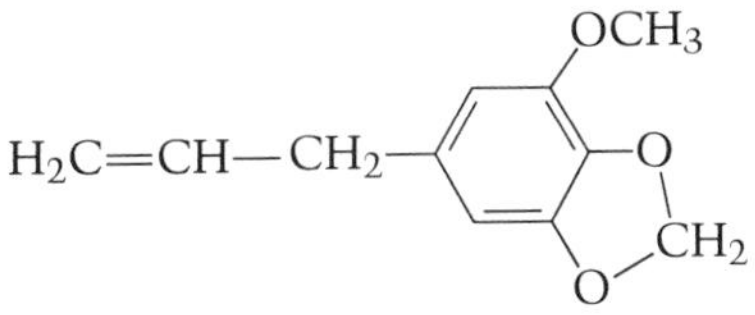

H_2C=CH—CH_2— [ring with OCH_3, OCH_3, OCH_3] Elemicin

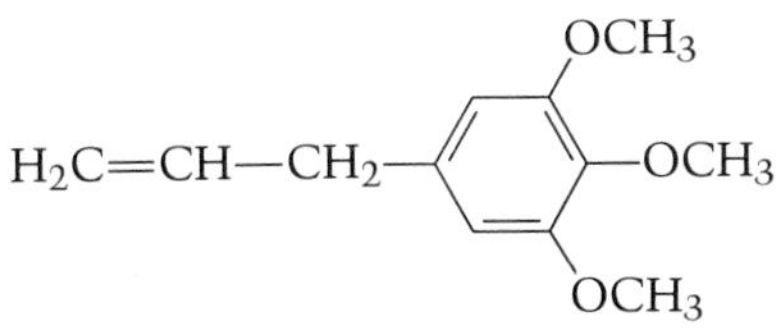

H_2N—CH—CH_2— [ring with OCH_3, OCH_3] DMA
|
CH_3

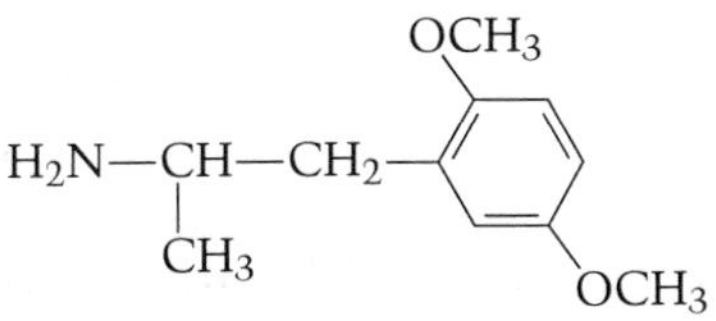

Mescaline (Peyote)

Peyote (*Lophophora williamsii*), a plant common to the southwestern United States and Mexico, is a spineless cactus with a small crown or "button" and a long root. For psychedelic use, the crown is cut from the cactus and dried to form a hard brown disc, frequently referred to as a mescal button. The dried button may later be softened in the mouth and swallowed. Often more than one button is ingested to obtain full psychedelic effectiveness. The buttons can also be prepared into cakes, tablets, or powder; the powder is water soluble and may be taken orally or by injection.

Historical Background   The use of peyote extends back for centuries—it is known to have been used in the religious rites of the Aztecs. Currently, peyote is the only psychedelic agent that has been sanctioned by the federal government for limited use. It is eaten as an important part of the religious practice of the Native American Church of North America, an organization that claims some one-quarter million members from Indian tribes throughout North America. In order to supply peyote to these Indians tribes, mail-order companies situated in desert regions in the southwestern United States sold the dried buttons at very low prices. In fact, as interest in peyote spread, these mail-order companies occasionally advertised in college newspapers during the late 1950s and early 1960s. In about 1960, interest in peyote became widespread. The interest among college students waned in the mid-1960s with the rising popularity of a much more powerful psychedelic drug, LSD. However, during the middle to late 1960s, as hostility toward LSD developed, hostility toward other psychedelic agents (including peyote) also increased, and laws were passed to control the availability of such drugs.

Members of the Native American Church regard peyote as sacramental, much as members of other churches regard bread and wine as sacramental. One must conclude that the use of peyote for religious purposes is not considered "abuse." Indeed, peyote is seldom abused by members of the Native American Church, and the Supreme Court of the United States has ruled that no federal control will interfere with freedom of religion, a ruling that allows the church to continue to use mescaline in religious services.

Pharmacological Effects   The initial research on the active ingredients of the peyote cactus was carried out near the end of the nineteenth century by German pharmacologists. In 1896, mescaline (Figure 9.2) was identified as the active ingredient in peyote. Despite identification of the active ingredient, however, the chemical structure of mescaline was not elucidated until approximately 1918, when its resemblance to norepinephrine was recognized. More recently, because of this structural resemblance, a wide variety of synthetic mescaline and norepinephrine derivatives have been synthesized, and those that may have methoxy ($-OCH_3$) additions to the benzene ring (on amphetamine) usually have psychedelic properties. Why methoxylation of the benzene ring adds psychedelic properties is not clear, but it is thought that at higher doses (for example, at doses higher than those that exert amphetamine-like behavioral effects), these drugs can stimulate presynaptic serotonin receptors (see the following discussion) and thus exert LSD-like psychedelic effects.

Taken orally, mescaline is rapidly and completely absorbed, and significant concentrations within the brain are usually achieved within 30 to 90 minutes. The effects of a single dose of mescaline persist for approximately 12 hours. The drug does not appear to be metabolized before excretion.

Presumably because of its resemblance to norepinephrine, low doses of mescaline produce effects similar to those observed during the fight/flight/fright syndrome: dilation of the pupils, increased blood pressure and heart rate, an increase in body temperature, EEG and behavioral arousal, and other excitatory symptoms, which are also similar to those produced by amphetamine. However, such actions are not the primary effects sought with mescaline. As one writer put it:

Interest in mescaline centers on the fact that it causes unusual psychic effects and visual hallucinations. The usual oral dose (5 mg/kg) in the average normal subject causes anxiety, sympathomimetic effects, hyperreflexia of the limbs, static tremors, and vivid hallucinations that are usually visual and consist of brightly colored lights, geometric designs, animals and occasionally people; color and space perception is often concomitantly impaired, but otherwise the sensorium is normal and insight is retained.[2]

DOM, MDA, TMA, MMDA, and DMA are structurally only slightly different from mescaline and, as might be expected, they produce effects similar to those produced by mescaline; their effects are amphetamine-like at low doses and LSD-like at higher doses. They differ from mescaline, however, in that they are considerably more toxic than mescaline as doses are increased. Mescaline itself is usually not considered to be very toxic, even in high doses. However, the behavioral responses to the synthetic mescaline derivatives rapidly progress as the dose is increased from behavioral excitation and sensory hallucinations to gross hyperactivity and hyperexcitability, with accompanying disturbances of body function—effects resembling amphetamine toxicity more closely than the sensory disturbances induced by mescaline. High doses produce tremors that may eventually lead to convulsive movements and prostration, which may be followed by death. Because these synthetic compounds are not commercially available through legitimate sources, there is no standardization of dosage or purity. With mescaline, this seems to present little problem because of its wide margin of safety, but with the more toxic synthetic mescaline derivatives, the safety range is lower and overdoses may occur much more frequently.

Absorption between these agents differs significantly. For example, DMT is ineffective when taken orally and must be smoked, sniffed, or injected to be effective.

Compounds sold on the street as mescaline are often not mescaline but LSD or one of the synthetic mescaline derivatives. Users must be careful (*caveat emptor*) because higher doses of any of these substitutes can be dangerous. Much work remains to be done to determine the safety, dose ranges, and toxicities of these synthetic derivatives of mescaline.

Myristin and Elemicin

Myristin and elemicin are two active ingredients in nutmeg and mace that are responsible for the psychedelic action of these spices. Nutmeg and mace, both readily available in grocery stores, are obtained, respectively, from the dried seed and seed coat of the nutmeg tree (*Myristica fragans*). Nutmeg and mace are occasionally encountered as drugs of abuse when no other compounds are available. Ingestion of large amounts (between 1 and 2 teaspoons, usually brewed in tea) may, after a delay of 2 to 5 hours, induce euphoria and changes in sensory perception, including visual hallucinations, euphoria, acute psychotic reactions, and feelings of depersonalization and unreality.

Considering the close structural resemblance of myristin and elemicin to mescaline (Figure 9.2), these psychedelic actions are not unexpected. The problem with nutmeg and mace, however, is that they induce many unpleasant side effects, including vomiting, nausea, and tremors. Once people have tried nutmeg or mace for its psychedelic action, the side effects usually dissuade them from trying it a second time. Further discussion of myristin intoxication may be found in the symposium edited by Efron.[3]

Psychedelics Acting on Serotonin Neurons

In Appendix II, we discuss the role of serotonin (5-hydroxytryptamine, or 5-HT) as a neurotransmitter actively involved in the regulation of body temperature, sleep, and sensory perception. Interest in the actions of serotonin in the brain arose in the late 1950s when it was found that reserpine (see Chapter 8), in addition to decreasing the levels of norepinephrine in the brain, also decreased serotonin levels. Theories arose that some types of mental illness could be caused by abnormalities of transmission between serotonin neurons. These theories were supported by the observation that a number of hallucinogenic compounds were found structurally to resemble serotonin. Figure 9.3 shows that dimethyltryptamine (DMT), bufotenin, psilocin, and psilocybin resemble serotonin in the same way that amphetamine, mescaline, myristin, and the synthetic mescaline derivatives resemble norepinephrine. Even LSD and harmine are structurally similar to serotonin. When the serotonin psychedelics are compared with the norepinephrine psychedelics, it appears that the former induce more powerful emotional and sensory experiences but seldom induce the behavioral excitation, mania, and psychosis of amphetamine.

Although LSD and related drugs exert several actions in the brain, the most prominent involve stimulation of presynaptic receptors for serotonin and a reduction in the turnover rate of serotonin in the brain, most prominently in the forebrain and midbrain. LSD and serotonin are both inhibitory when applied to neurons in these areas, and such inhibition may underlie psychedelic actions. Haloperidol (Haldol) and chlorpromazine (Thorazine) block the psychedelic actions of LSD and related drugs, probably by binding to these same receptors and blocking the effects of the psychedelics (in a manner similar to the action of naloxone, which blocks the analgesic and respiratory effects of opiate narcotics). Therapy with haloperidol or chlorpromazine is frequently successful but is certainly not specific, universally predictable, or a panacea for bad trips. Occasionally, such treatment might fail if the LSD that produced the bad experience were adulterated with other drugs—or were not LSD at all, but a concoction of assorted drugs that might produce bizarre effects.

Lysergic Acid Diethylamide (LSD)
In the 1960s and early 1970s, lysergic acid diethylamide (LSD) became one of the most remarkable and controversial drugs known. LSD, in doses that are so small that they might even be considered infinitesimal, is capable of inducing remarkable psychological changes with relatively few alterations in the general physiology of the body. This absence of physiological effects distinguishes LSD from the naturally occurring psychedelics.

Figure 9.3

Structural formulas of serotonin (a chemical transmitter) and six psychedelic drugs. These six drugs are structurally related to serotonin and are thought to exert their psychedelic actions through alterations of serotonin synapses in the brain. Although LSD is structurally much more complex than serotonin, the basic similarity of the two molecules is apparent.

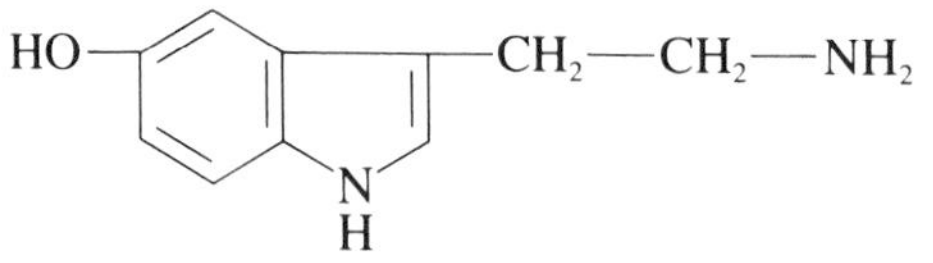

Serotonin

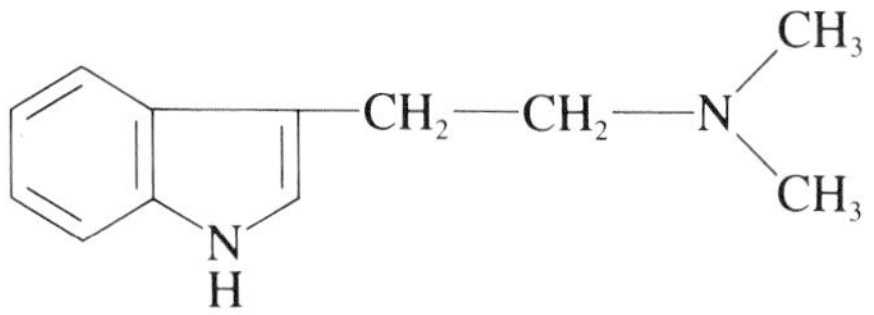

DMT

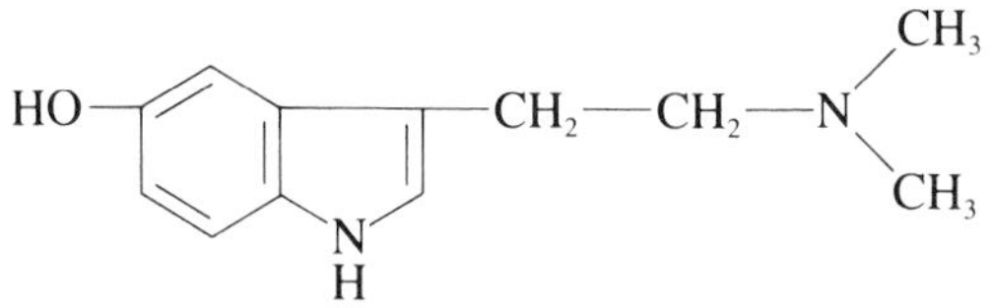

Bufotenin

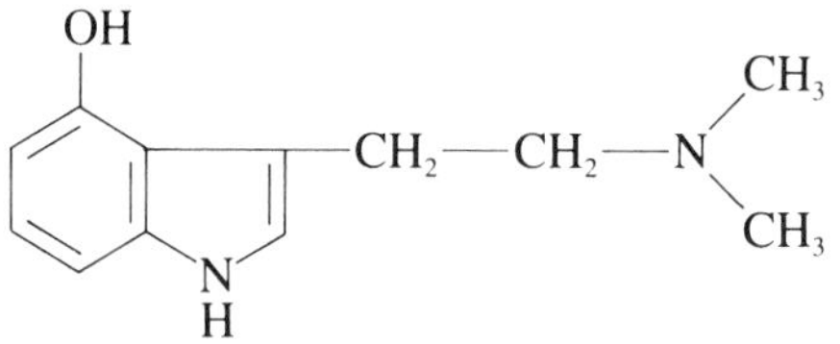

Psilocin

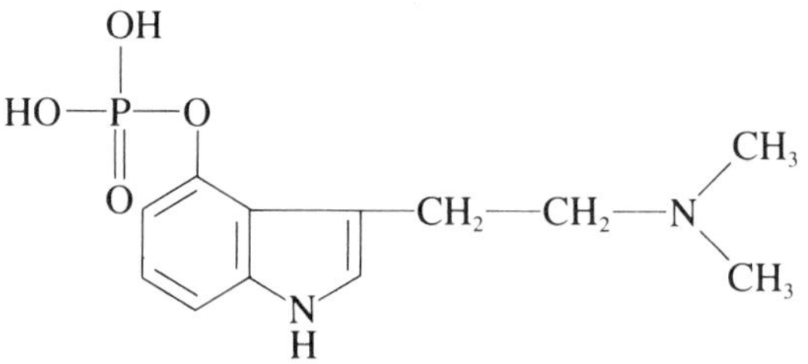

Psilocybin

Figure 9.3 (*continued*)

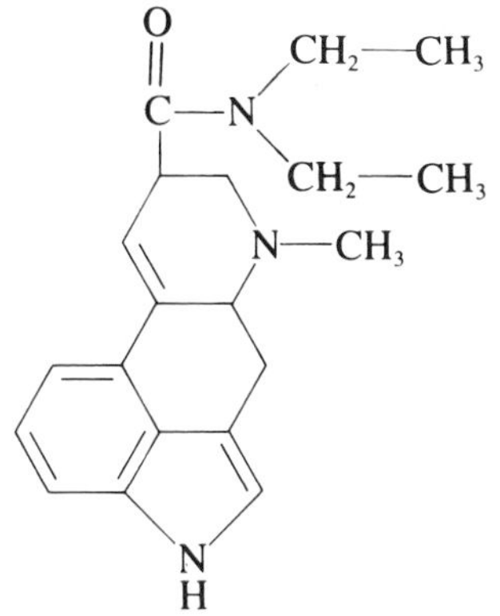

LSD

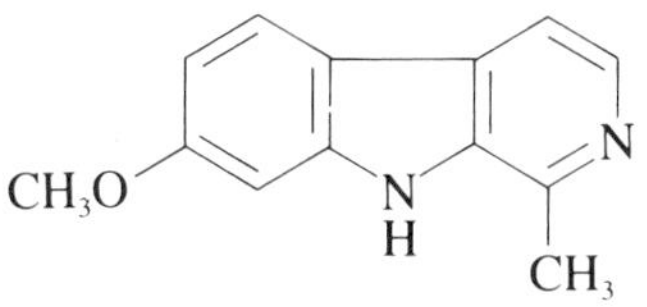

Harmine

Historical Background   LSD was first synthesized in 1938 by Albert Hoffman, a chemist at the Sandoz Laboratories in Basel, Switzerland. The compound was developed as part of an organized research program seeking to investigate the possible therapeutic uses of a group of compounds obtained from ergot, a natural product derived from a fungus (*Claviceps purpurea*) that grows as a parasite on rye in grainfields of Europe and North America. The active products extracted from ergot are derivatives of lysergic acid. The pharmacological actions of these lysergic acid derivatives do not usually include hallucinations but do include constriction of blood vessels (which restricts blood flow to the limbs, causing gangrene) and increased contraction of the uterus. Therapeutically, ergot alkaloids are used in the treatment of migraine headache and to control postpartum hemorrhage.

Early pharmacological studies of LSD in animals failed to reveal anything unusual, and the compound was almost forgotten. The psychedelic action was neither sought nor expected because most derivatives of ergot are not psychoactive. LSD remained on the laboratory shelf unnoticed from 1938 until 1943, when Dr. Hoffmann had an unusual experience that he later described as follows:

In the afternoon of 16 April, 1943, . . . I was seized by a peculiar sensation of vertigo and restlessness. Objects, as well as the shape of my associates in the laboratory, appeared to undergo optical changes. I was unable to concentrate on my work. In a dreamlike state I left for home, where an irresistible urge to lie down overcame me. I drew the curtains and immediately fell into a peculiar state similar to drunkenness, characterized by an exaggerated imagination. With my eyes closed, fantastic pictures of extraordinary plasticity and intensive color seemed to surge toward me. After two hours this state gradually wore off.[4]

Hoffmann correctly suspected that his experience must have resulted from accidental ingestion of LSD. He decided to take some of the compound under controlled conditions and to describe the experience more completely. Using the dose of other drugs as a guide, he administered what seemed like a miniscule dose (only 0.25 milligram, orally). We now know that this dose is many times that required to induce psychedelic effects in most individuals. As a result of this miscalculation, the response was quite spectacular:

After 40 minutes, I noted the following symptoms in my laboratory journal: slight giddiness, restlessness, difficulty in concentration, visual disturbances, laughing. . . . Later: I lost all count of time. I noticed with dismay that my environment was undergoing progressive changes. My visual field wavered and everything appeared deformed as in a faulty mirror. Space and time became more and more disorganized and I was overcome by a fear that I was going out of my mind. The worst part of it being that I was clearly aware of my condition. My power of observation was unimpaired. . . . Occasionally, I felt as if I were out of my body. I thought I had died. My ego seemed suspended somewhere in space, from where I saw my dead body lying on the sofa. . . . It was particularly striking how acoustic perceptions, such as the noise of water gushing from a tap or the spoken word, were transformed into optical illusions. I then fell asleep and awakened the next morning somewhat tired but otherwise feeling perfectly well.[5]

Four years later, the results of a clinical investigation of LSD in human subjects essentially confirmed Dr. Hoffmann's original experience. LSD became something of a laboratory and clinical curiosity. In 1949, the first study of LSD in North America in humans was conducted, and, during the 1950s, large quantities of LSD were distributed to pharmacologists and physicians throughout the world for research purposes. A significant impetus to this research was the thought that the effects of LSD might constitute a model psychosis that would provide some insight into the biochemical or physiological processes of mental illness and their treatment.

Subsequently, it was demonstrated that LSD mimicked the transmitter action of serotonin, an observation that led to the hypothesis that serotonin might somehow be involved in mental illness. Thus, through the 1950s, LSD was regarded as a tool that might be used to help acquire an understanding of psychoses. LSD has been used as an adjunct to psychotherapy by some therapists to aid patients in verbalizing their problems and in gaining some insight into the underlying causes of the illness, a use that is still much debated.

This early work with LSD on human volunteers was conducted in large medical centers, so the experiments introduced the LSD experience into medical schools and colleges where subjects were paid to participate. LSD propagandists began to appear in the late 1950s and early 1960s.

The drug reached a peak of popularity in the late 1960s, after which its use appeared to decrease markedly. Considering the long history of other psychedelic drugs, it is unlikely that the recreational use of LSD will ever completely disappear. It is quite clear, however, that the use of LSD in medicine and in psychotherapy will be limited. In the laboratory, these agents will continue to be used to help neuroscientists unravel some of the mysteries of the brain, especially those associated with the role of serotonin as a synaptic transmitter.

Absorption, Distribution, Metabolism, and Excretion   LSD is usually taken orally and is rapidly absorbed. The compound is seldom administered by injection. Since the doses of LSD are so small that several doses could be placed on the head of a pin, the drug is often added to other substances, such as sugar cubes, that may be more easily handled. LSD is rapidly and efficiently distributed throughout the body, easily diffuses into the brain, and readily crosses the placenta. It appears that the largest amounts of LSD in the body may be found in the liver, where the compound is metabolized before it is excreted. Relatively small levels of the drug are found in the brain, although the compound is so potent that only a few micrograms (for example, 25 micrograms, or one-millionth of an ounce) are needed to induce psychedelic effects.

Taken orally, LSD has a rapid onset of action (between 30 and 60 minutes) and its effects persist for approximately 10 or 12 hours.

The extreme potency of LSD, and thus the small quantity of metabolites, implies that only miniscule amounts can be detected in the urine. Conventional urine screening tests are inadequate for such detention. Thus, when LSD use is suspected, urine is collected (up to 30 hours after ingestion) and a radioimmunoassay is performed to determine its presence.

Pharmacological Effects   Although the LSD experience is characterized primarily by psychological alterations (see the following discussion), there are subtle physiological changes that occur. LSD causes a slight increase in body temperature, dilates the pupils, slightly increases the heart rate and blood pressure, produces sweating and chills, increases levels of glucose (sugar) in the blood, occasionally produces "goose pimples," headache, nausea, vomiting, and other effects that, although noticeable, seldom interfere with the psychedelic experience and are seldom serious.

LSD is known to possess a low level of toxicity. Deaths due to the direct effects of LSD overdose have not been reported, although fatal accidents and suicides are known to occur during periods of LSD intoxication. There is no evidence that permanent brain damage may be induced, even by repeated administration of high doses. Thus, although the drug is nonlethal, both short- and long-term alterations in the psyche of the user and possible adverse effects on the fetus[6] must be considered. The social complications arising from LSD use should also be considered.

Psychological Effects   Although the physiological alterations produced by LSD are usually quite minor and predictable, the psychological effects are not. They may be influenced by a variety of factors, including the personality of the user, his or her expectation of what the drug will produce, previous use of LSD and psychoactive drugs, attitudes toward use of LSD or any other illicit drug, motivations for using the drug, the setting in which the drug is administered, and the individuals with whom the user will interact during the LSD experience. The psychological effects induced by LSD are not necessarily directly related to the dose that is administered, because many of the psychological alterations induced are relatively unaffected by increases or decreases in dosage.

Because of these variables, it is difficult to predict the exact psychological experience that will be felt by an individual user on a given occasion. Thus, it is quite difficult to describe the essentials of the experience by listing the intensity of responses. Nevertheless, these responses include alterations in mood and emotion in which laughter or sorrow may easily be evoked, even simultaneously. Both euphoria and dysphoria can be experienced, even by the same individual during the same trip. The principal psychological effects involve perceptual changes, especially visual hallucinations and distortions.

As stated by Jaffe:

. . . visual illusions, wavelike recurrences of perceptual changes (e.g., micropsia, macropsia), and affective symptoms may occur. There may be difficulty in locating the source of a sound; the user may be hypervigilant or withdrawn, or may alternate between these states. With many subjects there is a fear of fragmentation or disintegration of the self. Afterimages are prolonged, and the overlapping of present and preceding perceptions occurs.

Some subjects recognize these confluences, whereas others elaborate them into hallucinations. In contrast to naturally occurring psychoses, auditory hallucinations are rare. Synesthesias, the overflow from one sensory modality to another, may occur. Colors are heard and sounds may be seen. Subjective time is also seriously altered, so that clock time seems to pass extremely slowly. The loss of boundaries and the fear of fragmentation create a need for a structuring or supporting environment; and, in the sense that they create a need for experienced companions and an explanatory system, these drugs are "cultogenic." During the "trip," thoughts and memories can vividly emerge under self-guidance or unexpectedly, to the user's distress. Mood may be labile, shifting from depression to gaiety, from elation to fear. Tension and anxiety may mount and reach panic proportions. After about 4 to 5 hours, if a major panic episode does not occur, there may be a sense of detachment and the conviction that one is magically in control.[7]

Objects that are visualized may be seen in strange, distorted ways, with clear-cut shapes and brilliant colors. The descriptions of the original LSD trip experienced by Hoffmann are probably the most lucid and exciting ever presented, possibly because the chemist had no preconceived notions about what to expect.

Tolerance and Dependence   *Tolerance* (a need to increase the dose in order to obtain the same effect) of both the psychological and physiological alterations induced by LSD readily develops. *Cross-tolerance* between LSD and other psychedelic agents, such as mescaline and psilocybin, may also develop. An individual who has developed tolerance to LSD will usually show a diminished response to mescaline or psilocybin. Cross-tolerance between LSD and marijuana has not been demonstrated.

Physical dependence on LSD does not develop, even when the drug is used repeatedly over a prolonged period of time. In fact, most heavy users of the drug say that they ceased using LSD because they tired of it, had no further need for it, or had had enough. Even when the drug is discontinued because of concern about bad trips or about physical or mental harm, withdrawal signs are not exhibited.

It appears that *psychological dependence* may occur in those few individuals who have become preoccupied with the drug. Normally, however, such preoccupation seems to run its course and is self-limiting. Most users eventually cease using LSD and return to other less potent psychedelic agents or to the more traditional sedative-hypnotic compounds such as alcohol or marijuana.

Adverse Reactions and Toxicity   The adverse reactions and toxicities attributed to LSD generally fall into four categories: (1) the effects on the psychological state of the user, (2) the possibility of permanent damage to the brain, (3) the possible effects on the fetus when the drug is taken by a pregnant woman, and (4) the deleterious effects upon society in general as a result of widespread use.

Concerning effects on the psychological state of the user:

> Unpleasant experiences with LSD are relatively frequent and may involve an uncontrollable drift into confusion, dissociative reactions, acute panic reactions, a reliving of earlier traumatic experiences, or an acute psychotic hospitalization. Prolonged nonpsychotic reactions have included dissociative reactions, time and space distortion, body image changes, and a residue of fear or depression stemming from morbid or terrifying experiences under the drug. . . . With the failure of usual defense mechanisms, the onslaught of repressed material overwhelms the integrative capacity of the ego, and a psychotic reaction results. It appears that this [LSD-induced] disruption of long-established patterns of adaption may be a lasting or semipermanent effect of the drug.[8]

LSD also reduces one's normal ability to control emotional reactions, and drug-released perceptions can become so intense that they overwhelm one's ability to cope.

Whether long-term, frequent, high-dose use of LSD results in discernible damage to the brain has not been determined, although it is generally agreed that experimental use of LSD on only a few occasions does not induce physical damage. When normal individuals are given a battery of psychological tests and then are given LSD and are reexamined 6 months later, no residual psychological damage resulting from the drug experience is evident. In fact, these individuals may show increases in anesthetic appreciation. Because LSD can remove normal defense (or coping) mechanisms, however, it may precipitate psychotic episodes that normally would have remained suppressed. Such psychotic episodes may require long-term therapy.

There is also the possible problem of persistent flashbacks, which may recur weeks or even months later. The mechanism underlying them is unknown, but it is thought to involve long-lasting impairment of psychological defense mechanisms, with periodic emergence of repressed feelings.[9]

"Flashbacks," are a puzzling phenomenon; they occur in more than 15 percent of users. Commonly precipitated by use of marihuana, anxiety, fatigue, or movement into a dark environment, "flashbacks" may persist intermittently for several years after the last exposure to LSD. They are exacerbated by the use of phenothiazines.

In some individuals the use of psychedelics can precipitate serious depressions, paranoid behavior, or prolonged psychotic episodes. Whether such episodes would have occurred without the drug is not clear. Prolonged psychotic episodes following repeated use of LSD tend to resemble naturally occurring schizophreniform psychotic states, and the prognosis appears to be similar (see Vardy and Kay, 1983). There is the possibility that repeated use of LSD can induce subtle deficits in the capacity for abstract thinking.[10]

The question of possible hazard to the fetus when LSD is taken by a pregnant woman also remains unanswered. Laboratory evidence indicates that *extremely high* doses of LSD may cause chromosome breakage. However, similar chromosome breakage may be induced by caffeine, aspirin, many other drugs, x-rays, fever, and viral infections. Even if LSD *in normal doses* should increase the rate of chromosome breakage, the user or any offspring will not necessarily be affected. In fact, clinical data indicate that the incidence of fetal abnormalities occurring in offspring of LSD users is the same as that of the normal population. While there is *some* evidence of increased incidence of structural abnormalities in infants born of parents who use LSD, the variety of other drugs also used by these same parents makes it impossible to blame one specific compound. The state of nutrition and lack of prenatal care must also be considered in such cases.

Psychoactive drugs (including LSD) *do* cross the placental barrier and have free access to the developing fetus. One should be aware that LSD or any other psychoactive agent may have some as yet undetermined effect on offspring. While current data indicate that the risk is small, the possibility has not been excluded.

Fears of long-term damage to *society* caused by widespread use of LSD appear to be unsubstantiated. The use of the drug has been decreasing, presumably because many who used the drug no longer do so. There is ample evidence to indicate that LSD induces tolerance to its several effects, but it does not create physical dependence. Psychological dependence may occur to some extent, since the psychological alterations induced by LSD may lead to a compulsion to reuse the drug. Most users, however, eventually cease taking it and return to less potent agents. Thus, despite extreme potency and unusual psychedelic effects, the social use of other psychoactive drugs, such as alcohol, nicotine, amphetamine, barbiturates, tranquilizers, caffeine, and the opiates, should cause more concern.

Dimethyltryptamine (DMT)

LSD closely resembles serotonin, and the psychedelic effects of LSD are thought to result by mimicking the presynaptic activity of serotonin neurons. There are various other naturally occurring psychedelic compounds that also resemble serotonin and are capable of producing LSD-like effects on the user. One such agent is dimethyltryptamine, DMT (Figure 9.3).

DMT is not extensively used in the United States, but it is widely used in other parts of the world. It is an active principle of various South American snuffs, such as cohoba (prepared from the beans of the *Piptadenia peregrina*) and yopo (a similar product from the West Indies). DMT is partly responsible for the hallucinations and confusional syndrome that follow inhalation of these powders, but the presence of the drug bufotenin (to be discussed) also contributes to the effect. Unlike LSD, DMT is not absorbed into the bloodstream when taken orally and therefore is usually inhaled through the lungs either as a powder or as a smoke.

The psychedelic properties of DMT appear to result predominantly from alterations in visual perception or the occurrence of true hallucinations. Euphoria and behavioral excitability often accompany the sensory alterations. The duration of action of DMT is extremely short, usually only an hour or two—hence its slang name, "businessmen's LSD."

Little information is currently available about the development of tolerance to or dependence upon DMT, but it is expected that it would differ little from LSD. Cross-tolerance between LSD and DMT is likewise predicted.

Psilocybin and Psilocin

The structures of psilocybin and psilocin, presented in Figure 9.3, closely resemble each other and those of DMT, LSD, and serotonin. Psilocybin and psilocin are two psychedelic agents found in at least 15 species of mushrooms belonging to the genera *Psilocybe, Panaeolus,* and *Conocybe.* These mushrooms grow throughout much of the world, including Central America and the Northwestern portion of the United States.[11] *Psilocybe mexicana* (also referred to as *Teonanacatl* or *God's Flesh*) has a long and colorful history of religious and sacramental use throughout Central America.

As noted previously, psilocin and psilocybin are the two major psychoactive drugs in the mushroom, and they are approximately 200 times less potent than LSD. Unlike DMT, psilocin and psilocybin are effectively absorbed when taken orally, and the mushrooms are eaten raw in order to induce psychedelic effects. It is difficult to know how much psilocybin and/or psilocin is contained in any particular mushroom. There is a great variation in potency among the different species of mushrooms as well as significant differences between mushrooms of the same species. For example, the usual oral dose of *Psilocybe semilanceata* ("Liberty Caps") may range from 10 to 40 mushrooms, while the dose for *Psilocybe cyanescens* may be only 2 to 5 mushrooms. Thus, the species must be properly identified to determine proper dosage. In addition, there are some extremely toxic species of mushrooms that are *not* psychoactive and that superficially resemble those that contain psilocybin and psilocin. Thus, to avoid unpleasant experiences, one must be familiar with all hallucinogenic and poisonous species of mushrooms.

For a long while psilocin and psilocybin were both thought to be pharmacologically active. However, as Figure 9.3 shows, the two compounds differ only in that psilocybin contains a molecule of phosphoric acid. After the mushroom is ingested, phosphoric acid is apparently removed from psilocybin, producing psilocin, the active psychedelic agent.

Although the psychedelic effects of *Psilocybe mexicana* have long been part of Indian folklore, the first detailed description of *Psilocybe* intoxication was not obtained until 1955, when Gordon Wasson, a New York banker, traveled through Mexico, mingled with native tribes, and was allowed to participate in a *Psilocybe* ceremony and eat the magic mushroom. Of the mushroom, Wasson said:

> It permits you to travel backwards and forward in time, to enter other planes of existence, even to know God. . . . Your body lies in the darkness, heavy as lead, but your spirit seems to soar and leave the hut, and with the speed of thought to travel where it listeth, in time and space, accompanied by the shaman's singing . . . at least you know what the ineffable is, and what ecstasy means. Ecstasy! The mind harks back to the origin of that word. For the Greeks, *ekstasis* meant the flight of the soul from the body. Can you find a better word to describe this state?[12]

The hallucinations and distortions of time and space are similar to those produced by LSD. The duration of action of *Psilocybe*, however, is much shorter (between 2 and 4 hours) than that of LSD. Cross-tolerance occurs between psilocybin, LSD, and also mescaline. Like LSD, side effects always precede development of the psychedelic action. Users feel symptoms associated with the fight/flight/fright response concomitantly with the psychological effects so vividly described by Wasson.

Psilocybin is not as potent as LSD, and it is somewhat easier to adjust the dose to reach a desired level of drug effect. Low doses of psilocybin (up to 4 or 5 milligrams) induce a pleasant experience with mental relaxation. Higher doses (to 15 milligrams) induce perceptual alterations, with occasional hallucinations. Further description of the psilocybin mushroom experience is offered by Weil.[13]

Bufotenin

Earlier in this chapter, we discussed *Amanita muscaria* and two of its psychoactive drugs, ibotenic acid and muscimol. *Bufotenin* is another drug that is found in *Amanita*, although the amounts are small. More significant amounts of bufotenin may be obtained from the secretion of the skin and parotid glands of toads. Bufotenin may also be found (as is DMT) in the seeds of the tree *Piptadenia peregrina*, which grows in Haiti and Venezuela. These seeds are pulverized and inhaled as snuff. Such preparations are referred to by various names, including yopo, parica, epena, and cohoba.

From Figure 9.3, one may note the close similarity of bufotenin to psilocin, DMT, psilocybin, LSD, and serotonin. Thus, it is not unexpected that the symptoms of intoxication following inhalation of a smoke or powder containing bufotenin are similar to the effects produced by other serotonin psychedelics. The fight/flight/fright responses are induced, followed by a period of excitation, followed finally by a state of stupor and sleep. Pharmacologically, bufotenin (in doses of 1 to 16 milligrams) may induce visual distortions together with a feeling of relaxation and light-weightedness. Hallucinations may or may not occur.

The side effects of bufotenin (increased blood pressure and heart rate, blurred vision, increased muscle tone, and so on) are greater than those produced by psilocybin or DMT and are often quite bothersome. Thus, bufotenin is more toxic than psilocybin and induces deficits of motor function with ataxia (staggering), minor paralysis, and muscular rigidity. Because these side effects may be frightening to the user, the drug is remarkably uncomfortable to take and such effects might be confused with hallucinations.

Ololiuqui (Morning Glory)

Ololiuqui is yet another naturally occurring agent used by Central and South American Indians, both as an intoxicant and as a hallucinogen. The drug is used ritually as a means of communicating with the supernatural, as are extracts of most plants that contain drugs of psychedelic potency. Use of ololiuqui seeds in Central and South America was first described by the Spaniard Hernandez who stated that "when the priests wanted to commune with their Gods . . . [they ate ololiuqui seeds and] a thousand visions and satanic hallucinations appeared to them."[14]

The seeds were analyzed in Europe by Albert Hoffmann and several ingredients were identified. One ingredient was lysergic acid amide (*not* lysergic acid diethylamide, LSD). The lysergic acid amide that Hoffmann identified is approximately one-tenth as active as LSD as a psychoactive agent. However, considering the extreme potency of LSD, lysergic acid amide is still quite potent.

Accompanying the psychedelic action of ololiuqui are the usual side effects of the serotonin psychedelics: nausea, vomiting, headache, increased blood pressure, dilated pupils, sleepiness, and so on. These side effects are usually quite intense and serve to limit the recreational usefulness of ololiuqui. Ingestion of 100 or more seeds produces sleepiness, distortion of perception, hallucinations, and confusion. Flashbacks have been reported but are infrequent.

Harmine

Harmine is a psychedelic agent obtained from the seeds of *Peganum harmala*, a plant native to the Middle East. These seeds have been used for centuries. Intoxication is usually accompanied by nausea and vomiting, sedation and, finally, sleep. The psychic excitement experienced consists of visual distortions similar to those induced by LSD. Harmine has been relatively well studied in animals, and the reader is referred to Longo's discussion of the drug.[15]

Psychedelic Anesthetics

In the late 1950s and early 1960s, two injectable anesthetic agents were introduced into medicine. They differ markedly from other general anesthetics and sedative-hypnotics in that they more closely resemble the psychedelic compounds. These drugs are phencyclidine (Sernyl) and ketamine (Ketalar).

Phencyclidine was synthesized in 1956 and was recommended for clinical trials as an anesthetic in humans in 1957. Earlier investigations of its effects in animals revealed a potent analgesic (pain-relieving) activity and its potential use as a nonbarbiturate, nonnarcotic, intravenous anesthetic agent. However, reports obtained from patients after surgery noted a number of quite severe reactions upon waking from anesthesia. These reactions included agitation, excitement, disorientation, and "hallucinatory" phenomena. In 1965, further human clinical investigation of phencyclidine was discontinued and the compound was marketed commercially as a veterinary anesthetic, primarily for use in primates. The structurally related anesthetic, ketamine (see Figure 9.4), was subsequently developed. Ketamine induced a similar state of anesthesia, but the psychedelic reactions were much less severe. Ketamine was therefore marketed as an anesthetic agent for human use.

In 1967, small amounts of phencyclidine became available through the drug culture, and the drug was referred to in that year as the "PeaCe Pill" (PCP). There was then a sharp decline in phencyclidine use between the years 1971 and 1975, and most PCP during this period was available as a component of various illicit drug mixtures. In 1975, however, there was a resurgence in illicit phency-

Figure 9.4

Structural formulas of phencyclidine and ketamine.

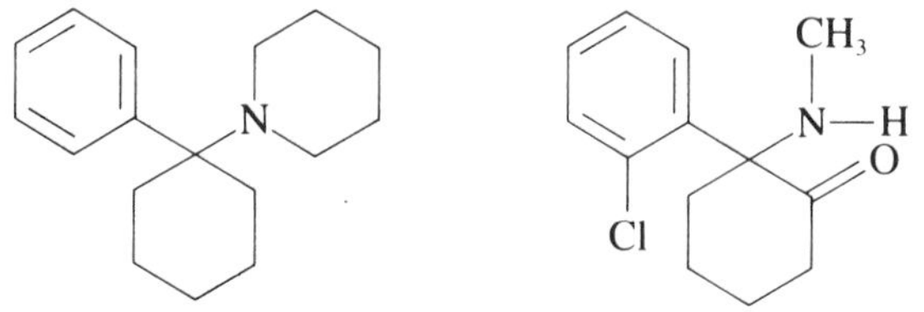

Phencyclidine (Sernyl)   Ketamine (Ketalar)

clidine use and it became one of the most abused drugs in the United States. By the 1980s, the use of PCP had peaked and it has now decreased markedly.

Phencyclidine has appeared on the illicit market in powder, tablet, leaf mixture, and 1 gram "rock" crystal forms. Phencyclidine found on parsley, mint, or other leaves is usually in the form of a "joint." Phencyclidine is commonly sold as "crystal," "angel dust," "hog," "PCP," "THC," "cannabinol," or "horse tranquilizer." The most persistent misrepresentation is "THC." When sold as "crystal" or "angel dust" (terms also used for methamphetamine), the drug is usually available in concentrations varying between 50 and 100 percent. When purchased under other names or in concoctions, the amount of phencyclidine drops to a range of 10 to 30 percent. Phencyclidine is usually taken orally, by smoking, snorting, or by intravenous injection. Powdered forms are generally sprinkled on "joints" or sometimes snorted.

PCP is well absorbed, whether it is taken orally or smoked. When smoked, peak effects occur in about 15 minutes, with about 40 percent of the dose appearing in the bloodstream. Oral absorption is slower; maximal blood levels are reached in about 2 hours. The elimination of half-life of PCP averages about 18 hours, but it varies widely.

About 90 percent of PCP is metabolized and its metabolites are excreted in the urine. Positive urine assay for PCP is assumed to indicate PCP use within the previous week. Blood and saliva tests for PCP can also be used. False-positives for PCP are common and, therefore, a positive assay requires secondary confirmation.

The pharmacology of phencyclidine is complicated. This compound (and its close relative, ketamine) does not induce anesthesia the same way the sedative-hypnotics do. Phencyclidine and ketamine are frequently referred to as "dissociative anesthetics" because patients may feel dissociated from themselves and from their environment. In humans, phencyclidine appears to be unique among all anesthetics studied. This drug induces an unresponsive state with amnesia (loss of memory), although the eyes remain open (blank stare) and the patient appears to be awake. Significant depression of either respiration or blood pressure is not produced by either phencyclidine or ketamine in anesthetic doses. Toxic doses of these agents may produce severe agitation, muscle rigidity, and generalized seizure activity. Used illicitly, low doses of phencyclidine produce mild agitation, euphoria, disinhibition, or excitement in a patient who appears grossly "drunk" and has a blank stare. The patient may be rigid and unable to speak. In many cases, however, the patient is communicative, although he or she does not respond to pain (these drugs are potent analgesics). In higher doses, a state of coma or stupor in which the eyes remain open is induced. Blood pressure is usually elevated but respiration is not depressed. The patient may recover from this state within 1 to 4 hours, although a confusional state may last for 8 to 72 hours.

Massive oral "overdoses," involving up to 1 gram of street-purchased material, have been reported to result in prolonged periods of stupor or coma. This state may last for several days and may be marked by potentially lethal depression of respiration, intense seizure activity, and increased blood pressure. Following this period of stupor, a prolonged recovery phase marked by confusional delusion may last for up to 2 weeks. In a few cases, this confusional state may be followed by a psychosis lasting several weeks to a few months.

Chronic users of phencyclidine frequently present themselves in hospital emergency rooms with psychiatric problems such as paranoid psychosis, severe depression, anxiety, or concern about brain damage. Phencyclidine psychosis is a leading cause of psychiatric admissions. Whether this drug indeed causes these problems or whether persons with a particular type of personality are attracted to high-dose or prolonged phencyclidine abuse because they already have one of these underlying problems is as yet unclear.

Treatment of overdosage is symptomatic and is directed at protecting the patient and others from the effects of impaired behavior and judgment and at supporting vital functions. Hastening excretion by continuous gastric suction and acidification of the urine can substantially shorten the half-life of the drug but can also increase the risk of renal failure. . . . Hypersalivation may require suction, respiratory depression may require artificial ventilation, and fever may require external cooling. Convulsions have been treated with diazepam and hypertension with hydralazine. "Talking down" is not helpful, and clinicians advise isolation of patients from external stimuli to the degree compatible with support of vital functions and control of violent or self-destructive behavior. Where possible, four or five burly aides are superior to mechanical restraints. . . . Coma may be preceded or followed by delirium, paranoia, and assaultive behavior, and clinical arrangements must take this into consideration. A psychotic phase may last for several weeks after a single dose of phencyclidine.[16]

The major risks associated with PCP use result from behavioral toxicities or toxic reactions. Behavioral toxicities include falling, drowning, burns, driving accidents, aggressive or violent behavior, and so on. These seem to occur as a result of impaired perception or delusional beliefs. There also appears to be a marked tendency toward violence, attributable to the drug itself and to the frame of mind created in the user. The toxic reactions to PCP are manifested as acute intoxication, acute psychosis, or coma from overdose. The intoxicated state is manifested by agitation, confusion, excitement, "blank stare" appearance, violent behavior, analgesia, and amnesia.

Self-inflicted injuries and injuries sustained during the application of physical restraints are frequent because intoxicated individuals are unaware of their surroundings and sometimes are unaware of or unresponsive to pain. Such injuries account for many of the injuries and deaths associated with PCP intoxication. Respiratory depression, generalized seizure activity, and pulmonary edema have all been implicated. PCP has been implicated in a number of deaths by drowning. Apparently the PCP user readily loses his orientation while immersed and drowns, sometimes in very shallow water. Other reported causes of death include violent behavior, automobile accidents, and suicide. For additional readings on phencyclidine, recent volumes are recommended.[17–22]

The mechanism underlying the psychedelic, analgesic, and amnesic effects of phencyclidine and ketamine are unknown and probably involve interactions with several transmitter systems. They potentiate dopamine, serotonin, and norepinephrine neurons, although traditional antagonists do not block their effects. They also bind to certain opiate receptors (the sigma receptor) in the limbic system (especially the hippocampus), although naloxone does not antagonize their effects.[23]

This multiplicity of actions provides researchers with a most interesting tool with which one may study the mechanisms of mental illness. While the personality changes associated with LSD use are somewhat similar to those induced by phencyclidine, many of the other features of phencyclidine psychosis are not common to other psychedelic drugs. In addition, there are reports that phencyclidine may both activate and mimic schizophrenic psychoses. Some individuals have developed classic schizophrenia following phencyclidine psychoses. These observations suggest a relationship between the pharmacology of phencyclidine and the biochemistry of schizophrenia.

Notes

1. M. E. Jarvik, "Drugs Used in the Treatment of Psychiatric Disorders," in L. S. Goodman and A. Gilman, eds., *The Pharmacological Basis of Therapeutics*, 4th ed. (New York: Macmillan, 1970), p. 195.
2. S. G. Potkin, F. Karoum, L. W. Chuang, et al., "Phenethylamine in Paranoid Chronic Schizophrenia," *Science* 206 (1979): 470.
3. D. H. Efron, ed., *Ethnopharmacologic Search for Psychoactive Drugs*, Public Health Service (Washington, D.C.: U.S. Government Printing Office, 1967), pp. 188–201.
4. *Interim Drug Report of the Commission of Inquiry into the Nonmedical Use of Drugs*, Gerald LeDain, chairman (Ottawa: Information Canada, 1970), p. 58.
5. *Interim Drug Report of the Commission of Inquiry into the Nonmedical Use of Drugs*, Gerald LeDain, chairman (Ottawa: Information Canada, 1970), pp. 58–59.
6. L. P. Finnegan and K. O'B. Fehr, "The Effects of Opiates, Sedative-Hypnotics, Amphetamines, Cannabis, and Other Psychoactive Drugs on the Fetus and Newborn," in O. J. Kalant, ed., *Research Advances in Alcohol and Drug Problems*, vol. 5. (New York: Plenum Press, 1980), pp. 653–723.
7. J. H. Jaffe, "Drug Addiction and Drug Abuse," in A. G. Gilman, L. S. Goodman, T. W. Rall, and F. Murad, eds., *Goodman and Gilman's The Pharmacological Basis of Therapeutics*, 7th ed. (New York: Macmillan, 1985), p. 564.
8. G. G. Dimijian, "Contemporary Drug Abuse," in A. Goth, ed., *Medical Pharmacology*, 11th ed. (St. Louis: Mosby, 1984), p. 356.
9. G. G. Dimijian, "Contemporary Drug Abuse," in A. Goth, ed., *Medical Pharmacology*, 11th ed. (St. Louis: Mosby, 1984), p. 357.
10. J. H. Jaffe, "Drug Addiction and Drug Abuse," in A. G. Gilman, L. S. Goodman, T. W. Rall, and F. Murad, eds., *Goodman and Gilman's The Pharmacological Basis of Therapeutics*, 7th ed. (New York: Macmillan, 1985), p. 565.
11. J. Ott, *Hallucinogenic Plants of North America* (Berkely: Wingbow Press, 1979).
12. M. E. Crahan, "God's Flesh and Other Pre-Columbian Phantastica," *Bulletin of the Los Angeles County Medical Association* 99 (1969): 17.
13. A. Weil, *The Marriage of the Sun and the Moon* (Boston: Houghton Mifflin, 1980).
14. Quoted in E. M. Brecher and *Consumer Reports* editors, *Licit and Illicit Drugs* (Mt. Vernon, N.Y.: Consumers Union, 1972), p. 345.
15. V. C. Longo, *Neuropharmacology and Behavior* (San Francisco: W. H. Freeman and Co., 1972), pp. 136–141.
16. J. H. Jaffe, "Drug Addiction and Drug Abuse," in A. G. Gilman, L. S. Goodman, T. W. Rall, and F. Murad, eds., *Goodman and Gilman's The Pharmacological Basis of Therapeutics*, 7th ed. (New York: Macmillan, 1985), pp. 566–567.

17. D. H. Clouet, ed., "Phencyclidine: An Update," National Institute of Drug Abuse, Research Monograph No. 64, Department of Health and Human Services, Publication No. (ADM) 86-1443 (Washington, D.C.: U.S. Government Printing Office, 1986).
18. S. M. Pittel and M. C. Oppendahl, "The Enigma of PCP," in R. L. Dupont, A. Goldstein, and J. O'Donnell, eds., *Handbook on Drug Abuse* (Washington, D.C.: National Institute on Drug Abuse and Office of Drug Abuse Policy, 1979), pp. 249–254.
19. R. H. Cravey, D. Reed, and J. L. Ragle, "Phencyclidine-Related Deaths: A Report of Nine Fatal Cases," *Journal of Analytical Toxicology* (Sept.–Oct. 1979): 199–201.
20. D. O. Clardy, R. H. Cravey, B. J. MacDonald, S. J. Wiersema, D. S. Pearce, and J. L. Ragle, "The Phencyclidine-Intoxicated Driver," *Journal of Analytical Toxicology* 3 (Nov.–Dec. 1979): 238–241.
21. E. F. Domino, "Neurobiology of Phencyclidine—An Update," in R. C. Peterson and R. C. Stillman, eds., *PCP Phencyclidine Abuse: An Appraisal*, National Institute on Drug Abuse (Washington, D.C.: U.S. Government Printing Office, 1978), pp. 18–43.
22. O. Aniline and F. N. Pitts, Jr., "Phencyclidine (PCP): A Review and Perspectives," *CRC Critical Review of Toxicology* 10 (1982): 145–177.
23. R. S. Zukin and S. R. Zukin, "A Common Receptor for Phencyclidine and the *Sigma* Opiates," in J. M. Kamenka, E. F. Domino, and P. Geneste, eds., *Phencyclidine and Related Arylcyclohexylamines: Present and Future Applications* (Ann Arbor: NPP Books, 1983), pp. 107–124.

CHAPTER 10

Marijuana

The Ancient Drug of Cannabis

This ancient drug has sedative, euphoriant, and hallucinogenic properties. The hemp plant *Cannabis sativa* grows throughout the world and flourishes in most temperate and tropical regions. One of humanity's oldest cultivated nonfood plants, it appears to have originated in Asia. The earliest written reference to *Cannabis sativa* dates from approximately 2700 B.C. The active compound, Δ^9-tetrahydrocannabinol (hereafter referred to as THC), is most concentrated in the resin obtained from the flowers of the female plant.

Names for *Cannabis* products include *marijuana, hashish, charas, bhang,* and *ganja. Hashish* and *charas* are the most potent preparations, consisting of the dried resinous exudate of the female flowers. *Bhang* is slightly less potent, consisting of dried leaves and flowers of the plant. *Ganja* refers to the resinous mass of the crushed leaves. *Marijuana* refers to any product containing *Cannabis* plant parts or extract therefrom that induces physical and psychic changes in humans. The THC concentration in marijuana varies widely, usually from 0.5 to 11 percent. THC concentrations in other preparations varies from 10 to greater than 50 percent. Note that THC is the active ingredient in each product; only the concentration and the purity vary.

Classification

Tetrahydrocannabinol (THC) is a difficult compound to classify. At low-to-moderate doses, THC is a mild sedative-hypnotic agent resembling alcohol and the antianxiety agents (chlordiazepoxide, diazepam, and meprobamate) in its pharmacological effects. Unlike the sedative-hypnotics, however, higher doses of THC may (in addition to sedation) produce euphoria, hallucinations, and heightened sensation, effects similar to a mild LSD experience. Also unlike the sedatives, high doses of THC do not produce anesthesia, coma, or death. Similarly, there appears to be little cross-tolerance between THC and LSD on one hand or between THC and the sedative-hypnotic compounds on the other. Thus, the THC contained in the various preparations of *Cannabis* is only superficially related to either the sedatives or the psychedelics.

The courts often classify the products from *Cannabis sativa* with the opiates as narcotics. As is well known and appreciated today, marijuana and hashish are *not* narcotics and are pharmacologically quite distinct from them. *Cannabis* products are currently used in the United States chiefly in the form of marijuana, which has approximately a 1 to 10 percent concentration of THC. Potent *Cannabis* products (usually hashish) are not as frequently encountered, and, even when they are, only very small quantities are used. It is only at high doses of THC that *Cannabis* resembles the psychedelics in its pharmacological effects. Thus, at least for the present discussion, THC will be classified as a unique psychoactive drug. The structure of THC does not resemble that of any known or suspected chemical transmitter, and its mechanism of action remains unknown.

Historical Background

The history of *Cannabis sativa* from about 2700 B.C. until the nineteenth century still remains obscure. Marijuana was primarily used as a mild intoxicant; it is somewhat milder than alcohol and much less useful for religious and psychedelic experiences than the opiates or the naturally occurring psychedelics. Although products from *Cannabis sativa* were claimed to have a wide variety of medical uses, none of these uses seemed to persist for very long, and even today few are documented.

Cannabis sativa is a rather new entry into Western culture. In the American colonies, the plant was widely grown in Virginia in the 1700s, presumably for its fiber, which was used for rope. Even George Washington grew hemp, presumably for its fiber, but possibly also for its medicinal and other properties.

Hemp cultivation in the United States flourished for many years and then declined with the introduction of more profitable crops such as cotton and the importation of cheap hemp from the Far East. Periodically, however, hemp is still grown commercially in this country. During World War II, for example, cultivation was expanded in order to provide hemp when imports were severely limited. However, hemp need not be cultivated because *Cannabis sativa* grows wild and does not need to be tended.

Marijuana, at least until the beginning of the twentieth century, was not widely used either in therapy or for recreation. This does not imply that its psychoactive properties had not been discovered (they had been), but they had not attracted the attention of the larger society. Its use was primarily restricted to the "less desirable" element. In the early 1920s, the news media decided that marijuana was evil and was being used in the underground. In 1926, a New Orleans newspaper exposed the "menace of marijuana," claiming an association between marijuana and crime, and laws were subsequently passed in Louisiana to outlaw its use. Slowly, during the next 5 years, other newspapers took up the call, and more states began to pass laws against marijuana.

Probably the greatest impetus to the outlawing of marijuana was provided in the early 1930s by the Commissioner of Narcotics, Harry Anslinger, who had an intense interest in encouraging the states and the Bureau of Narcotics to enforce vigorously the laws against the drug. During the next few years, marijuana began to be looked upon as a narcotic, an agent responsible for crimes of violence, and a great danger to public safety. These attitudes were popularized through the 1930s by numerous news articles that served to convince the public that marijuana was indeed evil. By approximately 1940, the country was convinced that marijuana was a "killer drug" and a potent narcotic that induced crimes of violence, led to heroin addiction, destroyed the individual, and in general was one of the great social menaces.

The campaign against marijuana and the emotion that it generated continued through the 1950s. The use of marijuana was still primarily restricted to the lower classes of society, for it was not often encountered by average citizens or their children. Then, in the late 1950s and early 1960s, marijuana and other psychoactive drugs became widely used by middle- and upper-class youth. Through the 1960s, marijuana use by American youth increased steadily. Marijuana experimentation did not explode with the rapidity that LSD use rose, and its wide use did not really develop until the late 1960s and early 1970s, when the use of LSD and other potent psychedelics had begun to decline.

It has been estimated that by 1972 at least 2 million Americans used marijuana daily. A 1974 survey found that in one high-use county in California, 20 percent of seventh-grade students reported having used marijuana at least once during the preceding year. The same survey noted that in 23-year-old men, 14 percent smoked marijuana daily during the preceding year. In this group, marijuana use exceeded the use of alcohol.

The number of people using marijuana increased steadily throughout the 1970s. The results of a 1977 National Survey on drug use, presented in Figure 10.1, showed that young adulthood (the period between 18 and 25) is the peak period of marijuana use. Sixty percent of the 18- to 25-year-olds reported having used marijuana at some time in their lives. Over one in four 18- to 25-year-olds had used marijuana in the month preceding the survey. Marijuana use was closely correlated with increasing age through the period of young adulthood, with use falling precipitously in individuals over the age of 35. If one takes these percentages of *Cannabis* users and extrapolates them to the general population, 43 million Americans had tried marijuana as of spring 1977. About 16 million Americans were currently using the drug (that is, had used it during the month previous to the 1977 survey).

Figure 10.1

Marijuana (or hashish) experience by age: lifetime prevalence and use in past month, 1977. [From Secretary of Health, Education, and Welfare, *Marihuana and Health,* 7th Annual Report to the U.S. Congress (Washington, D.C.: U.S. Government Printing Office, 1977), p. 6.]

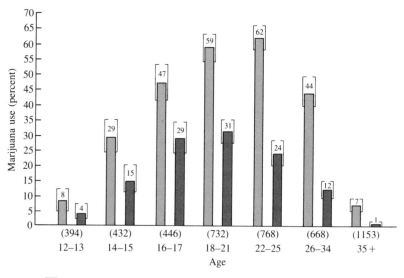

Table 10.1

Percentage of high-school seniors nationwide responding to a confidential questionnaire who said they had used drugs within the past 30 days.

	'75	'76	'77	'78	'79	'80	'81	'82	'83	'84	'85	'86
Marijuana, hashish	27.1	32.2	35.4	37.1	36.5	33.7	31.6	28.5	27.0	25.2	25.7	23.4
Cocaine	1.9	2.0	2.9	3.9	5.7	5.2	5.8	5.0	4.9	5.8	6.7	6.2
Alcohol	68.2	68.3	71.2	72.1	71.8	72.0	70.7	69.7	69.4	67.2	65.9	65.3

SOURCE: University of Michigan Institute for Social Research. Conducted for the National Institute on Drug Abuse, 1987.

A 1986 survey (Table 10.1) confirmed earlier studies, which note that marijuana smoking has been steadily declining among high-school seniors since the peak period of use from 1977 to 1979. Disquieting, however, was the confirmation that cigarette smoking has not declined; alcohol use has only slightly declined; and cocaine use has increased dramatically. Marijuana use is still rare in individuals over the age of 50. Daily marijuana use in high-school seniors was down from a peak of 11 percent in 1978 to 4 percent in 1986.

Thus, the escalation in marijuana use noted during the 1970s appears to have leveled off and has probably reached a level of chronic use that may not change markedly in the near future. Thus, the use of other, more potent psychoactive drugs (such as cocaine) may become the object of focus.

Administration and Absorption

Most marijuana grown in the United States has a THC content that varies tremendously and may range from near zero to as much as 10 or 11 percent. These figures are important for the discussion (in the following section) of the pharmacological effects of *Cannabis*.

In the United States, THC is usually administered in the form of a hand-rolled marijuana cigarette, the average cigarette containing between 1 and 2 grams of plant material. Thus, if a marijuana cigarette contained 1.5 grams of plant material with a THC content of 2 percent, the cigarette would contain approximately 0.030 gram (30 milligrams) of THC. Since THC is usually administered by smoking marijuana, the quantity of drug actually absorbed into the bloodstream varies considerably with the previous smoking experience of the user, the time the smoke is held in the lungs, and the number of other users of the same cigarette.

Usually, individuals who have smoked marijuana several times before can hold the smoke in their lungs longer than can novices, allowing a longer time for THC to be absorbed into the bloodstream before the smoke is exhaled. Similarly, individuals with a habit of inhaling the smoke of tobacco cigarettes usually can hold marijuana smoke in their lungs longer than can nonsmokers. The fewer individuals with whom the marijuana cigarette is shared, the more THC is available to each smoker. In general, approximately one-half of the THC present in a marijuana cigarette is actually available in the smoke. Thus, if a cigarette contained 30 milligrams of THC, about 15 milligrams would be available in the smoke. But it is extremely unlikely that one individual smoking one cigarette would be able to absorb 100 percent of the available THC in that cigarette. In practice, the amount of THC absorbed into the bloodstream from the social smoking of one cigarette is probably much lower.

As discussed in Chapter 1, the absorption of inhaled drugs is rapid and complete. The onset of action of THC is usually within minutes after smoking begins and peak concentrations in plasma occur within 10 to 30 minutes. Unless more is smoked, the effects seldom last longer than 2 or 3 hours. THC is also absorbed when administered orally, but the absorption is slow and incomplete. Administered orally, the onset of action usually takes 3 to 60 minutes, with peak effects occurring 2 to 3 hours after ingestion. Effects persist for 3 to 5 hours or even longer. THC is approximately three times more effective when smoked than when taken orally. Since marijuana and hashish are crude preparations of plants and are not soluble in water, they should not be administered by injection. Indeed, injection of any crude product of *Cannabis sativa* or any other plant is extremely dangerous. It should be noted that what is sold on the street as "THC" virtually never contains THC but may be any of a number of other psychedelic agents.

Distribution, Metabolism, and Excretion

Because THC is only very slightly soluble in water, once it enters the bloodstream and is distributed to the various organs of the body, it tends to be deposited in the tissues, especially those that have significant concentrations of fatty material. Because THC is soluble in fat, it readily penetrates the brain; the blood-brain barrier does not appear to hinder its passage. THC may also be found in significant concentrations in the liver, kidneys, spleen, lungs, and even in the testes. Similarly, THC readily crosses the placental barrier and reaches the fetus. Unlike the opiates, THC achieves levels in the brain comparable to those found in other tissues.

THC is almost completely metabolized to less active products before it is excreted. This metabolism is accomplished primarily in the liver but may also occur in other tissues, such as the lungs. Because it is so rapidly metabolized and distributed, practically no THC is found in urine.

Unlike most psychoactive drugs, the metabolites of THC are excreted not only in the urine but also in the feces. After the initial period of intoxication, THC levels fall rapidly over about an hour to a low level (due to a high solubility in body fat) that persists for days. As can be deduced, metabolism is quite slow, indeed, an elimination half-life of about 1 week has been postulated. This tends to prolong and intensify the activity of subsequently smoked marijuana and may at least partially explain why regular users achieve a "high" more quickly, more easily, and with less drug than do intermittent users (a phenomenon formerly and probably mistakenly called "reverse tolerance"). As noted in Chapter 1, if a drug has an elimination half-life of 1 week, it would take about 6 weeks to eliminate 98 percent of the drug originally ingested.

Since only the metabolites of THC are found in urine, detection tests for THC focus primarily on isolating such metabolites as 9-carboxy-THC, which is known to be excreted in the urine. Such detection methods are complex and involve either one of the immunoassays, chromatography, or spectrometry. Acute or occasional use is detected for about 1 to 3 days. Chronic smokers (even if only 2 to 3 times weekly) will have persistently positive urine tests for THC metabolites. A heavy smoker who stops smoking may have positive urine tests for about 1 month after cessation. Thus, a positive urinalysis can indicate recent use as well as use that occurred several weeks earlier; multiple sampling may be necessary to differentiate the results. As stated by Hawks and Chiang:

A single positive urine test does not mean that the person was under the influence of marijuana at the time the urine specimen was collected. A true-positive urine test means only that the person providing the specimen used marijuana in the recent past, which could be hours, days, or weeks depending on the specific use pattern.[1]

Pharmacological Effects

Within the last few years much information about the pharmacological effects of THC has become available. Research has been done on a variety of species, including mice, rats, cats, monkeys, and pigeons. Although these species obviously differ markedly from humans, and people do not always react the same way to a drug as an animal does, drugs that produce similar effects in several species of animals will likely exert similar effects in humans. If THC were to decrease behavioral activity in rats, mice, monkeys, and pigeons, it would probably do the same thing in people.

Effects on Animals

In almost all animal species, THC induces sedation and decreases both spontaneous motor activity and behavioral responses to painful stimuli. In addition, it decreases body temperature, calms aggressive behavior, potentiates the effects of barbiturates and other sedatives, blocks convulsions, depresses reflexes, and exerts other effects similar to those produced by the sedative-hypnotic compounds. In primates, specifically, it produces sedation, decreases aggression, decreases the ability to perform complex behavioral tasks, seems to induce hallucinations, and appears to cause temporal distortions. Social interactions (such as allogrooming) appear to increase in frequency.

Effects on People

The commonly observed responses to the acute use of either orally administered or smoked marijuana are seen as changes in the functioning of both the CNS and the cardiovascular system. Increases in pulse rate and slight increases in blood pressure are commonly encountered. Blood vessels of the cornea also dilate, resulting in the bloodshot eyes usually associated with indulgence in alcohol. THC users frequently report increased appetite, dry mouth, occasional dizziness, increased visual and auditory perception, and some nausea. Taste, touch, and smell may be enhanced, time perception altered, and an increased sense of well-being, mild euphoria, relaxation, and relief from anxiety are felt.

As described by Jaffe:

> Most commonly there is an increased sense of well-being or euphoria, accompanied by feelings of relaxation and sleepiness when subjects are alone; where users can interact, sleepiness is less pronounced and there is often spontaneous laughter. . . . Short-term memory is impaired, and there is a deterioration in capacity to carry out tasks requiring multiple mental steps to reach a specific goal. This effect on memory-dependent, goal-directed behavior has been called "temporal disintegration," and is correlated with a tendency to confuse past, present, and future, and with depersonalization—a sense of strangeness and unreality about the self.
>
> Balance and stability of stance are affected even at low doses, effects that are more apparent when the eyes are closed. Decreases in muscle strength and hand steadiness can be demonstrated. Performance of relatively

simple motor tasks and simple reaction times are relatively unimpaired until higher doses are reached. More complex processes, including perception, attention, and information processing, which are involved in driving and flying, are impaired by doses equivalent to one or two cigarettes; the impairment persists for 4 to 8 hours, well beyond the time that the user perceives the subjective effects of the drug. The impairment produced by alcohol is additive to that induced by marihuana.

Marihuana smokers frequently report increased hunger, dry mouth and throat, more vivid visual imagery, and a keener sense of hearing. Subtle visual and auditory stimuli previously ignored may take on a novel quality, and the nondominant senses of touch, taste, and smell seem to be enhanced. Yet, in usual social doses, marihuana decreases empathy and the perception of emotions in others; clarity of sequential dialogue is impaired, and irrelevant ideas and words intrude into the stream of communication. Altered perception of time is a consistent effect of cannabinoids. Time seems to pass more slowly—minutes may seem like hours.[2]

Higher doses of THC can induce delusions, paranoia, hallucinations, confusion and disorientation, altered sensory perception, and increasing anxiety. As doses are further increased, these drug effects intensify, with more vivid hallucinations, delusions, and increasing disorientation.

Jaffe states:

Higher doses of Δ^9-THC can induce frank hallucinations, delusions, and paranoid feelings. Thinking becomes confused and disorganized; depersonalization and altered time sense are accentuated. Anxiety reaching panic proportions may replace euphoria, often as a result of the feeling that the drug-induced state will never end. With high enough doses, the clinical picture is that of a toxic psychosis with hallucinations, depersonalization, and loss of insight; this can occur acutely or only after months of use. Most users are able to regulate their intake in order to avoid the excessive dosage that produces these unpleasant effects. . . . Because of the high prevalence of marihuana use, dysphoric reactions and psychiatric emergencies as a result of smoking marihuana are no longer uncommon. Use of marihuana may also cause an acute exacerbation of symptomatology in stabilized schizophrenics, and it is one of the common precipitants of "flashbacks" in former users of LSD.[2]

Psychiatric emergencies as a result of smoking marijuana, however, are extremely uncommon. Indeed, if one comes to an emergency room with a toxic psychosis purported to be due to "THC," the most likely cause was phencyclidine, not THC.

Chronic use of marijuana increases the risk of untoward effects. Thus, the continuing trend toward greater use of more potent preparations by younger individuals is of concern. Though daily and multiple daily use is common, use of tobacco is much more prevalent. Because inhalation is by far the most common route of administration,[3] an analysis of the gaseous and particulate components of both marijuana and tobacco smoke (Table 10.2)[4] is particularly relevant. Note that with the exception of THC in marijuana and nicotine in tobacco, both inhalants are remarkably similar, except the marijuana smoke contains about 50 percent more carcinogens. In determining the significance of this, remember that the average cigarette smoker consumes 10 to 20 times more tobacco than the average marijuana smoker consumes cannabis; the marijuana smoker, on the other hand, inhales deeper and holds the smoke in the lungs

Table 10.2

Comparison of gaseous and particulate components of marijuana and tobacco smoke.

	Marijuana cigarette	Tobacco cigarette
Gas phase analysis		
Carbon monoxide (vol %)	3.99	4.58
(mg)	17.6	20.2
Carbon dioxide (vol %)	8.27	9.38
(mg)	57.3	65.0
Ammonia (μg)	228	178
HCN (μg)	532	498
Isoprene (μg)	83	310
Acetaldehyde (μg)	1200	980
Acetone (μg)	443	578
Acrolein (μg)	92	85
Acetonitrile (μg)	132	123
Benzene (μg)	76	67
Toluene (μg)	112	108
Dimethylnitrosamine (ng)	75	84
Methylethylnitrosamine (ng)	27	30
Particulate matter analysis		
Phenol (μg)	76.8	138.5
o-Cresol (μg)	76.8	24
	17.9	24
m-,p-cresol (μg)	54.4	65
2,4- and 2,5-dimethylphenol (μg)	6.8	14.4
Cannabidiol (μg)	190	—
Δ^9 THC (μg)	820	—
Nicotine (μg)	—	2850
Naphthalene (ng)	3000	1200
l-methylnaphthalene (ng)	6100	3650
2-methylnaphthalene (ng)	3600	1400
Benzo(a)anthracene (ng)	75	43
Benzo(a)pyrene (ng)	31	22.1

SOURCE: D. Hoffman, K. D. Brunnemann, G. B. Gori, and E. L. Wynder, "On the Carcinogenicity of Marijuana Smoke," *Recent Advances in Phytochemistry* 9 (1975): 63–81.

longer. Chronic use of marijuana, therefore, should profoundly affect the lungs (see side effects and toxicity).

Chronic use by certain individuals means maintaining a constant state of intoxication. Such behavior by itself causes particular risks. As Cohen states,

Being stoned during much of one's waking hours is particularly undesirable during the formative years when critical coping techniques should be mastered. When preadolescents and adolescents use marijuana, and not just marijuana, to distance themselves from the problems and frustrations of their existence, they do themselves a substantial disservice. They deprive themselves of learning time and may, as a result, never learn the strategies for living this admittedly difficult life.[5]

A "fringe benefit" of marijuana research has been the extensive study of its therapeutic potential. THC exhibits mild analgesic properties, decreases epileptic seizures, decreases the pressure of fluid within the eyes, decreases the resistance in the airways of the lung, and is an antivomiting agent for cancer patients receiving chemotherapy. Marijuana thus has potential usefulness in treating pain, epilepsy, glaucoma, and asthma.

At present, marijuana must still be considered a remarkably nonlethal compound. No deaths directly attributable to its use have been reported, although there has been some question concerning deaths following intravenous injection of crude, nonsterile preparations of marijuana or hashish, which may be unrelated to the THC content. Such use of marijuana products is to be condemned. However, when injected or inhaled there is an extremely large safety margin between the recreational and the toxic or lethal doses of pure THC.

Psychological Effects

As described previously, the usual subjective effects of normal, social doses of marijuana consist of subtle mood alterations resembling daydreaming or mild sedative-hypnotic drug intoxication—alterations frequently imperceptible to the novice or the nonsmoking observer.

At higher doses of THC (several cigarettes or moderate doses of hashish taken orally), the reactions mentioned previously become intensified, though individuals are still in control of themselves and changes in their behavior may not be noticeable to an observer. Individuals experience intensification of emotional responses and alterations in sensation resembling mild sensory distortions or even mild hallucinations. In the current use of marijuana in the United

States, such effects are seldom sought by the social smoker but more frequently by those few who use the drug to induce a pronounced state of sensory distortion.

With even higher doses one may experience extremely vivid hallucinations and psychedelic phenomena that include distortions in body image, loss of identity, sensory hallucinations, and fantasies similar to those induced by LSD, although less intense and probably more similar to the experience induced by the milder psychedelic compounds such as mescaline.

High-dose experiences induce frank hallucinations, delusions, and paranoid feelings. Thinking becomes confused and disorganized; depersonalization and altered time sense are accentuated. Anxiety reaching panic proportions may replace euphoria, often as a result of the feeling that the drug-induced state will never end. With high enough doses, the clinical picture is that of a toxic psychosis, with hallucinations, depersonalization, and loss of insight.

Thought and motor activity are barely impaired at low, usual, social doses of THC but significantly impaired at higher doses. It is important to note, however, that these effects are normally achieved only with unusually large amounts of the drug, amounts that are more clearly related to the dosages that decrease spontaneous motor activity in animals.

Thus, there are marked differences in the effects induced by usual social doses of marijuana and those induced by higher doses. At social doses, effects consist of a mild sedative action most closely resembling a state of daydreaming. From this, one would tend to classify marijuana as a sedative, resembling alcohol or the other sedative-hypnotic agents. Marijuana, however, does not dull sensation as does alcohol but may induce mild alterations in perception. There is little cognitive or motor dysfunction induced by the drug, but it may alter a person's ability to drive an automobile safely. Gross impairments of driving ability seem to occur only after high or extremely high doses of THC. Even then, such impairment may be less than that observed during alcohol intoxication. Nevertheless, driving while under the influence of marijuana should probably be discouraged, just as is driving while under the influence of alcohol. It has been demonstrated that smoking marijuana in socially used doses causes significant deterioration of simulated instrument flying ability in experienced pilots for at least 2 hours.[6] Therefore, acute marijuana intoxication should be considered incompatible with the performance of complex tasks such as automobile or airplane operation.

It is now well documented that the effects of marijuana and alcohol on driving are additive.[7] Increasing concern is being expressed about the behavioral effects resulting from the combined use of marijuana and other drugs. In a recent survey of 20- to 30-year-old males, it was reported that nearly 50 percent of regular marijuana users combined its use with that of alcohol.[8] This combined use of marijuana and alcohol produces greater impairment in the performance of complex tasks than does the use of either drug in similar amounts by itself.[9] It is quite likely that the combined use of marijuana and other drugs, particularly alcohol, will continue to increase. Urgently needed are research projects to evaluate the behavioral and physical effects of the combined use of marijuana and other drugs and to determine the relationship between the blood levels of the several drugs and the degree of impairment to be expected in the execution of highly integrated psychomotor tasks such as driving.

Side Effects and Toxicity

THC is remarkably nonlethal, with perhaps the widest safety margin between recreational and lethal levels of any available psychoactive drug. Although there are few consequences associated with the *acute* use of marijuana, it now appears that *chronic* use is associated with significant toxicity. The impact of these toxicities (and potential toxicities) has been examined, so far, on the lungs, the heart, the brain, and the endocrine and reproductive systems.[10–11]

Reports of altered lung function show evidence of bronchial irritation and inflammation, airway narrowing with increased reactivity to irritants (as in asthma), reduced macrophage and ciliary activity (leading to reduced ability to clear the lungs of inhaled particulate matter), and signs of early stages of emphysema. These pulmonary changes should not be surprising because they result from the persistent and repetitive inhalation of the gases and particulate products comprising marijuana smoke (Table 10.2). The pulmonary effects are absent when marijuana is taken orally, and THC seems even to act beneficially by relaxing the smooth muscles of the lungs.

Aside from its irritant effects, the obvious question is whether marijuana smoke causes lung cancer. There is currently little evidence to rule out that likelihood, especially since marijuana smoking starts at an early age and many users are increasing the frequency of their smoking. It is possible that we are in a prodromal phase of cannabis-induced lung cancer. (See Table 10.2 for a comparison of marijuana and tobacco smoke.) Cellular changes consistent with early carcinous stages are found in bronchial biopsies in heavy marijuana smokers and in a variety of animal models.

On the positive side, only a small percentage of cigarette smokers develop lung cancer[12] and even then usually only after high-dose

(1–2 packs per day) long-term use (20–50 years). Few individuals use marijuana to this extent, though future trends in smoking habits are difficult to predict. The combined smoking of marijuana and tobacco is inadvisable because heavy smokers of both substances develop significant abnormalities of their bronchial airways. These abnormalities are uncommon in those who smoke only tobacco or marijuana, and they are absent in nonsmokers of either substance.

As concluded by Dimijian:

> The neoplastic potential of marijuana smoking has been inadequately researched. No reliable data are available on the incidence of carcinoma of the lung and upper respiratory passages in cannabis users. Studies have suggested, however, that marijuana smoke may prove carcinogenic and that a combination of marijuana and tobacco smoking may have greater carcinogenicity than either alone.[13]

Of some concern is the possibility that marijuana adversely effects the heart. That there is a significant increase in heart rate after smoking has been well documented, but this increase appears to be free of adverse consequences. In patients with existing impairment of heart function, however, the use of marijuana may precipitate chest pain (angina pectoris). Because most marijuana use is confined to individuals younger than 35 years of age (Figure 10.1), individuals with impairment of heart function are rare. In the future, this finding may prove to be of considerable significance if marijuana use expands to include older populations or if today's younger users continue their use as they progress into middle life. Even now, however, it seems prudent to warn patients who may have impaired heart function not to use marijuana, nor to combine marijuana and alcohol.

Neither physiological nor anatomical abnormalities of the brain have been convincingly demonstrated after chronic use of marijuana. One persistent concern is the loss of the work ethos and a possible loss of goal direction. Such concerns arose in the early 1970s with the observation of some American armed forces enlisted men who used high doses of hashish on a chronic basis and exhibited apathy, dullness, impaired judgment, loss of interest in personal appearance, poor hygiene, and some loss of memory. Such effects were reversed when drug use was discontinued. Today this situation, which arises from long-term, high-dose use of cannabis, is called *amotivational syndrome* or *burnout* and is characterized by mental dulling, emotional blunting, and loss of drive and goal directedness.[14] Though marijuana is not the only factor involved, it most likely contributes.

As stated by Cohen:

That some people become ambitionless and sluggish under the influence of a considerable amount of *Cannabis* should not be surprising. THC is a CNS depressant and chronic daytime intoxication with any sedative will demotivate people. The fact that it takes weeks to years for the process to reverse itself is more difficult to explain, and the long retention time of THC in lipids like brain tissue does not directly resolve the issue.[14]

As stated by Jaffe:

Chronic marihuana users may exhibit apathy; dullness; impairment of judgment, concentration, and memory; and loss of interest in personal appearance and pursuit of conventional goals. This has been called the "amotivational syndrome." It is clear that this may be due in part to factors other than the use of cannabis, and it is difficult to know the contribution of drug use in any given case. Cessation may lead to gradual improvement over a period of several weeks. . . . At present there is no evidence to suggest that any personality changes are due to irreversible organic brain damage. The possibility of an adverse effect of frequent or chronic low levels of intoxication on developing personality cannot be dismissed.[15]

The question of whether heavy *Cannabis* use produces long-term effects on the brain remains unanswered. The fact that juveniles are often heavy users causes increased concern. Their brains are still developing and some fear this puts them at higher risk than older individuals who consume the drug. However, two reports concluded that marijuana intoxication has no significant effect on motivation or on cognitive or psychomotor performance.[16,17] The National Commission on Marijuana and Drug Abuse concluded that "if heavy long-term marijuana use is linked to the formation of this complex of social, psychological, and behavioral changes in young people, then it is only one of many contributing factors."[18]

Evidence has recently implicated long-term marijuana use with a degree of immunosuppression, which may render the smoker susceptible to infections, diseases, or cancer. While data in this area are controversial, and implications unproved, marijuana smoking in some circumstances can partially suppress immunity. The clinical significance of this is not known, although it should also be noted that other depressant drugs such as alcohol, barbiturates, benzodiazepines, and anticonvulsants share this immunosuppressive action.

Evidence of *Cannabis*-induced suppression of sexual functioning and reproduction is being gathered. Some studies have demonstrated that chronic use of marijuana in the male can reduce levels of the hormone testosterone[15,19] (Chapter 12) and inhibit sperm formation. Reductions in male fertility and sexual potency, however, have not been reported. Alcohol also reduces testosterone levels. In females, the hormones FSH (follicle stimulating hormone) and LH (leutenizing hormone) are reduced by marijuana. Menstrual cycles can be affected and anovulatory cycles have been reported.[20] Because marijuana freely crosses the placenta, it probably should not be used during pregnancy.

Tolerance and Dependence

It was previously thought that physical dependence on THC did not develop, and, indeed, this appears to be true in recreational users of the drug.[21] Drug withdrawal symptoms, however, are seen in some individuals exposed repeatedly to high doses:

> Abrupt discontinuation of cannabinoids after chronic use of high dosage is followed by irritability, restlessness, nervousness, decreased appetite, weight loss, and insomnia. There is a rebound increase in REM sleep, which is suppressed by marihuana. Tremor, increased body temperature, and chills may also occur. This syndrome, observed under laboratory conditions when high doses of the drug have been used every few hours for several weeks, is relatively mild, begins within a few hours after cessation of drug administration, and lasts about 4 to 5 days. The relationship between this relatively mild syndrome and cannabis-seeking behavior, if any, is unclear.[22]

Tolerance to *Cannabis* is well substantiated in humans and animals. It is thought to result from an adaption of the brain to the continuous presence of the drug rather than from an increased rate of elimination. Soldiers returning from the Far East demonstrated that experienced users were able to tolerate quantities of the drug that were toxic to individuals accustomed to using less. The practical application is that experienced, frequent users of marijuana experience less pronounced physiological and psychological changes at a constant level of use than would less experienced users. This finding leaves little doubt that under conditions of heavier, more regular use, tolerance to THC does develop. Such heavy, long-term use is, however, still only infrequently encountered in this country. Thus, as Szara states,

> I think it is justified to conclude at this point that the development of cannabis-type tolerance and physical dependence—as different from the opiate type—is a theoretical possibility, but its practical significance in a naturalistic setting—if any—is probably slight. . . . In conclusion, the results of studies presented in this volume [*The Pharmacology of Marijuana*] appear to justify the position taken by the *Fourth Marijuana and Health Report:*

Occasional use may impair perception, cognition, and driving ability but does not lead to detectable physical or mental health consequences. Everyday light use is already suspected of producing some deleterious effects and heavy daily use undoubtedly has some consequences in the function of pulmonary, hormonal, and central nervous systems. Exactly what these consequences are and how significant remain the subject of further extensive investigations.[23]

The daily use of low doses does not produce a clinically significant degree of tolerance, unlike that seen in abusers who use high doses. Some degree of cross-tolerance between alcohol and THC has been observed in rats, but there is no cross-tolerance between THC and the psychedelic drugs.[22]

Marijuana and Public Safety

The first reports causally linking the use of marijuana to aggression, violence, and crime appeared during the 1930s. It was felt (with little factual basis) that marijuana led to antisocial acts, to crimes of violence and aggression, and even to the use of opiates.

As the Commission on Marijuana and Drug Abuse stated in 1972:

> In the absence of adequate understanding of the effects of the drug, . . . largely unsubstantiated stories profoundly influenced public opinion and gave birth to the stereotype of the marijuana user as physically aggressive, lacking in self-control, irresponsible, mentally ill and, perhaps most alarming, criminally inclined and dangerous. . . . Now, more than 30 years later many observers are skeptical about the existence of a cause-effect relationship between marijuana use and antisocial conduct.[24]

Major government reports conclude that there is no scientific proof that marijuana use itself is responsible for criminal behavior. There appears to be little or no relationship between marijuana and violent crime. Marijuana is much less likely than alcohol to produce aggressive behavior. If there is any relation between drug use and crime, other psychoactive drugs that produce aggressive behavior (such as alcohol or the amphetamines) are more likely responsible. As the National Commission on Marijuana and Drug Abuse pointed out:

> In essence, neither informed current professional opinion nor empirical research, ranging from the 1930s to the present, has produced systematic evidence to support the thesis that marijuana use, by itself, either invariably or generally leads to or causes crime, including acts of violence, juvenile delinquency, or aggressive behavior. Instead the evidence suggests that so-

ciolegal and cultural variables account for the apparent statistical correlation between marijuana use and crime or delinquency.[25]

The greatest danger to public safety today probably involves driving a car while in a state of acute intoxication. This danger increases dramatically if alcohol has also been ingested.

Conclusions

Based on the previous discussion, what should be society's response to the known pharmacology of marijuana? There is now enough information on the pharmacological and toxicological effects of marijuana to begin formulating new legal policy. Many states, in fact, have already done this by removing felony penalties for simple possession of small amounts. As the National Commission on Marijuana and Drug Abuse reported in 1972, "The State is obliged to justify restraints on individual behavior."[26] Therefore, if the state is to maintain harsh marijuana laws, it should justify their severity.

Perhaps the most conservative course of action might be for society to oppose the widespread use of marijuana as part of an attempt to discourage the use of *all* psychoactive drugs (at least insofar as they might endanger others), and refrain from punishing those who use marijuana (or at least mete out less severe punishment). Such a course of action was proposed by the National Commission on Marijuana and Drug Abuse, which recommended *only* the following changes in federal law:

—Possession of marijuana for personal use would no longer be an offense, but marijuana possessed in public would remain contraband subject to summary seizure and forfeiture.

—Casual distribution of small amounts of marijuana for no remuneration, or insignificant remuneration not involving profit, would no longer be an offense.[24]

The Commission further recommended that a plea of marijuana intoxication shall not be a defense to any criminal act committed under its influence, nor shall proof of such intoxication constitute a negation of specific intent.[27]

These changes would essentially "decriminalize" the possession of marijuana in all states, and individuals apprehended with small quantities would no longer be subject to a punishment that many regard as more severe than the offense. The product would *not* be legalized, the state would continue to discourage its use, but those in possession of small amounts would not be subject to punishment.

Though marijuana is not a "killer weed," it is *not* an innocuous substance, devoid of toxicity. The legal statutes should protect users, nonusers who might be affected by intoxicated users, and juveniles who might not be able to make rational decisions concerning the risks and benefits of the drug. It is up to society to determine the extent and mechanism through which protection is offered.

The explosive increase in marijuana use seen in the 1970s now appears to have leveled off, and it may be reaching a point of social acceptance or tolerance. States that have not yet "decriminalized" marijuana possession are recognizing the reality of widespread marijuana use and are considering decriminalization. It is also becoming clear that there is little evidence to support the contention that marijuana use displaces the use of alcohol and other psychoactive drugs. Those who use marijuana are also likely to use alcohol, often simultaneously.[8] The more heavily the user smokes marijuana, the greater the likelihood that he or she has used or will use other drugs. Such drug use may be related to a "drug-use proneness" and involvement with other drug users rather than to the characteristics of marijuana per se.

It appears, then, that society is accepting and tolerating (although not yet approving) the social use of marijuana as a recreational drug. Legal guidelines for recreational use and limitations, however, are still far from decided.

Notes

1. R. L. Hawks and C. N. Chiang, "Examples of Specific Drug Assays," in "Urine Testing for Drug Abuse," NIDA Research Monograph No. 73 National Institute on Drug Abuse, (Washington, D.C.: U.S. Government Printing Office, 1986), p. 87.

2. J. H. Jaffe, "Drug Addiction and Drug Abuse," in A. G. Gilman, L. S. Goodman, T. W. Rall, and F. Murad, eds., *Goodman and Gilman's The Pharmacological Basis of Therapeutics*, 7th ed. (New York: Macmillan, 1985), p. 559.

3. S. Cohen, "Adverse Effects of Marijuana: Selected Issues," in *Research Developments in Drug and Alcohol Use, Annals of The New York Academy of Science* 362 (1981): 119.

4. D. I. Hoffman, K. D. Brunemann, G. B. Gori, and E. L. Wynder, "On the Carcinogenicity of Marijuana Smoke," *Recent Advances in Phytochemistry* 9 (1975): 63–81.

5. S. Cohen, "Adverse Effects of Marijuana: Selected Issues," in *Research Developments in Drug and Alcohol Use, Annals of The New York Academy of Science* 362 (1981): 120.

6. J. D. Blaine, N. P. Meacham, D. S. Janowsky, M. Schoor, and L. P. Bozzetti, "Marihuana Smoking in Simulated Flying Performance," in M. C. Braude and S. Szara, eds., *The Pharmacology of Marijuana*, vol. 1 (New York: Raven Press, 1976), pp. 445–447.

7. See H. Klonoff, "Marijuana and Driving in Real-Life Situations," *Sci-*

ence 186 (25 October 1974): 317–324 and R. W. Hansteen, D. Miller, L. Lonero, L. D. Reid, and B. Jones, "Effects of Cannabis and Alcohol in Automobile Driving and Psychomotor Tracking," *Annals of the New York Academy of Sciences* 282 (1976): 240–256.

8. "National Survey on Drug Abuse: Main Findings, 1982," U.S. Department of Health and Human Services (Washington, D.C.: U.S. Government Printing Office, 1983), pp. 27–42.

9. R. E. Willette, ed., *Drugs and Driving,* National Institute on Drug Abuse, monograph No. 11, (Washington, D.C.: U.S. Government Printing Office, 1977).

10. K. O. Fehr, and H. Kalant (eds.), *Cannabis and Health Hazards* (Toronto: The Addiction Research Foundation, 1983.)

11. R. T. Jones, "Cannabis and Health." *Annual Review of Medicine* 34 (1983): 247–258.

12. *The Health Consequences of Smoking: The Changing Cigarette,* A Report of the Surgeon General (Washington, D.C.: U.S. Government Printing Office, 1981), pp. 81–85.

13. G. G. Dimijian, "Contemporary Drug Abuse," in A. Goth, ed., *Medical Pharmacology,* 11th ed., (St. Louis: Mosby, 1984), p. 346.

14. S. Cohen, "Adverse Effects of Marijuana: Selected Issues," in *Research Developments in Drug and Alcohol Use, Annals of The New York Academy of Science* 362 (1981): 123.

15. J. H. Jaffe, "Drug Addiction and Abuse," in A. G. Gilman, L. S. Goodman, T. W. Rall, and F. Murad, eds., *Goodman and Gilman's The Pharmacological Basis of Therapeutics,* 7th ed. (New York: Macmillan, 1985), p. 560.

16. P. J. Lessin and S. A. Thomas, "Assessment of the Chronic Effects of Marihuana on Motivation and Achievement: A Preliminary Report," in M. C. Braude and S. Szara, eds., *The Pharmacology of Marihuana,* vol. 2 (New York: Raven Press, 1976), pp. 681–683.

17. R. L. Dornbush, A. M. Freedman, and M. Fink, eds., "Chronic Cannabis Use," *Annals of the New York Academy of Sciences* 282 (1976): 1–57.

18. R. L. Dornbush, A. M. Freedman, and M. Fink, eds., "Chronic Cannabis Use," *Annals of the New York Academy of Sciences* 282 (1976): 76 (fn. 7).

19. R. C. Koldny, P. Lessin, G. Toro, W. H. Masters, and S. Cohen, "Depression of Plasma Testosterone with Acute Marihuana Administration," in M. C. Braude and S. Szara, eds., *The Pharmacology of Marihuana,* vol. 1 (New York: Raven Press, 1976), pp. 217–225.

20. B. Mantilla-Plata and R. D. Harbison, "Influences of Alteration of Tetrahydrocannabinol Metabolism on Tetrahydro-Cannabinol-induced Teratogenesis," in M. C. Braude and S. Szara, eds., *The Pharmacology of Marihuana,* vol. 2 (New York: Raven Press, 1976), pp. 733–742.

21. Secretary of Health, Education, and Welfare, *Marihuana and Health,* 7th Report to the U.S. Congress (Washington, D.C.: U.S. Government Printing Office, 1977).

22. J. H. Jaffe, "Drug Addiction and Drug Abuse," in A. G. Gilman, L. S. Goodman, T. W. Rall, and F. Murad, eds., *Goodman and Gilman's The Pharmacological Basis of Therapeutics,* 7th ed. (New York: Macmillan, 1985), p. 561.

23. S. Szara, in M. C. Braude and S. Szara, eds., *The Pharmacology of Marihuana,* vol. 2 (New York: Raven Press, 1976), p. 690.

24. National Commission on Marihuana and Drug Abuse, *Marihuana: A*

Signal of Misunderstanding, R. P. Shafer, Chairman (New York: Signet, 1972), p. 85.

25. National Commission on Marihuana and Drug Abuse, *Marihuana: A Signal of Misunderstanding,* R. P. Shafer, Chairman (New York: Signet, 1972), p. 94.

26. National Commission on Marihuana and Drug Abuse, *Marihuana: A Signal of Misunderstanding,* R. P. Shafer, Chairman (New York: Signet, 1972), p. 159.

27. National Commission on Marihuana and Drug Abuse, *Marihuana: A Signal of Misunderstanding,* R. P. Shafer, Chairman (New York: Signet, 1972), p. 191.

CHAPTER 11

Neurological Drugs

Previous editions of this text focused primarily on drugs that are classified as psychoactive and, therefore, are frequently subject to abuse. However, because there is increasing interest in the broader scope of drug action, this chapter extends our discussion of neuropharmacology, covering five types of drugs not included in previous editions. These agents include antiepileptic drugs, antiparkinsonian drugs, drugs to treat spasticity and muscle spasms, nonnarcotic analgesics, and local anesthetics.

Antiepileptic Drugs

Seizures are manifestations of electrical disturbances of the brain. The term *epilepsy* refers to CNS disorders characterized by seizures of rapid onset, relatively brief duration, and with a tendency toward chronic recurrence. The prevalence of epilepsy within our society is exhibited by approximately 5 individuals per 1000 population.

Most seizure disorders do not spontaneously disappear and they are only occasionally amenable to surgical therapy. Indeed, drug therapy of epilepsy is the only widely applicable, effective mode of treatment. To aid in drug treatment, the various types of seizure disorders are broadly classified into two groups: generalized seizures and partial seizures, with multiple subdivisions of each type (Table 11.1). Indeed, it is imperative that the type of seizure is characterized accurately because drug therapy for this disorder is quite selective.

Mechanism of Action

Table 11.2 lists the available antiepileptic drugs and the years during which they were introduced. Although the exact mechanisms of

Table 11.1

Classification of epileptic seizures

Seizure type		Characteristics
I. Partial seizures (focal, local seizures)	A. Simple partial seizures	Various manifestations, without impairment of consciousness, including convulsions confined to a single limb or muscle group (*Jacksonian motor epilepsy*), specific and localized sensory disturbances (*Jacksonian sensory epilepsy*), and other limited signs and symptoms depending upon the particular cortical area producing the abnormal discharge
	B. Complex partial seizures	Attacks of confused behavior, with impairment of consciousness, with a wide variety of clinical manifestations, associated with bizarre generalized EEG activity during the seizure but with evidence of anterior temporal lobe focal abnormalities even in the interseizure period in many cases
	C. Partial seizures secondarily generalized	
II. Generalized seizures (convulsive or nonconvulsive)	A.1. Absence seizures	Brief and abrupt loss of consciousness associated with high-voltage, bilaterally synchronous, 3-per-second spike-and-wave pattern in the EEG, usually with some symmetrical clonic motor activity varying from eyelid blinking to jerking of the entire body, sometimes with no motor activity
	A.2. Atypical absence seizures	Attacks with slower onset and cessation than is usual for absence seizures, associated with a more heterogeneous EEG
	B. Myoclonic seizures	Isolated clonic jerks associated with brief bursts of multiple spikes in the EEG
	C. Clonic seizures	Rhythmic clonic contractions of all muscles, loss of consciousness, and marked autonomic manifestations
	D. Tonic seizures	Opisthotonus, loss of consciousness, and marked autonomic manifestations

Table 11.1 (*continued*)

Classification of epileptic seizures

Seizure type		Characteristics
II. Generalized seizures (convulsive or nonconvulsive)	E. Tonic-clonic seizures (grand mal)	Major convulsions, usually a sequence of maximal tonic spasm of all body musculature followed by synchronous clonic jerking and a prolonged depression of all central functions
	F. Atonic seizures	Loss of postural tone, with sagging of the head or falling

SOURCE: [T. W. Rall and L. S. Shleifer, "Drugs Effective in the Therapy of the Epilepsies," in A. G. Gilman, L. S. Goodman, T. W. Rall, and F. Murad, eds., Goodman and Gilman's *The Pharmacological Basis of Therapeutics*, 7th ed. (New York: Macmillan, 1985), p. 447.]

Table 11.2

Antiepileptic drugs available in the United States.

Year introduced	Generic name	Trade name
1912	phenobarbital	Luminal
1935	mephobarbital	Mebaral
1938	phenytoin	Dilantin
1946	trimethadione	Tridione
1947	mephenytoin	Mesantoin
1949	paramethadione	Paradione
1951	phenacetamide	Phenurone
1952	metharbital	Gemonil
1953	phensuximide	Milontin
1954	primidone	Mysoline
1957	methsuximide	Celontin
1957	ethotoin	Peganone
1960	ethosuximide	Zarontin
1968	diazepam	Valium
1974	carbamazepine	Tegretol
1975	clonazepam	Clonopin
1978	valproic acid	Depakene
1981	clorazepate	Tranxene
	lorazepam	Ativan

SOURCE: Modified from R. M. Julien, "Antiepileptic Drugs," in N. T. Smith and A. N. Corbascio, eds., *Drug Interactions in Anesthesia*, 2d ed. (Philadelphia: Lea & Febiger, 1986), p. 246.

action of antiepileptic drugs remain obscure, two general ways exist in which drugs might exert their antiepileptic actions. First, drugs might act directly on a site of abnormal electrical activity within the brain to decrease its excitability. Second, drugs might act on adjacent nonepileptic neurons to limit their involvement in the spread of seizure activity that occurs at a site distant from the abnormal electrical discharge. Most currently available antiepileptic drugs appear to act primarily (or at least in part) by the second mechanism; that is, they limit the spread of epileptic activity. Postulated mechanisms include stabilizing the membranes of normal neurons and reinforcing the activity of inhibitory neurons, which serve to increase the inhibitory functions of the brain. Indeed, current research aimed at developing new antiepileptic drugs is focused on agents that may selectively reinforce the functional activity of GABA neurons in a manner similar to that produced by the benzodiazepines (Chapter 3). As discussed in the following section, certain of the benzodiazepines are among the more effective antiepileptic drugs available.

Structure-Activity Relationships

The majority of antiepileptic drugs belong to one of a relatively small number of chemical classes (Table 11.2), many of which have already been discussed. The *barbiturates* are the oldest of these drugs and, until recent years, these and the *hydantoins* [of which phenytoin (Dilantin) is the prototype] were the most widely used antiepileptic compounds. More recently, several *benzodiazepines* have been found to be exceedingly useful. Older drugs that are structurally similar to either the barbiturates or the hydantoins (but are slightly altered to make them chemically unique) and that are used in the treatment of epilepsy include the *succinimides*, the *oxazoladines*, and *primidone* (Mysoline). Finally, two newer agents are structurally dissimilar but, nevertheless, are effective in treating seizures: *carbamazepine* (Tegretol) and *valproic acid* (Depakene). Carbamazepine structurally resembles both phenytoin and imipramine, while valproic acid exerts specific actions at GABA synapses. Structures of representative drugs are shown in Figure 11.1.

Plasma levels of antiepileptic drugs can be determined by chemical assay and a correlation can be made with the level at which seizures are controlled. Indeed, by measuring drug concentrations in plasma, a physician may be assisted in finding the optimal pharmacological treatment for controlling seizures. Continuing progress in this area has led to seizure control in approximately 50 percent of epileptic patients and significant improvement in at least half of those remaining. Ongoing search for new drugs and improved tech-

Figure 11.1

Representative drugs used in the treatment of epilepsy.

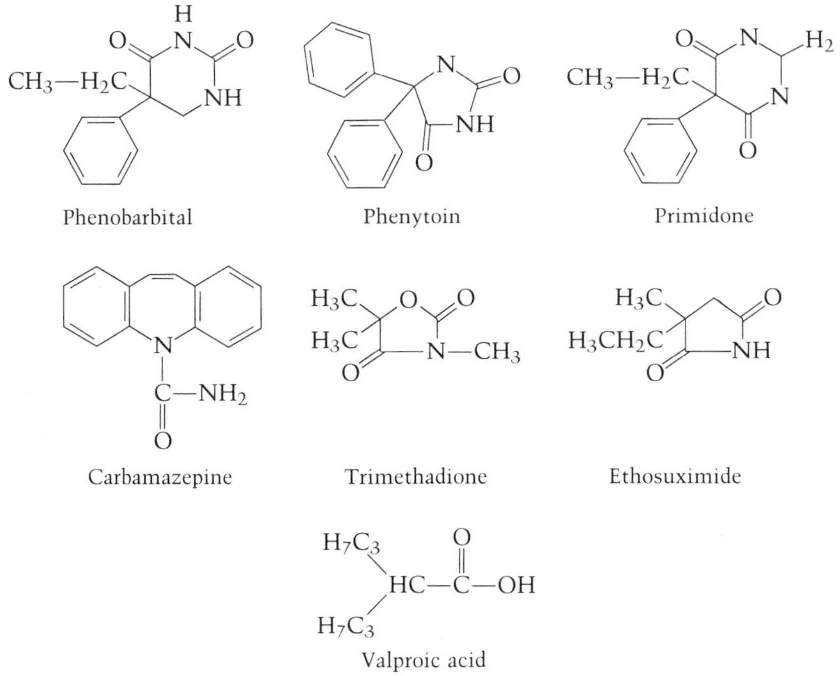

Phenobarbital

Phenytoin

Primidone

Carbamazepine

Trimethadione

Ethosuximide

Valproic acid

niques to monitor drug therapy is promising for the treatment of those patients who do not respond to currently available therapies.

Barbiturates

The pharmacology of the barbiturates was presented in Chapter 3: the barbiturates presumably exert antiepileptic effects as a result of general depression of the CNS. Phenobarbital was the first widely effective antiepileptic drug (introduced in 1912), replacing the more toxic agent, bromide, which had been used for many years earlier. Two other barbiturates are occasionally used for treating epilepsy: mephobarbital (Mebaral) and metharbital (Gemonil).

Because of their relative lack of toxicity, these drugs are still being used despite the fact that more effective, more specific, and less sedating antiepileptic agents are now available. The barbiturates are primarily useful for treating generalized seizures, but they are much less effective in persons who experience partial seizures. The durations of action of these drugs are quite long, so doses can be administered only once each day. The primary disadvantages of giving these drugs to children are the behavioral hyperactivity and interference with learning ability that follow. *Primidone* (Mysoline) is an antiepileptic agent that is structurally very similar to phenobarbital (Figure 11.1). Primidone is metabolized to phenobarbital, which might well be the major active form of the drug.

Hydantoins

Phenytoin (Dilantin), introduced in 1938, is the prototype hydantoin anticonvulsant, and it is still one of the most widely used and effective of the available antiepileptic drugs. It is used primarily for major motor seizures. At an effective dose level, it produces less sedation than occurs with the barbiturates. Phenytoin appears to act by exerting a stabilizing effect on neuronal membranes, limiting their involvement in the spread of seizure activity. The drug is slowly, but completely, absorbed orally and has a half-life of about 24 hours, which allows for once a day administration. Thus, daytime sedation can be minimized if the patient takes the full daily dose at bedtime.

Although the sedative effects of phenytoin are lower than those of the barbiturates, other toxicities are more significant. Ataxia (postural instability with staggering) and nystagmus are quite common. The drug interferes with vitamin D metabolism, and alterations of calcium metabolism and bone formation may occur. Hypertrophy of the gums occurs and results in gingival and dental problems. Hirsutism (abnormal growth of hair) is common and quite annoying to female patients. If phenytoin is administered to pregnant patients, fetal abnormalities frequently occur. Despite these toxicities, however, phenytoin is widely used and reasonably well tolerated for the long-term control of seizures. Failure to respond to phenytoin at therapeutic blood levels usually indicates the need to add additional drugs to the prescribed regimen.

Benzodiazepines

The pharmacology of the benzodiazepines was presented in Chapter 3. Of available agents, clonazepam (Klonopin) and clorazepate (Tranxene) are frequently used for the treatment of seizures, especially drug-resistant patients or those who suffer from seizure types that are difficult to treat. Diazepam (Valium) and midazolam (Versed) are administered intravenously to control status epilepticus rapidly (an emergency situation characterized by rapidly recurring, intense seizures).

Benzodiazepines inhibit the spread of seizures by facilitating GABA neurotransmission (Chapter 3 and Appendix II). The toxicity of benzodiazepines is relatively low (Chapter 3). Because these drugs are used frequently for treatment of chronic seizures in children, drug-induced personality changes and learning disabilities must be carefully sought and evaluated.

Miscellaneous Antiepileptic Drugs

Carbamazepine (Tegretol) and *valproic acid* (Depakene) are two of the newest antiepileptic drugs. Carbamazepine is structurally related to the tricyclic antidepressants. Its profile of effectiveness is similar to that of phenytoin, although carbamazepine is also quite effective in the treatment of psychomotor types of epilepsy (a seizure type not affected by phenytoin). Possibly because of its structural resemblance to imipramine, its sedative effects are much lower than those of the other antiepileptic agents. The primary limitations of carbamazepine include rare, but potentially serious, alterations in the cellular composition of blood, presumably secondary to effects on the bone marrow.

Valproic acid is a simple organic compound (Figure 11.1) that was approved for use in patients with epilepsy in 1978. It suppresses a wide variety of seizure types and is quite effective in petit mal seizures in children. The drug augments the postsynaptic action of GABA on its receptors within the nervous system. Valproic acid is rapidly absorbed, but its short half-life necessitates divided daily dosage. The drug is particularly effective in patients in whom other drug therapy has failed; and seizure reductions have been observed in the majority of such patients. About 75 percent of epileptic patients respond favorably to the drug. Serious toxicities associated with valproic acid are rare, although gastric upset is observed in a large percentage of patients at the beginning of drug therapy.

Older, seldom used antiepileptic agents include such compounds as acetazolamide (Diamox), the oxazolidinediones trimethadione (Tridione) and paramethadione (Paradione), and the succinimides ethosuximide (Zarontin), methsuximide (Celontin), and phensuximide (Milontin).

For the interested reader, general principles regarding the choice of drugs for the treatment of epileptic seizures are listed in the readings located at the end of this chapter.[1-4]

Antiparkinsonian Drugs

Parkinson's disease affects approximately 500,000 persons in the United States alone, with most cases occurring in persons over the age of 55 years. Although the cause of parkinsonism remains unknown, it is clear that it results from an alteration in the function of dopamine-secreting neurons within the basal ganglia of the brain (Appendix II). At its simplest, functional activity of the basal ganglia is determined by a balance of dopamine-secreting (inhibitory) and acetylcholine-secreting (excitatory) neurons. In 1960, it was reported that patients with parkinsonism demonstrated a marked deficiency of dopamine in their basal ganglia. Subsequent work has led to the hypothesis that parkinsonism may be caused by a loss of dopamine neurons within the basal ganglia. Thus, therapy is aimed at restoring these levels of dopamine and, as an additional effect, antagonizing the excitatory effects of the acetylcholine neurons that remain and function unopposed by dopaminergic inhibitory neurons.[5-6]

Pharmacological Treatment of Parkinsonism

Levo-DOPA   Because the loss of dopamine is the primary deficiency in patients with Parkinson's disease, it was postulated that replacement of the dopamine might ameliorate the symptoms of the disease. However, dopamine does not cross the blood-brain barrier into the brain from the blood. Therefore, it is not useful therapeutically. However, DOPA (DihydroxyPhenylAlanine) (Appendix II, Figure II.5) has been found to be the immediate precursor of dopamine, and this compound does cross the blood-brain barrier. Administered orally, levo-DOPA (an isomer of naturally occurring DOPA) is rapidly absorbed and converted to dopamine in the blood. Although only small amounts of levo-DOPA penetrate the blood-brain barrier and are converted to dopamine within the brain, even those small amounts are effective in alleviating the symptoms of parkinsonism. The remaining high levels of dopamine in the systemic circulation produce nausea, vomiting, cardiac arrhythmias, and blood pressure alterations. Thus, such therapy, although effective, is obviously not optimal, and some method is needed to reduce the high levels of dopamine in the systemic circulation while maintaining sufficient quantities in the brain.

Referring to the biosynthetic pathway of dopamine (Appendix II), one sees that the enzyme *DOPA decarboxylase* is necessary for the conversion of DOPA to dopamine. Thus, by inhibiting this enzyme in the systemic circulation (but not the brain), systemic biotransformation of the drug should be reduced, with a concomitant reduction in dopamine levels and thus in side effects. In other words, if this DOPA-decarboxylase inhibitor did not cross the blood-brain barrier, then the DOPA that crossed the blood-brain barrier into the brain could still be converted to dopamine and the symptoms of parkinsonism would be relieved without the same degree of systemic effects. An example of such a peripherally restricted DOPA-decarboxylase inhibitor is the drug *carbidopa* (available in combination with levodopa as *Sinemet*). Combination of carbidopa with levo-DOPA allows a greater portion of the levo-DOPA to reach the CNS where it is biotransformed in the brain to dopamine. Thus, the current treatment of parkinsonism relies heavily on this combination of levo-DOPA with carbidopa.

Adverse Effects   Administration of levo-DOPA, even with carbidopa, has adverse effects. Nausea, vomiting, abnormal involuntary muscle movements, and psychiatric disturbances can still occur. The drug must be used with caution in patients with hypertension or cardiac disease.

Other Drugs for Parkinsonism

Amantadine (Symmetrel)   Amantadine is an antiviral agent primarily used for the prevention of certain types of influenza (flu). Several years ago, it was reported that amantadine would relieve the symptoms of parkinsonism. The mechanism responsible for such action is unclear, but the drug probably releases dopamine from whatever dopamine neurons remain within the patient's basal ganglia. Amantadine also appears to potentiate the therapeutic effects of levodopa, although such potentiation is not consistent. Thus, amantadine is much less effective than levodopa for long-term relief of the symptoms of parkinsonism. Adverse effects include slurred speech, ataxia, gastric distress, hallucinations, confusion, and nightmares.

Anticholinergic Drugs   Prior to the introduction of levodopa, use of the anticholinergic drugs comprised the most effective treatment for the symptoms of parkinsonism. These drugs apparently worked by blocking the excitatory cholinergic (acetylcholine) neurons that persist in the basal ganglia following degeneration of the inhibitory dopamine neurons. Representative agents include trihexyphenidyl (Artane), procylidine (Kemadrin), and biperiden (Akineton). Significant side effects include blurred vision, constipation, urinary retention, mental confusion, and delerium. Today, these agents are used only when levodopa therapy has failed or has been suboptimal.

Antihistamines   Diphenhydramine (Benadryl) and other histamine blocking agents have long been used to treat the symptoms of parkinsonism. Efficacy is presumably achieved because of the anticholinergic side effects produced by these drugs. With the advent of levodopa, antihistamines are seldom used today for this purpose.

Bromocriptine (Parlodel)   Bromocriptine (an ergot derivative) is structurally similar to dopamine. It is a potent stimulant of dopamine receptors, which has led to its occasional use with levodopa in the management of patients who do not respond adequately to levodopa therapy alone. Dopamine-like side effects are produced and include gastric distress, cardiac arrhythmias, hypertension, hallucinations, and behavioral arousal.

Drugs Used to Treat Spasticity and Muscle Spasms

Spasticity is a term that refers to abnormal increases in skeletal muscle tone: increases that result from a dysfunction in the CNS.[7-8] Reflexes are hyperactive because the regulation of motor control is lost. There are multiple causes of spasticity, some of which include head injury, stroke, multiple sclerosis, spinal cord trauma, and cerebral palsy. The most effective agents for controlling spasticity include two drugs that act predominantly within the CNS, baclofen (Lioresal) and diazepam (Valium), and one, dantrolene (Dantrium), which acts directly on skeletal muscles.[9]

Baclofen
Baclofen (Lioresal) is a derivative of GABA (Figure 11.2). It reduces muscle tone and muscle spasm by altering the transmission of reflexes that travel through the polysynaptic reflex loops located in the spinal cord. This may occur as a result of stimulation of GABA receptors, which inhibits the release of glutamic acid and aspartic acid, the excitatory amino acid transmitters (Appendix II).

Baclofen appears to be more effective than either diazepam or dantrolene in relieving spasms. It is well absorbed orally and has a relatively short half-life in plasma, necessitating multiple daily doses. Side effects include drowsiness, lassitude, dizziness, ataxia, and muscle weakness.

Diazepam (Valium)
As discussed in Chapter 3, diazepam is a benzodiazepine that exerts its effects by facilitating GABA neurotransmission. It is somewhat less effective than baclofen in relieving spasticity. Sedation and ataxia are the primary limiting side effects of diazepam.

Figure 11.2

Structure of GABA and three drugs used in the treatment of spasticity. Note the resemblance of baclofen to GABA.

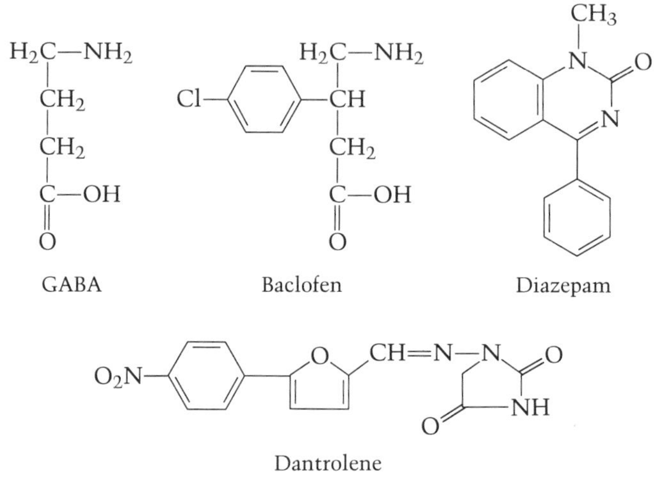

GABA

Baclofen

Diazepam

Dantrolene

Dantrolene (Dantrium)

Dantrolene is unique among the antispastic agents because it acts directly on skeletal muscle.[10] Its site of action is unlike that of the neuromuscular blocking agents, which produce complete muscle paralysis by blocking postsynaptic receptors at the neuromuscular junction. Dantrolene acts at a site within the muscle fiber itself and interferes with the release of calcium ions from the sarcoplasmic reticulum, blocking excitation/contraction coupling, and therefore interfering with the primary process of muscle contraction. Unfortunately, this process is not specific for hypertonic (spastic) muscles, and a generalized muscle weakness is produced. Such weakness tends to limit patient compliance in taking the drug, which negates the improvements the drug can produce (that is, patients who take dantrolene generally feel "weak").

When anesthesia is administered, dantrolene is the drug of choice in alleviating a rare but previously fatal syndrome termed *malignant hyperthermia*, which occurs in certain genetically predisposed individuals.[11] This syndrome only occurs once every 10,000 times that an anesthetic is given and is triggered by certain anesthetic agents; it involves the drug-induced, massive release of calcium from the sarcoplasmic reticulum, an action that is effectively blocked by an intravenous infusion of dantrolene.

Side effects of dantrolene include muscle weakness, drowsiness, and diarrhea. In rare instances, an allergic-type destruction of the liver can occur that can be fatal.

Therapeutic Status

As stated by Bianchine:[12]

There is no completely satisfactory form of therapy for alleviation of skeletal muscle spasticity. While drugs such as baclofen, diazepam and dantrolene are capable of providing variable relief of spasticity in given circumstances, troublesome muscle weakness, adverse effects on gait and a variety of other side effects minimize their overall usefulness.

Muscle Spasms

In everyday life, a variety of situations can produce acute muscle spasm and pain. Numerous drugs have been employed to provide temporary, symptomatic relief of such discomfort. These drugs include anti-inflammatory analgesics (such as aspirin), sedative "muscle relaxants" (such as diazepam and meprobamate), heat, and massage. In general, all have limited usefulness but do provide some relief until the natural healing process occurs. The combination of time, rest, and physical therapy, combined with the pharmacological provision of analgesia and sedation are all of benefit.

Nonnarcotic Analgesics

The nonnarcotic analgesics are a group of chemically unrelated drugs (Figure 11.3) that produce both analgesic and anti-inflam-

Figure 11.3

Chemical structures of anti-inflammatory analgesics.

Aspirin   Ibuprofen

Phenylbutazone   Indomethacin   Acetaminophen

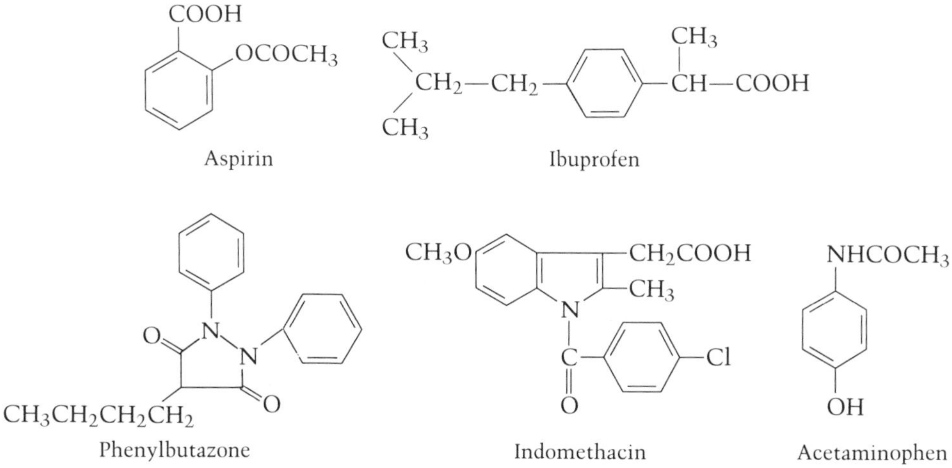

matory effects by inhibiting the synthesis and release of prosta-glandins.[13-14] The effects produced by these drugs include (1) a re-duction of inflammation (anti-inflammatory effect), (2) a reduction in body temperature during fever (antipyretic effect), (3) a reduction in pain without sedation (analgesic effect), and (4) an inhibition of platelet aggregation (anticoagulant effect).

Drugs classified as nonnarcotic analgesics include aspirin and other salicylates, ibuprofen, acetaminophen, indomethacin, and phenylbutazone.

Many of these drugs are used to reduce both the inflammation and the pain associated with arthritic disease. Gastric irritation serves to limit the long-term usefulness of these compounds.

Aspirin

In the United States, about 10 to 20 thousand tons of aspirin are consumed each year; it is our most popular analgesic. Despite (or perhaps because of) this widespread use, aspirin is one of our most effective analgesic, antipyretic, and anti-inflammatory agents. It is most effective for low-intensity pain, and one should note that these drugs do not act on opiate receptors within the CNS (Appendix II).

The antipyretic (fever-reducing) effect of aspirin appears to act by inhibiting prostaglandin synthesis in the hypothalamus, a struc-ture in the brain that modulates body temperature (Appendix III).

Aspirin increases oxygen consumption by the body, increasing carbon dioxide production—an effect that stimulates respiration. Therefore, overdose with aspirin is often characterized by marked increases in respiratory rate, which cause the overdosed individual to appear to pant. This occurrence results in other, severe, metabolic consequences that are beyond the present discussion.

Aspirin exerts important effects on blood coagulation. For blood to coagulate, platelets must first be able to aggregate; and prosta-glandins appear to be necessary for that occurrence. (Platelets are small components of the blood that, following vessel injury, adhere to injured vascular membranes, forming an initial plug over which a blood clot eventually forms to limit bleeding from a lacerated blood vessel.) Aspirin can inhibit platelet aggregation, reducing the for-mation of intravascular clots. Low doses of aspirin (for example, one tablet daily) are now widely used for prophylaxis against strokes and heart attacks, which can be caused by atherosclerosis, intravascular clotting, or emboli formation on either artificial or damaged heart valves.

Side effects of aspirin are common; gastric upset occurs most frequently. In addition, poisoning with aspirin occurs thousands of times each year and such poisoning can be fatal. Mild intoxication can produce ringing in the ears, auditory and visual difficulties, mental confusion, thirst, and hyperventilation. More serious toxicity produces severe disturbances in body metabolism, and these disturbances can lead to severe cardiac and kidney dysfunction.

Acetaminophen

Acetaminophen (Tylenol) is an effective alternative to aspirin as an analgesic and antipyretic agent. However, its anti-inflammatory effect is minor and not clinically useful. It is commonly felt that acetaminophen may have fewer side effects than aspirin, but it should be noted that an acute overdose (either accidental or intentional) may produce severe or even fatal liver damage. Acetaminophen does not inhibit platelet aggregation and therefore is not useful for preventing vascular clotting.

Side effects of acetaminophen are generally fewer than those of aspirin; the drug produces less gastric distress and less ringing in the ears. However, as stated previously, overdose can lead to severe damage to the liver.

Acetaminophen has been proved to be a reasonable substitute for aspirin when analgesic or antipyretic effectiveness is desired, especially in patients who cannot tolerate aspirin. This might include patients with peptic ulcer disease or gastric distress or those in whom the anticoagulant action of aspirin might be undesirable.

Ibuprofen

Ibuprofen (Advil, Motrin) is a relatively new aspirinlike analgesic, antipyretic, and anti-inflammatory agent. Compounds similar to ibuprofen include *naproxen* (Naprosyn, Anaprox) and *fenoprofen* (Nalfon). Of these three drugs, only ibuprofen is available without a prescription.

All three of these compounds are effective analgesics, anti-inflammatory agents, and antipyretics. These actions presumably occur secondary to drug-induced inhibition of prostaglandin synthesis. The incidence and severity of side effects produced by these agents are somewhat lower than those of aspirin, but gastric distress and the formation of peptic ulcers have been reported. Like aspirin and unlike acetaminophen, these compounds inhibit platelet aggregation and thus they interfere with the clotting process. These drugs should therefore be used with caution in patients with peptic ulcer disease or bleeding abnormalities. At the present time, ibuprofen is not recommended for use by pregnant women or by women who are breast-feeding their infants.

Phenylbutazone

Phenylbutazone (Butazolidin) is an older, effective anti-inflammatory agent that was used widely at one time to relieve the inflammation associated with rheumatoid arthritis. However, significant toxicities have limited its long-term usefulness. Unlike most of the other anti-inflammatory drugs, its half-life is quite long (about 2 days).

Most patients who take phenylbutazone experience some degree of toxicity, usually in the form of gastric distress and skin rashes. More severe toxicities include ulcer formation, allergies, liver and renal dysfunction, and a variety of quite severe abnormalities in various types of blood cells. At the present time, phenylbutazone is considered to be a secondary choice of treatment for the symptoms of rheumatoid arthritis and other similar disorders.

Indomethacin

Indomethacin (Indocin) is an effective anti-inflammatory drug that is used primarily for the treatment of rheumatoid arthritis and similar disorders. Like phenylbutazone, its use is limited because of its toxicities. Indomethacin is analgesic and antipyretic as well as being anti-inflammatory. Indeed, its clinical effects closely resemble those of aspirin. Side effects occur in about 50 percent of the patients taking indomethacin, with gastric dysfunction being most prominent. Paradoxically, drug-induced headache limits its use in many patients. Other toxicities are rare but potentially serious.

Indomethacin-induced toxicities limit its routine use, except in certain arthritic patients who have not responded to other types of therapy.

Local Anesthetics

Local anesthetics are drugs that temporarily interrupt the conduction of electrical impulses in nerve tissue.[15–17] An *ideal* local anesthetic should not irritate the tissues to which it is applied; it should not cause any damage to nerve structures; it should not be toxic after it is absorbed from the site of injection into the bloodstream; and it should have a predictable duration of action. It should be noted that none of the available local anesthetics meet all of these requirements. Also, reversibility of action is mandatory because normal nerve conduction must be regained after the drug has been eliminated from the body's tissues.

Mechanism of Action

Local anesthetics block the conduction of nerve impulses by acting directly on nerve cell membranes. At appropriate concentrations, sensory, autonomic, and motor nerve fibers can all be completely, yet reversibly, blocked. As discussed in Appendix I, the neuronal membrane is a semipermeable, lipid-protein structure that separates sodium and potassium ions across the membranes, maintaining a resting electrical potential of 75–90 mV. Thus, the interior side of the membrane is negatively charged relative to its exterior side. Transient fluctuations occur in the sodium-ion permeability as electrical impulses are conducted through the axons of the neuron. However, when the axons are at rest, the channels through which the sodium ions travel are blocked by calcium ions. Thus, the prevailing theory holds that local anesthetics act by displacing calcium ions from the inner surface of the neuronal membrane, blocking the sodium channels and preventing the depolarization-induced movement of sodium ions across the membranes. This action blocks the process of depolarization and nerve-impulse propagation.

Classification

The chemical structure of local anesthetics is comprised of three parts: each molecule includes an aromatic ring, an intermediate chain, and a nitrogen-containing portion (Figure 11.4). The aromatic ring accounts for the fat solubility of the anesthetic; and the nitrogen-containing portion (the amine portion) accounts for its water

Figure 11.4

Structural formulas of procaine and lidocaine, illustrating the three-part structure of each. Reproduced from R. M. Julien, *Understanding Anesthesia* (Stoneham, MA: Butterworth Publishers, 1984), p. 121, with permission of the publisher.

Three-part structure	Aromatic ring	Intermediate chain	Amine portion
Procaine			
Lidocaine			

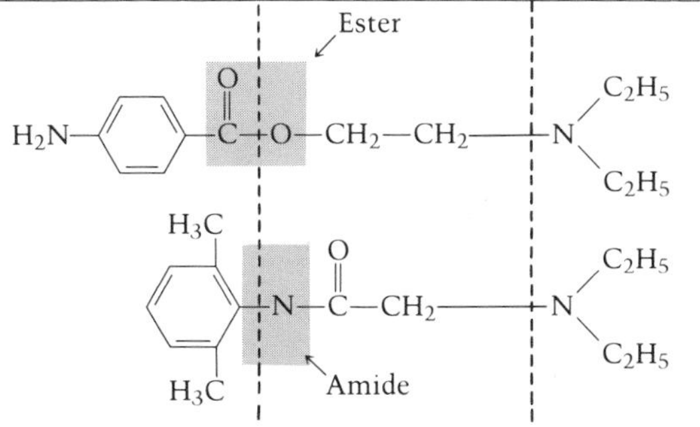

solubility. Changes in either portion alter the fat-water distribution of the drug and thus affect its duration of action. The intermediate chain can be comprised of either an ester or an amide. Anesthetics that contain ester intermediate chains are metabolized in the plasma by an enzyme called *plasma cholinesterase,* whereas anesthetics that contain an amide intermediate chain are metabolized by enzymes in the liver. The metabolic end product of the ester-type anesthetics is para-aminobenzoic acid, a compound that contributes to the development of allergic reactions in a small percentage of patients. However, allergic reactions to the amide-type of local anesthetics are extremely rare. Table 11.3 classifies local anesthetics by their intermediate chain as well as by their potencies and durations of action. With the exception of tetracaine, the ester-type of local anesthetics are less potent and have a shorter duration of action than the amide-type. Note that as potency increases, toxicities (discussed in the following section) also increase.

Uses of Local Anesthetics
Local anesthetics are used to reversibly block the conduction of nerve impulses through the nerve fibers that lie close to the point of injection. Therefore, they are used to provide local anesthesia when injected into the skin, to block major nerve trunks distal to the site of injection prior to surgery, or when injected into the spinal canal (as a spinal or epidural anesthetic), to produce complete sen-

Table 11.3

Classification of local anesthetics.

Generic name	Trade name	Class	Onset	Potency	Toxicity	Duration (min)
Low potency, short duration of action						
Procaine	Novocain	Ester	Moderate	1	1	60
Chloroprocaine	Nesacaine	Ester	Fast	1	1	45
Intermediate potency and duration of action						
Lidocaine	Xylocaine	Amide	Fast	2	2	120
Mepivacaine	Carbocaine	Amide	Moderate	2	2	150
High potency, long duration of action						
Tetracaine	Pontocaine	Ester	Slow	10	10	180
Bupivacaine	Marcaine	Amide	Moderate	10	10	200 +
Etidocaine	Duranest	Amide	Moderate	6	6	200 +

SOURCE: R. M. Julien, *Understanding Anesthesia* (Menlo Park, Calif.: Addison-Wesley, 1984), p. 121.

sory and motor blockade prior to surgery or for relief of the pain associated with labor and delivery.

Side Effects and Toxicities

Following their injection near nerve fibers, local anesthetics are slowly absorbed into the bloodstream. If concentrations in the plasma achieve sufficient levels, effects can occur both in the brain and within the cardiovascular system.

In the brain, local anesthetics initially produce sedation, dizziness, and light-headedness. As levels in the brain increase, toxicities are associated with slurred speech, muscular twitching, and convulsions with loss of consciousness. This toxicity can be reduced by administering a benzodiazepine such as diazepam, although in some cases mechanical support of ventilation may be necessary.

Local anesthetics can produce significant effects on the cardiovascular system. At low doses, local anesthetics are mild cardiac depressants and are clinically useful in treating certain types of cardiac arrhythmias. Lidocaine, for example, decreases the electrical excitability of the heart and decreases both the rate at which electrical impulses are conducted and the force with which the heart muscle contracts. At high doses, these depressant effects can lead to hypotension and cardiovascular collapse. The most cardiotoxic of the currently available local anesthetics are the long-acting amide-anesthetics bupivacaine and etidocaine.

All local anesthetics cross the placenta, which is a matter of concern when these drugs are used for pain relief during labor and delivery. However, no adverse effects appear to result from such placental transport.

Notes

1. American Medical Association, "Antiepileptic Drugs," in *Drug Evaluations*, 6th ed. (Chicago: American Medical Association, 1986), pp. 169–195.
2. T. W. Rall and L. S. Schleifer, "Drugs Effective in the Therapy of the Epilepsies," in A. G. Gilman, L. S. Goodman, T. W. Rall, and F. Murad, eds., *Goodman and Gilman's The Pharmacological Basis of Therapeutics*, 7th Ed. (New York: Macmillan, 1985), pp. 446–472.
3. D. M. Woodbury, J. K. Penry, and C. E. Pippenger, eds., *Antiepileptic Drugs*, 2d ed. (New York: Raven Press, 1982).
4. H. H. Jasper, A. A. Ward, and A. Pope, eds., *Basic Mechanisms of the Epilepsies* (Boston: Little Brown, 1969).
5. American Medical Association, "Drugs Used in Extrapyramidal Movement Disorders," in *Drug Evaluations*, 6th ed. (Chicago: American Medical Association, 1986), pp. 203–219.

6. J. R. Bianchine, "Drugs for Parkinson's Disease, Spasticity, and Acute Muscle Spasms," in A. G. Gilman, L. S. Goodman, T. W. Rall, and F. Murad, eds., *Goodman and Gilman's The Pharmacological Basis of Therapeutics*, 7th ed. (New York: Macmillan, 1985), pp. 473–486.

7. B. Bishop, "Spasticity: Its Physiology and Management," *Physical Therapy* 57 (1977): 371–401.

8. R. R. Young and P. J. Delwaide, "Spasticity, Parts 1 and 2," *New England Journal of Medicine* 304 (1981): 28–33, 96–99.

9. J. R. Bianchine, "Drugs for Parkinson's Disease, Spasticity and Acute Muscle Spasms," in A. G. Gilman, L. S. Goodman, T. W. Rall, and F. Murad, eds., *Goodman and Gilman's The Pharmacological Basis of Therapeutics*, 7th ed. (New York: Macmillan, 1985), pp. 486–490.

10. R. M. Pinder, et al. "Dantrolene Sodium: Review of Pharmacological Properties and Therapeutic Efficacy in Spasticity," *Drugs* 13 (1977): 3–23.

11. G. A. Gronert, "Malignant Hyperthermia," *Seminars in Anesthesia* 2 (1983): 197–204.

12. J. R. Bianchine, "Drugs for Parkinson's Disease, Spasticity, and Acute Muscle Spasms," in A. G. Gilman, L. S. Goodman, T. W. Rall, and F. Murad, eds., *Goodman and Gilman's The Pharmacological Basis of Therapeutics*, 7th ed. (New York: Macmillan, 1985), p. 488.

13. R. J. Flower, S. Moncada, and J. R. Vane, "Analgesic-Antipyretics and Anti-Inflammatory Agents: Drugs Employed in the Treatment of Gout," in A. G. Gilman, L. S. Goodman, T. W. Rall, and F. Murad, eds., *Goodman and Gilman's The Pharmacological Basis of Therapeutics*, 7th ed. (New York: Macmillan, 1985), pp. 674–715.

14. B. B. Brown, Jr., "Pharmacology of Local Anesthesia," in A. Goth ed., *Medical Pharmacology*, 11th ed. (St. Louis: C. V. Mosby, 1984), pp. 408–416.

15. J. M. Ritchie and N. M. Green, "Local Anesthetics," in A. G. Gilman, L. S. Goodman, T. W. Rall, and F. Murad, eds. *Goodman and Gilman's The Pharmacological Basis of Therapeutics*, 7th ed. (New York: Macmillan, 1985), pp. 302–321.

16. R. M. Julien, *Understanding Anesthesia* (Menlo Park, Ca.: Addison Wesley, 1984), pp. 119–124.

17. R. H. deJong, *Local Anesthetics* (Springfield, Ill.: C. C. Thomas, 1977).

CHAPTER 12

Birth Control and Fertility

How Drugs Modify Reproductive Systems

Neurons interact with one another through the liberation of chemical transmitters, which are also called neurohormones (see Appendix II). The transmitters are liberated from one neuron, diffuse across a narrow synaptic cleft, and act on the postsynaptic membrane of the next neuron. These chemical transmitters are called neurohormones because, by definition, a hormone is a substance that is released by one cell and then travels some distance before exerting its effect upon a different organ or structure. The neurohormones travel a very short distance from their site of release to their site of action (in the range of 200 Å). The other normal hormones of the body (compounds such as the estrogens, insulin, thyroid hormone, growth hormone, testosterone, and so on) are released into the bloodstream and are transported in the blood to target organs that are a great distance away.

In addition to this physiological similarity between hormones and neurotransmitters, the brain exerts a regulatory role over the synthesis and release of both. For example, the estrogens are female hormones released from the ovaries but regulated by another hormone released from the hypothalamus, which has a receptor for the estrogens and is therefore sensitive to their level in the blood. When estrogen levels are low, the hypothalamus releases a hormone that ultimately results in stimulation of the ovaries, which results in the production and release of estrogens. Birth-control pills, which contain a synthetically produced estrogen and a synthetically produced progesterone called a progestin, prevent conception largely as a result of the actions of the two drugs on these receptors in the hypothalamus. Thus, estrogens exert prominent effects on the hypothalamus and this "hormone feedback loop" is the mechanism through which the levels of estrogen in the body are regulated.

The Female Reproductive System and How It Is Modified by Drugs

Figure 12.1 illustrates the principal organs of the human female reproductive system. These organs include the ovaries, the fallopian tubes, the uterus, and the vagina. The reproductive process involves the development of one ovum or several ova (eggs) in the ovaries. Once developed, a single ovum is released into the abdominal cavity. The ovum is not lost in the abdominal cavity because, in close proximity to the ovaries, extensions of the fallopian tubes called fimbriae (see Figure 12.1) gather the ovum into the opening of the fallopian tube, down which it is transported into the uterine cavity. If the ovum has been fertilized by a sperm (usually in its passage down the fallopian tube), it implants itself in the body of the uterus, where it develops into a fetus and a placenta.

The Monthly Ovarian Cycle
After puberty and the development of ovarian function, the normal sex life of a female is characterized by monthly rhythmic changes

Figure 12.1

Principal organs of the female reproductive system.

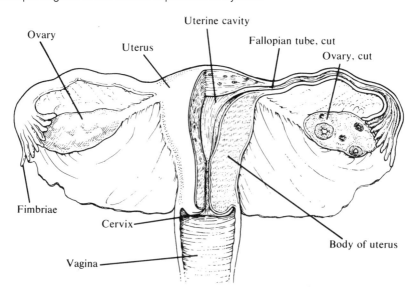

in the secretion of various sex hormones, together with corresponding changes in the activity of the female sexual organs themselves. The duration of this cycle averages 28 days but may vary from 20 days to as long as 45 days.

In order to accomplish the two most important aims of this cycle—the development and release of a single ovum, and the proliferation of a uterine endometrium that is prepared for the implantation of a fertilized ovum—a coordinated sequence of hormonal events must occur. This sequence of events is illustrated in Figure 12.2. At the beginning of the cycle, the levels of both the estrogens and progesterone in the blood are low, the endometrium that was built up during the preceding cycle begins to slough, and a several-day period of menstruation occurs. Because these levels of estrogens and progesterone are low, the cells in the hypothalamus begin to release two hormones: FSH-releasing factor (FSHRF) and LH-releasing factor (LHRF). These two hormones are transported in the blood from the hypothalamus to the pituitary gland, where they induce the release of FSH (follicle-stimulating hormone) and LH (luteinizing hormone). In response to the FSH in the blood, a variable number of ovarian follicles (each containing an ovum) begin to enlarge. After 5 or 6 days, one of these ovarian follicles begins to develop more rapidly than the others, and the ovum begins to mature.

This maturing ovum then begins to release small quantities of estrogens into the circulating blood. These estrogens act to inhibit the further secretion of FSHRF from the hypothalamus and therefore to inhibit the further release of FSH from the pituitary gland. This inhibition results in the regression of the other follicles that also had started to develop. The secretion of estrogens by the one maturing ovum and the follicle in which it is contained reaches a peak just before mid-cycle (day 14). Near the end of this preovulatory phase, LH is released from the pituitary gland under the stimulus of LHRF and prepares the ovarian follicle for ovulation by stimulating it to grow rapidly and swell to the point where it eventually ruptures and the developed ovum is released. This is referred to as the time of *ovulation*. LH is necessary for the final preovulatory development of the follicle and subsequent ovulation. Without LH (even with large quantities of FSH), the follicle will not rupture and ovulation is inhibited. (The pharmacological importance of this activity is discussed in the following section.)

After ovulation, the ovum is gathered by the fimbriae into one of the fallopian tubes, where fertilization by a sperm is generally conceded to occur. The ovum (whether fertilized or not) then enters the uterine cavity. The follicle from which the ovum was released changes and becomes a structure called a *corpus luteum*, which secretes both progesterone and estrogens. These hormones, released

Figure 12.2

Sequence of events in brain, ovaries, and uterus during the monthly ovarian cycle in females. *FSH,* follicle-stimulating hormone; *FSHRF,* FSH-releasing factor; *LH,* luteinizing hormone; *LHRF,* LH-releasing factor; *E,* estrogen; *P,* progesterone. *Solid arrows,* stimulation. *Dashed arrows,* inhibition.

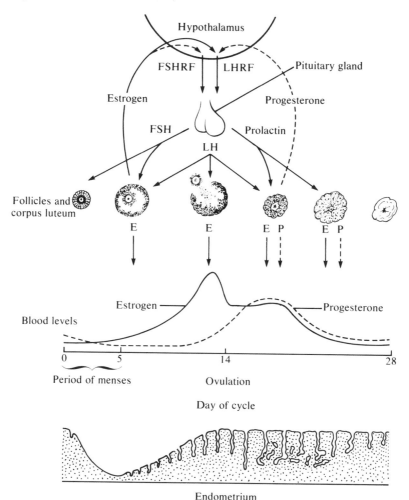

from the corpus luteum, maintain the uterus in a state that is conducive to the receipt of a fertilized ovum. This is accomplished by the maintenance of a highly vascular endometrial lining (or endometrium) on the wall of the uterine body. In addition, the estrogens and progesterone released from the corpus luteum act on the hypothalamus to inhibit the release of FSHRF and LHRF. During the next 10 days, the corpus luteum regresses and within about 12 days, it ceases to function. Estrogens and progesterone are no longer released by the corpus luteum, menstruation begins, and a new sexual cycle follows if fertilization did not occur. If the ovum is fertilized and implanted, the endometrium begins to secrete large quantities of hormones that act to maintain pregnancy and prevent menstrual sloughing.

Birth-Control Pills (Oral Contraceptives)

Oral contraceptives are the most effective technique for preventing pregnancy. Most commonly, these compounds are mixtures of a synthetic estrogen (either *ethinyl estradiol* or *mestranol*) and a synthetic progesterone derivative (a "progestin," most commonly *norethindrone, ethynodiol, norethynodrel,* or *norgestrel*). Three preparations are available that contain only a progestin. Naturally occurring estrogens and progestins are not used because they are poorly absorbed when taken orally; however, the synthetic derivatives are well absorbed by this route.

The availability of orally absorbed estrogens and progestins provided the technology for the pharmacological control of ovulation as well as its prevention for as long as it is desired. The problem was to develop appropriate combinations of estrogen and progestin that would effectively suppress ovulation, while producing only minimal side effects with prolonged use. Excessive amounts produce abnormal menstrual bleeding, whereas insufficient amounts might not completely inhibit the release of FSHRF and LHRF and might result in an unwanted pregnancy. Today, four decades after the introduction of these agents, we are still searching for the ideal oral contraceptive. All but three of the oral contraceptive products currently available are combination products (consisting of an estrogen and a progestin) in the form of low-dose, regular, or variable-dose preparations. The low-dose combination pills contain 30–35 micrograms of ethinyl estradiol and afford a reasonable compromise between the toxicities produced by too much estrogen and the bothersome breakthrough bleeding that results from too little estrogen. Table 12.1 lists these preparations. The regular-dose products contain 50 micrograms of ethinyl estradiol; their use is diminishing rapidly in favor of the lower-dose products that appear to be equally effective in preventing pregnancy while causing only modest increases in breakthrough bleeding. A small number of products contain greater than 50 micrograms of estrogen (usually mestranol), and these products are used even less frequently (most are among the earliest products marketed). The variable-dose products have been introduced relatively recently and are either "biphasic" or "tri-

Table 12.1

Oral contraceptives available in the United States.

Trade name	Manufacturer	Composition			
		Progestin	mg	Estrogen	μg
Brevicon	Syntex	Norethindrone	0.5	Ethinyl estradiol	35
Demulen 1/35	Searle	Ethynodiol	1.0	Ethinyl estradiol	35
Demulen 1/50	Searle	Ethynodiol	1.0	Ethinyl estradiol	50
Enovid-E	Searle	Norethynodrel	2.5	Mestranol	100
Enovid-5	Searle	Norethynodrel	5.0	Mestranol	75
Enovid-10	Searle	Norethynodrel	9.85	Mestranol	150
Loestrin-1/20	Parke-Davis	Norethindrone	1.0	Ethinyl estradiol	20
Loestrin-1.5/30	Parke-Davis	Norethindrone	1.5	Ethinyl estradiol	30
Lo/Ovral	Wyeth	Norgestrel	0.3	Ethinyl estradiol	30
Micronor	Ortho	Norethindrone	0.35	—	—
Modicon	Ortho	Norethindrone	0.50	Ethinyl estradiol	35
Nordette	Wyeth	Levonorgestrel	0.15	Ethinyl estradiol	30
Norinyl 1 & 35	Syntex	Norethindrone	1.0	Ethinyl estradiol	35
Norinyl-150	Syntex	Norethindrone	1.0	Mestranol	50
Norinyl-1/80	Syntex	Norethindrone	1.0	Mestranol	80

Norinyl-2	Syntex	Norethindrone	2.0	Mestranol	100
Norlestrin-1/50	Parke-Davis	Norethindrone	1.0	Ethinyl estradiol	50
Norlestrin-2.5/50	Parke-Davis	Norethindrone	2.5	Ethinyl estradiol	50
Nor-Q.D	Syntex	Norethindrone	0.35	—	—
Ortho-Novum 7/7/7	Ortho	Norethindrone	0.5, 0.75, 1	Ethinyl estradiol	35
Ortho-Novum 10/11	Ortho	Norethindrone	0.5, 1.0	Ethinyl estradiol	35
Ortho-Novum 1/35	Ortho	Norethindrone	1.0	Ethinyl estradiol	35
Ortho-Novum-1/50	Ortho	Norethindrone	1.0	Mestranol	50
Ortho-Novum-1/80	Ortho	Norethindrone	1.0	Mestranol	80
Ortho-Novum-2	Ortho	Norethindrone	2.0	Mestranol	100
Ovcon-35	Mead Johnson	Norethindrone	0.4	Ethinyl estradiol	35
Ovcon-50	Mead Johnson	Norethindrone	1.0	Ethinyl estradiol	50
Ovral	Wyeth	Norgestrel	0.5	Ethinyl estradiol	50
Ovrette	Wyeth	Norgestrel	0.075	—	—
Ovulen	Searle	Ethynodiol	1.0	Mestranol	100
Tri-Norinyl	Syntex	Norethindrone	0.5, 1, 0.5	Ethinyl estradiol	35
Tri-Levlin 30, 40, 30	Berlex	Levonorgestrel	0.5, 0.075, 0.125	Ethinyl estradiol	30, 40, 30
Triphasil 30, 40, 30	Wyeth	Levonorgestrel	0.5, 0.075, 0.125	Ethinyl estradiol	30, 40, 30

phasic", depending on the number of dosage variations that are possible for administration within a given month's cycle. These products are designed to reduce the total hormone content that is administered to the body throughout the menstrual cycle and, at the same time, to provide contraception comparable that obtained from products containing higher doses. At present, it is unclear whether these variable-dose products offer any significant benefits over the low-dose (30–35 microgram) preparations.

The three progestin-only pills are occasionally termed "mini pills", and the rationale for their use is discussed in the following section.

The combination oral contraceptives are taken for 21 days of the menstrual cycle (usually days 5–24, counting day 1 as the first day of menstruation). This is followed by 1 week without medication, toward the end of which withdrawal bleeding (menstruation) occurs. The progestin-only pills are taken daily and continuously.

Combination of Estrogens and Progestins

By combining an estrogen and a progestin, release of both FSH and LH is blocked, ovarian follicles do not develop, and no ovulation occurs. Two synthetic estrogens are used in the oral contraceptives. Natural estrogen cannot be used because it is not absorbed when administered orally. Adding an ethinyl group to estradiol (a natural estrogen) results in a compound that is orally absorbed. Thus, *ethinyl estradiol* is one commonly used estrogen. The second is *mestranol*, a compound that is converted in the body to ethinyl estradiol. While the estrogen inhibits the release of FSH, the progestin inhibits the release of LH, secondary to blocking the release of LHRF. In addition to this action on the hypothalamus, the progestin acts on the uterus to produce an endometrium that is hostile to implantation of a fertilized ovum. The protestin also thickens the normal mucus discharge of the cervix so that sperm cannot gain access to the uterus and fallopian tubes (where fertilization occurs). All of these actions tend to decrease the likelihood of conception and implantation.

Progestational Contraceptives

During the last few years, there has been increasing concern over the possibility that long-term use of the estrogens in the combination estrogen-progestin contraceptives might be harmful. These fears have prompted the use of continuous progestational therapy without concomitant administration of estrogens.

As is apparent from Figure 12.2, if a progestational agent is given alone, FSH would still be released from the pituitary gland and an ovarian follicle would still mature. It is felt, however, that the protestin would greatly decrease the release of LH from the pituitary gland (secondary, of course, to blocking the release of LHRF from the hypothalamus) and the possibility of ovulation occurring would be slight. If, however, some LH were released from the pituitary, ovulation might not be completely blocked and an ovum would occasionally be released. Pregnancy would not necessarily result because the progestin also alters the structure and consistency of the endometrial lining of the uterus and decreases the fluidity of the cervical mucus, which would restrict the passage of sperm into the fallopian tubes. Thus, although agents consisting only of progestin *do not* totally block ovulation, they do tend to impede the sperm. Even if fertilization should occur, the progestin tends to prevent implantation of the fertilized ovum into the endometrium.

This discussion of *tendencies*, however, illustrates that the administration of a product consisting only of progestin (of which three are currently available) is not quite as reliable as the administration of a combination product: statistics indicate an approximately three-fold increase in the incidence of unwanted pregnancies. For women who experience significant side effects with combination products, administration of progestin only affords better contraceptive protection than is afforded by foams, creams, jellies, or rhythm and is certainly far better than no contraception at all. Appendix VI includes comparison of pregnancy rates in women taking oral contraceptives with rates in women using other nonsurgical contraception.

Undesirable Effects of Estrogen and Progestins

The frequent, mild side effects induced by the contraceptive pill resemble those found in early pregnancy and are generally attributed to the estrogen in the combination products. These side effects are usually related to the dose, and products with less estrogen generally have milder side effects. These effects include nausea, occasional vomiting, headache, dizziness, weight gain, and discomfort in the breasts.

All may be alleviated if a product with *low* doses of estrogen (30 micrograms) or a product containing progestin only (Micronor, Nor-Q.D., or Ovrette) is taken. Breakthrough bleeding is a problem that appears to decrease with increasing doses of estrogen. As mentioned previously, the products that contain 30 micrograms of estrogen offer virtually complete contraceptive protection, a minimum of serious side effects, and an acceptable level of breakthrough bleeding. If spotting or breakthrough is excessive, however, additional small amounts of ethinyl estradiol (20 micrograms daily for 7 days) usually alleviate the problem.

Other side effects are generally not too bothersome and include weight gain and psychological changes that may result in depression in some individuals. These side effects are most frequently seen with the use of progestin-only pills or with an injection every 3 months (quarterly) of Depo-Medrol, a long-acting, injectable progestin. Vaginal infections appear to be more common and more resistant to treatment in women who take oral contraceptives than in women who do not.

When administration of these agents is stopped, normal cyclic periods often are not immediately resumed, an effect that may prove a problem if a woman stops taking the pill in the hope of becoming pregnant immediately. It may take several months or possibly, for some women, 1 or 2 years to reestablish a normal cycle, presumably because the hypothalamus, pituitary gland, and ovaries have been suppressed for a prolonged period of time. However, approximately 95 percent of women whose menstrual periods were normal before taking oral contraceptives resume normal periods within a few months after cessation of the drug. Indeed, in those women who discontinue oral contraceptives to become pregnant, 50 percent conceive within 3 months and, more important, after 2 years only 7 to 15 percent have failed to conceive.[1] Thus, there seems to be little or no increase in infertility in women who discontinue the use of oral contraceptives.

Serious side effects rarely occur as a result of the use of oral contraceptives. They include thrombophlebitis (the development of blood clots in the veins), pulmonary embolism (the lodging of a blood clot in the lungs), and cerebral thrombosis (the lodging of a blood clot in the brain). Current evidence indicates that the risk of death from these complications is about six times higher among users than among nonusers of birth-control pills (1.3 versus 0.2 deaths per 100,000 patients per year). However, the risk of death from all causes in pregnancy is 22.8 per 100,000 per year. Further discussion of the statistics involved may be found in the reviews by Murad and Hayes[2] and the American Medical Association.[3]

It may be pointed out that even though the occurrence of these toxicities is statistically greater than that observed in women who are not pregnant and not taking birth-control pills, they are usually conceded to be lower than those associated with pregnancy. This is not too surprising because the oral contraceptives essentially induce a state of pseudopregnancy—that is, the blood levels of estrogen and progesterone are elevated in the same manner that they would be during normal pregnancy. Likewise, during normal pregnancy, the hypothalamus and pituitary gland are both inhibited by the same negative-feedback mechanism that is induced by the estrogens and progestins contained in birth-control pills. Because of this hormonal resemblance to normal pregnancy and the small associated risk of vascular disorders, many women feel that alternative forms of contraception, if feasible, may be desirable.

Other serious side effects that occur only infrequently but that may necessitate discontinuation of the drug include liver dysfunction (jaundice), emotional depression, increases in blood pressure, increased incidence of heart attacks, and increased risk of gall bladder disease. There is little evidence to indicate that oral contraceptives increase the likelihood of cancer of the breast, ovaries, or uterus; in fact, recent data point to a protective effect of oral contraceptives against cancers in these organs.[4-7]

Because of the potential complications occasionally induced by oral contraceptives, strict controls have been placed on the labeling of these products. The Food and Drug Administration requires a statement that these compounds are not to be used where there may be suspicion of thrombophlebitis, danger of embolism, impaired liver function, undiagnosed uterine bleeding, known or suspected pregnancy, estrogen-dependent cancers, or cancers of the breast. Because most of these complications are related to the estrogen in the product, it seems reasonable to use preparations with the lowest possible dose of estrogen, that is, in the range of 30 micrograms per tablet. In addition, it is extremely important to discuss with the physician the possible problems, toxicities, limitations, and alternatives to the use of oral contraceptives before use is initiated.

Appendix VI is a modification of package insert material that the U.S. Government requires be given to every woman taking oral contraceptives. It outlines the risks and the benefits that accompany use of these preparations. Any woman contemplating use of oral contraceptives is advised to read this material carefully and decide for herself whether the risks outweigh the benefits received.

Alternatives to the Pill

Unfortunately, there are presently few *effective* alternatives to birth-control pills when a woman desires to avoid pregnancy. At the moment, the most effective contraceptive practices include the pill, male or female sterilization, or abstention. Diaphragms, condoms, or intrauterine devices (IUD) are only approximately 90 to 95 percent effective (Table 12.2). Even less effective are vaginal spermicides, the rhythm method, *coitus interruptus*, or douching. Thus, the most effective practices for *temporary* and *effective* prevention of unwanted pregnancy are the pill or abstention. Sterilization of either

Table 12.2

Pregnancies per 100 woman years

Contraception method	Range
Oral contraceptive pills, combination	1
Oral contraceptive pills, progestin only	2–3
Intrauterine device (IUD)	1–6
Diaphragm with spermicidal cream or gel	2–20
Condom	3–36
Spermicidal aerosol foams	2–29
Spermicidal gels and creams	4–36
Periodic abstinence ("rhythm")	
All types	1–47
Calendar method	14–47
Temperature method	1–20
Mucus method	1–25
No contraception	60–80

the male or female (although 100 percent effective) is *permanent* and should not be considered reversible.

When intercourse has occurred without contraceptive protection and pregnancy is not desired, certain pharmacological measures may be used to thwart an unwanted pregnancy. *Postcoital* techniques include high doses of estrogens, which are often referred to as "morning after" pills.[8] The best understood and most effective of such preparations contain large doses of diethylstilbestrol (about 25 milligrams); they are administered twice daily for 5 days. This type of drug apparently shortens the time a fertilized ovum takes to pass down the fallopian tube into the uterus, impairing its ability to implant and survive in the endometrial lining of the uterus. In other regimens, either ethinylestradiol is used (the oral contraceptive product Ovral; two tablets twice daily, 12 hours apart) or the conjugated estrogens are prescribed (Premarin; 2.5 mg twice daily for 5 days).

One should note that while such regimens use may be effective for contraception, their *routine* may be dangerous. When there is a great desire to avoid pregnancy, as in instances of rape and incest, however, they can be very useful. Severe nausea, vomiting, and breast tenderness are noted frequently following treatment.

Depot Preparations   Certain long-acting, injectable preparations can be used as contraceptive agents. Medroxyprogesterone acetate

(Depo-Provera), a long-acting injectable progestin, is the most studied and the most widely used contraceptive worldwide. A single dose of 100–400 mg injected intramuscularly every 3 to 6 months has proved effective. The advantages of this form of contraceptive include freedom from taking daily tablets, freedom from the side effects of estrogen (this is a progestin-only product, containing no estrogen), and the maintenance of normal FSH activity as a result. Depo-Provera inhibits ovulation by blocking the mid-cycle increase in LH, inducing thickening of the cervical mucus and inhibiting the development of the lush uterine endometrium that is necessary for the fertilized ovum to survive. Follicular development is not suppressed because the normal estrogen cycle cannot be prevented. The contraceptive protection is approximately equal to that afforded by the combination-type oral contraceptives. Disadvantages of this mode of therapy include breakthrough bleeding, weight gain, depression, headache, and abdominal bloating. Irregular menstrual cycles and spotting are quite common. Use of this technique has not been associated with an increased risk of cancer.

Great controversy has arisen concerning the use of Depo-Provera as a contraceptive. It is currently used in more than 70 countries, including such highly developed countries as Great Britain and many developing countries. In the United States, the drug has not been approved for use in contraception, although it is used for other purposes. Its use is particularly appropriate in patients who cannot tolerate other forms of contraception or in geographical areas where other contraceptive agents are not available. Uneducated or noncompliant patients are the best candidates for its use. In countries where these problems exist widespread and where population control is desired, a quarterly or semiannual injection has proved quite effective. Depo-Provera may also be appropriate in patients who are impaired intellectually or psychologically and in whom pregnancy might be unwise.

Agents That Increase Fertility
Women who desire to conceive but may not be able to do so need a compound to *increase* fertility. Infertility may be the result of any of many factors (physical or psychological) in either the male or the female. Certain types of physical infertility in the female are susceptible to pharmacological manipulation. One such pharmacological approach is a direct extension of the scheme illustrated in Figure 12.2.

When estrogen acts upon the hypothalamus, the release of FSHRF is inhibited, the release of FSH by the pituitary gland is decreased, and follicular development is inhibited. If the action of estrogen on the hypothalamus were blocked, FSHRF would be released, and this would be followed by the release of FSH from the pituitary gland; subsequently, one or more ovarian follicles would develop and eventually at least one ovum would be released. For a drug to be capable of blocking the inhibitory action of estrogen on the hypothalamus, it would necessarily have to be capable of attaching to the normal estrogen receptors (thus blocking the normal access of estrogen to the receptor) and yet cause no change in cellular behavior.

Clomiphene (Clomid), a compound frequently referred to as a "fertility pill," is such a drug. Clomiphene has been responsible for conception in many women who previously were unable to conceive. The drug has also been responsible for many multiple births; sometimes four or five ova are released and fertilized. The possibility of bearing more than one child is usually not a problem; frequently it is desired by couples who have not been able to conceive. Since clomiphene acts at the level of the hypothalamus, the pituitary gland and ovaries must be functional if the drug is to improve the chances of conception. The drug is ineffective when infertility is the result of a deficit in the male or when the female's infertility is due to pituitary or ovarian dysfunction.

Ordinarily, clomiphene is taken starting on day 5 of the menstrual period (day 1 being the first day of menses) and then taken daily for 5 days. The drug is stopped until the next menstrual cycle if the patient does not become pregnant. The procedure is then repeated, often with slowly increasing doses. A recent study indicates that approximately 35 percent of formerly infertile females become pregnant on clomiphene. Side effects of clomiphene include ovarian cysts (14 percent), multiple pregnancies (8 percent), and birth defects (2.4 percent). The incidence of birth defects in nontreated females is approximately 1 percent.

If a woman does not become pregnant after several trials on clomiphene, Pergonal (human postmenopausal hormone) and Follutein (chorionic gonadotropin) can be tried. Pergonal is FSH extracted from the urine of postmenopausal females. Follutein, a hormone produced by human placenta and extracted from the urine of pregnant women, exerts actions virtually identical to those of pituitary LH. Thus, sequential injection of Pergonal and then Follutein can, in anovulatory women, simulate normal FSH and LH release in the same manner that it occurs in fertile females. Pergonal is injected daily for 9–12 days, and after a day of rest, the woman receives a single injection of Follutein. Approximately 75 percent of women so treated will ovulate, and approximately 25 percent become pregnant.

The Male Reproductive System

Figure 12.3 illustrates some of the important structures of the male reproductive system. The testes are situated within the scrotal sac and are composed of great numbers of seminiferous tubules in which sperm cells are formed. When formed, the sperm cells empty into the epididymus, where they are stored and mature. The epididymus leads into a long duct (the vas deferens) and the sperm cells are transported through this duct into the seminal vesicles and the prostate gland. In the upper vas deferens, they are mixed with fluids from both the prostate gland and the seminal vesicles. During ejaculation, the prostate gland, the vas deferens, and the seminal vesicles all contract simultaneously so that the fluids and sperm cells are mixed and expelled through the ejaculatory duct and penis.

The actual neural control of arousal and of the male sexual act is extremely complicated, involving sensory input to the spinal cord and the brain and final coordination of motor activity to cause arousal with eventual ejaculation. The present discussion, however, is centered not so much on the act itself as on the hormonal regulation of the male reproductive system as a possible site of action of a male contraceptive.

Figure 12.3

Principal organs of the male reproductive system.

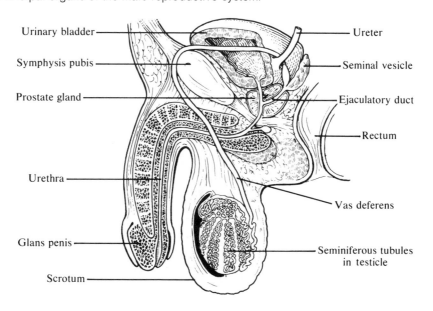

If a drug could be developed to serve as a male contraceptive, it would probably have to affect sperm production in the testes, sperm storage and maturation in the epididymus, sperm transport in the vas deferens, or the chemical constitution of the seminal fluid. All four processes are potentially susceptible to modification by drugs.

Hormonal Regulation of Male Fertility

The production of male sex hormones is closely controlled by hormones released by the hypothalamus and the pituitary gland (Figure 12.4). The most important male hormone is testosterone, which is formed in the testes by cells near the seminiferous tubules. The hormone is released into the bloodstream and distributed throughout the body. In general, testosterone is responsible for the distinguishing characteristics of the male: the development of male features, including distribution of body hair, the lower voice, muscular development, bone growth, and so forth.

Figure 12.4

Hormonal regulation of male fertility. *Solid arrows,* stimulation. *Dashed arrows,* inhibition. (See legend for Figure 12.2 for explanation of abbreviations.) Note that the brain (hypothalamus and pituitary gland) is involved in the control of male fertility, just as it is in the control of female fertility. Note also, however, that fertility in the male is not subject to periodic cycling as it is in the female.

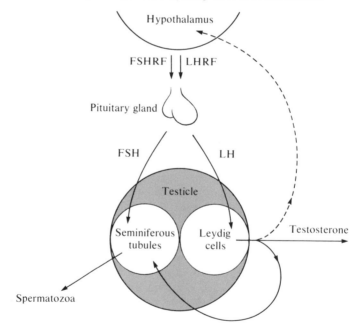

The production of testosterone is controlled by the hypothalamus. When testosterone levels in the blood decrease, LHRF is secreted from the hypothalamus and is carried in the blood to the pituitary gland, where it induces the release of LH, which then acts to promote the synthesis of testosterone in the testes. Testosterone, in turn, acts back on the hypothalamus to slow the rate of its own synthesis by blocking the release of LHRF.

The formation of sperm cells is controlled not by LHRF and LH but by FSH from the pituitary under the stimulus of FSHRF, which is released from the hypothalamus. In the absence of FSH, sperm cells will not be produced. However, FSH alone will not cause complete sperm cell formation. Testosterone (secreted under the influence of LH) is also apparently necessary. Thus, both FSH and LH must be secreted by the pituitary if sperm cells are to be produced.

Male Contraceptives

In the search for a male contraceptive, it would be necessary to interfere with sperm production by altering the hormonal cycle involving the hypothalamus, pituitary gland, and testes; to be useful clinically, the drug would have to leave the LHRF-LH-testosterone system intact so as not to interfere with virility and libido. To date, no satisfactory product has been developed. Products that *do* inhibit sperm production have been produced, but all have side effects of sufficient intensity to limit their usefulness. Such side effects include the inhibition of the secretion of testosterone, with resultant reduction of libido and virility. Since testosterone is necessary for the development of masculine characteristics, a drug that blocks testosterone synthesis would be undesirable. To date, no specific blocker of FSH activity has been developed. Similarly, no clinically acceptable drug has been found that alters sperm transport or viability.

The only currently effective contraceptive method in the male is vasectomy. At present, this surgical technique, by which a portion of the vas deferens is removed, should be considered to be permanent and irreversible. It may be seen from Figure 12.3 that the cutting of the vas deferens would interfere only with the *transport* of sperm cells from the epididymus to the ejaculatory duct. Vasectomy does not interfere with masculinity, with sexual activity, with sperm production, or with the production of testosterone and therefore does not interfere with male virility, libido, or function. Fluids are still secreted from the prostate gland and seminal vesicles into the ejaculatory duct and, during the sexual act, fluid is still expelled upon ejaculation. The only difference in function is that this fluid does not contain sperm cells.

At present, the primary limitation to vasectomy is that it is irreversible. Perhaps in the future a drug may be found that inhibits sperm production, storage, or transport or alters the properties of the seminal fluid so that the sperm cells are no longer viable—contraceptive actions exerted in such a way that, when the use of the drug is discontinued, sperm production is restored.

Notes

1. S. Linn et al., "Delay in Conception for Former Pill Users," *Journal of the American Medical Association* 247 (1982): 629–632.
2. F. Murad and R. C. Haynes, Jr., "Estrogens and Progestins," in A. G. Gilman, L. S. Goodman, T. W. Rall, and F. Murad, eds., *Goodman and Gilman's The Pharmacological Basis of Therapeutics,* 7th ed. (New York: Macmillan, 1985), pp. 1412–1439.
3. American Medical Association, "Contraceptive Agents," in *Drug Evaluations,* 6th ed. (Chicago: American Medical Association, 1986), pp. 711–733.
4. Division of Reproductive Health, Centers for Disease Control, Atlanta, "Oral Contraceptive Use and the Risk of Endometrial, Ovarian, and Breast Cancer" (3 articles), *Journal of the American Medical Association* 249 (1983): 1591–1595 (Breast), 1596–1599 (Ovarian), 1600–1604 (Endometrial).
5. L. Rosenberg et al., "Breast Cancer and Oral Contraceptive Use," *American Journal of Epidemiology* 119 (1985): 167–176.
6. D. R. Mishell, Jr., ed., "Update on Oral Contraceptives," *Journal of Reproductive Medicine* 30(Suppl.) (1985): 689–713.
7. N. S. Weiss and T. A. Sayvetz, "Incidence of Endometrial Cancer in Relation to Use of Oral Contraceptives," *New England Journal of Medicine* 302 (1980): 551–554.
8. A. A. Yuzpe, "Postcoital Contraception," *Clinical Obstetrics and Gynaecology* 11 (1984): 787–797.

CHAPTER 13

Drugs and Society

Priorities and Alternatives

As far back as recorded history, every society has used drugs that produce effects on mood, thought, and feeling. Moreover, there were always a few individuals who digressed from custom with respect to the time, the amount, and the situation in which these drugs were to be used. Thus, both the nonmedial use of drugs and the problem of drug abuse are as old as civilization itself.[1]

If we decide that we wish to reduce the level of drug abuse that exists in our society, we will find that our choice of methods is limited. Over the years, we have attempted to pass laws designed to limit the availability of drugs and to punish those users whom we determine to be dangerous to themselves or to society because of their drug use. Brecher,[2] in a now-classic text, describes the successes and failures that have resulted from this approach. When combined with strict enforcement, such an approach can reduce drug use by those who fear reprisal. But this approach creates problems of its own: Such problems are obvious and beyond the scope of this discussion.

Other techniques used in attempts to reduce drug use usually involve education combined with the development of negative attitudes from peers (for example, "Just say no!") or from elders (for example, "parent power"[3]). Although today we are realizing that such efforts have brought limited results, perhaps the problem is rooted in our basic approach, that is, maybe our goals are misguided and our efforts are uncoordinated. Perhaps it is time to ask *why* we as a society want to discourage drug abuse and misuse. Do we focus solely on drugs as "evil," as deleterious to the physical or psychological health of the user, as potentially dangerous to ourselves as a consequence of someone else's use of drugs, or more generally as a means by which the degradation of society has occurred because of widespread use? Perhaps all are true. Perhaps, however, the reality goes deeper, involving the core of our own sense of individual self-worth, self-respect, and dignity.

> One of the most excitingly heartening happenings today is the widening effort to restore the teaching of moral values in the nation's schools. The direness of the drug epidemic has provided immense immediate impetus.
>
> More Americans now realize the best vaccination to prevent drug addiction is inculcation of a sense of personal worth, personal integrity. Trying to inculcate a sense of moral values is as vital a task as any in our students' curricula.[4]

Applying this to the home situation, it is clear that the family can be centrally important in preventing drug misuse. Parental example, concern, influence, values clarification, open communication, and the teaching of self-responsibility are essential. Parental example should certainly include abstinence from cigarettes, moderation in alcohol use, and avoidance of driving after drinking. Parents can be positive educators if they provide a good role model, an accurate education, and examples of alternatives to the drug experience.

In society, we can undertake educational and legislative goals that seek both short- and long-term objectives, remembering the ultimate goal of improving personal self-worth, integrity, and dignity. To this end, education has been a classic and continuing effort.

The classic approach to teaching people about the actions of psychoactive drugs is to describe how the body absorbs, distributes, metabolizes, and excretes them; how the brain is organized and operates; how neuronal function is related to behavior; and finally how these functions are altered when the drugs are ingested. Such a scheme avoids many complications inherent in an emotion-laden approach to drug education. The facts provided leave no room for mystery.

Of course, such an approach provides explicit directions for people seeking to satisfy existing needs with drugs. This result has been amply demonstrated in comprehensive education programs that *increased* the extent of drug use rather than decreased it, contrary to our original expectations.[5] However, the goal of drug education is not only to decrease drug use, but to provide accurate information that will enable people to make intelligent decisions about their own use of and attitudes toward drugs. With such information, they can examine and modify their own risk-taking behavior.

The Objectives of Drug Education

The approach used in this book was not chosen with the goal of achieving an immediate impact on drug use in our society. Drug education cannot achieve such a goal, and large programs designed to eliminate or drastically reduce use of psychoactive drugs will probably all fail. Society will eventually learn about the effects of a given drug, but education may hasten this learning process and increase knowledge of the risk/benefit ratio that accompanies all drug use. Such knowledge will ultimately be disseminated into the community, and as a society learns of a drug's risks and benefits, a level of drug use (and abuse) will be established that relates to this knowledge. In short, it is hoped that, as a result of education, society will be able to place drugs in proper perspective. Education can function only to present the truth as far as it is known. Indeed, although solid facts *can* be misinterpreted, they will serve society best in the long run.

This factual approach is also taken in the hope of countering much of the magic, mysticism, and emotionalism that surrounds the psychoactive drugs. In many social circles, discussion of psychoactive drugs evokes a very emotional response. It is hoped that by this method of presentation, discussion of the actions of psychoactive drugs will be concentrated on the drugs themselves as chemical entities and as compounds that alter processes in the brain.

Now that the pharmacology of these drugs has been presented, one should be able to compare and contrast the pharmacological effects induced by the different compounds. For example, there is presently controversy about the different effects induced by drinking alcohol or smoking marijuana. Chapters 4 and 10 should provide sufficient background to compare the divergence of attitudes toward their use, a divergence that shows that people tend stoutly to defend their own pattern of drug use while condemning the use of different drugs by others. For example, an adult might attempt to justify his or her own alcohol use while attacking the use of marijuana by young adults. This same adult might even be relieved if the youth abandoned marijuana and adopted the adult pattern of alcohol use. The pharamacology of these two drugs suggests we should question the wisdom of such a shift.

While many consider that such psychoactive drugs as marijuana, LSD, amphetamine, and the barbiturates carry significant potential for toxicity, they overlook the fact that caffeine, nicotine, and alcohol are also psychoactive drugs with similar toxic potentials. Millions of people do not even consider these compounds to be drugs, despite the fact that they all have all the characteristics (the reinforcing properties and the negative health consequences) associated with illicit drugs. The pharmacology and toxicity of these drugs, detailed in Chapters 4 and 5, show that all exert powerful effects on the brain, peripheral nervous system, heart, and a variety of other body structures.

Practical and Immediate Efforts

Practical and immediate efforts to deter the use of drugs that cause the *most* harm to society and extract a multibillion dollar toll in loss of lives, health, and productivity *must* focus on *cigarettes* and *alcohol*. These substances should now—and in the future—be a major focus of educational, regulatory, and enforcement efforts.

In addition, we must meet the challenge of the sudden and episodic emergence of fashionable, potent, and dangerous drugs such as LSD, cocaine, methamphetamine, or "designer" derivatives of anesthetic narcotics. Such drugs will undoubtedly be stimulants (euphoriants), narcotics, or psychedelics and will wax and wane in popularity. Most resistant to educational and legislative efforts will be the long-term abuser of intravenous agents.

Cigarettes

The extent of people's dependence upon cigarettes, clearly illustrated by the inability of many individuals to abstain from smoking, is clear. The more serious toxicities associated with smoking (bronchial irritation, wheezing, chest pain, lung congestion, and lung cancer) have been examined. The toxic effects of smoking on the cardiovascular system—coronary heart disease, peripheral vascular arteriosclerosis, increases in heart rate and blood pressure, and possibly an increased predisposition to the formation of blood clots—have been shown as well. The effects on the developing fetus, including increased rates of abortion, stillbirths, and early postpartum death in infants born of mothers who smoked during pregnancy have been especially emphasized.

Cigarette smoking by *women* is reaching crisis proportions.[6-7] Lung cancer has surpassed breast cancer as the greatest cause of cancer deaths in women. In addition, the risk of fatal or nonfatal heart attacks in smokers of more than one pack of cigarettes per day is higher than 500 percent of the risk in nonsmokers.[8] Even in light smokers (1 to 4 cigarettes per day), the risk of heart attacks is more than doubled. Among heavy smokers, more than 80 percent of heart attacks are caused by smoking (Figure 13.1).

Finally, the worst consequences of smoking by women are the

Figure 13.1

Rates of total coronary heart disease (CHD) per 100,000 person-years (vertical scale) among women according to cigarette use and age. [W. C. Willett, A. Green, M. J. Stampfer, F. E. Speizer, G. A. Colditz, B. Rosner, R. R. Monson, W. Stason, and C. H. Hennekens, "Relative and Absolute Excess Risks of Coronary Heart Disease Among Women Who Smoke Cigarettes," *New England Journal of Medicine* 317 (Nov. 19, 1987): 1306].

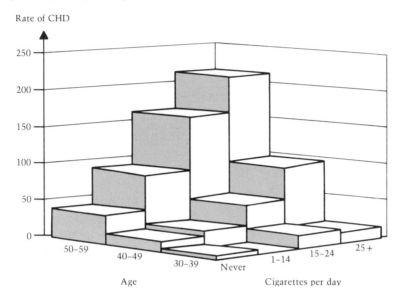

effects on reproduction and children. Some of these consequences have been discussed already. Less appreciated is the growing body of evidence that maternal smoking during pregnancy has long-term effects on children, affecting growth, intellectual and emotional development, and behavior.[6] There is now no doubt that cigarette smoking during pregnancy is incompatible with giving an unborn child the best chance of being normal both at birth and during later development.

The increase in cigarette smoking by women has been largely attributed to cigarette advertising:[7,9]

> Over the past half century and with remarkable consistency, tobacco advertising has linked smoking with women's emancipation and achievement of equality with men. Themes like "You've come a long way, baby" and the introduction of a new cigarette "For women who know the meaning of free" testify to the continuing marketing appeal of stressing independence and equal right to enjoyment.
>
> Marketing to women includes special packaging for feminine appeal, the introduction of "designer" cigarettes, and offering discounted women's

products with the purchase of a particular brand of cigarettes. Sponsorship of sporting events, the fastest growing use of the tobacco industry's marketing dollars, coupled with sports themes in cigarette advertisements, deceptively associates smoking with enhanced physical capacity.[9]

Therefore, if society is concerned about the social and health consequences of the recreational use of products containing psychoactive drugs, it would seem, from the pharmacological and toxicological data, that the use of cigarettes should be greatly discouraged. Certainly, the efforts of many dedicated workers in the American Heart Association, the American Cancer Society, the Respiratory Diseases Association, and others are evidence of increasing public concern. Recent restrictions on smoking in public places is another step in the right direction.

Cigarette smoking is clearly the most widespread example of drug dependence and the most preventable cause of disease and disability in this country. Fifty-six million Americans still smoke, and cigarettes cause more illness and death than any of the other drugs. The major problem that most people have with recognizing and accepting this fact is that most toxicities are delayed in onset, often until someone has smoked for 20 years or more, at which time much of the damage is irreversible. Toxicity that occurs in middle age leads to disability and greatly increased costs of both private and federal insurance.

The latest data show that annual health-related costs of cigarette smoking in the United States are greater than $53 billion. This estimate includes direct medical costs and salary losses for smokers who suffer from lung cancer, heart attacks, emphysema, and other respiratory illnesses. Persons over the age of 55 accounted for $13 billion of this amount. Losses of lifetime earnings of patients who died of diseases caused by smoking have been estimated at $21 billion. More than 350,000 deaths occur yearly as a result of smoking, resulting in 3.9 million person-years lost.

If 56 million American smokers are responsible for $53.7 billion in yearly medical and social costs, each smoker is responsible for a yearly expense of $1000 (53.7 billion divided by 56 million smokers). Thus, a person who smokes two packs of cigarettes daily (730 packs per year) incurs an average health-related cost of $1.37 for each pack of cigarettes he or she smokes, a cost that is probably conservative.

Given these facts and statistics, what should be our educational, legislative, and enforcement response? I would suggest the following as a beginning.

1. Continue educational efforts to warn people about the dangers and depict smoking as dangerous.

2. Encourage health-care providers (such as pharmacies) to cooperate by not selling cigarettes.

3. Designate all health-care facilities as "smoke free" areas.

4. Discontinue direct or indirect cigarette promotion to youth (those under 21 years). This effort should include cigarette sponsorship of athletic events, automobile races, youth-oriented music concerts, and so forth.

5. Because virtually all cigarette-dependent adults became dependent before the age of 21 years, sales and promotion to individuals below 21 years of age should be rigorously discouraged and enforced.

6. Eliminate "free sampling" of cigarettes.

7. Eliminate cigarette advertising and promotion on college campuses.

8. Continue to create smoke-free zones.

9. Regulate advertising to separate smoking from the youthful, macho, and avante-garde image currently portrayed.

10. Remove all government subsidies for tobacco growing.

11. Create a national cigarette health-care fund to contribute to health-care expenses of smokers. Based on current cost estimates, a surcharge of $1 per pack of cigarettes would help to fund the health-care costs incurred by cigarette-induced toxicities.

These criteria are not intended to establish a prohibition against smoking. Rather, their purpose is to highlight the health dangers of cigarettes, prevent development of dependency in youth, provide for future payment of medical costs incurred by smokers, remove the attractions of smoking, and dissipate the concept that cigarette smoking is compatible with a youthful, active, healthy lifestyle.

Alcohol

In addition to the focus on cigarettes, we should become equally concerned about the use of alcohol. As was illustrated in Chapter 4, alcohol is a sedative-hypnotic compound that, like all the sedatives, induces a state of behavioral disinhibition, which is manifested by a variety of behavioral patterns, including euphoria, aggression, hostility, and altered driving behavior. Alcohol is a powerful psychoactive agent that profoundly affects the behavior of the user as well as his or her social situation, including the social groups in which he or she operates.[10] Alcohol damages the brain, liver, pancreas, and other tissues to the extent at which it is the direct pathological cause of death in more than 31,000 Americans each year and an indirect cause of more than 37,000 deaths by accident or violence.[11] Fifty percent of our highway deaths involve alcohol, and the drug is a factor in 70 percent of homicides. Every year, the average American consumes 3 gallons of absolute alcohol. This is equivalent to a personal consumption of 591, 12-ounce cans of beer, 115 fifths of table wine, or 35 fifths of 80-proof whiskey, gin, or vodka. We pay about $90 billion per year for alcohol-related problems, including medical treatment of alcoholism, alcohol-related illness, and fetal alcohol syndrome. Also included in that figure are the costs due to loss of life, productivity, and property, including fire losses; crime; motor vehicle accidents; and social responses.

We are now beginning to recognize the toll that we, as a society, are paying for widespread, recreational alcohol use. A 1986 poll reported that 1 out of 4 families are troubled by alcohol, the highest incidence of problem drinking in 37 years. There are an estimated 10 million adult alcoholics in the United States and 7 million people are problem drinkers. Alcohol-related deaths each year account for at least 25 times more deaths than those caused by *all* illegal drugs combined.

Especially devastating are the injuries and fatalities to youth who correlate alcohol with social experiences and expectations. As portrayed in numerous commercials, we are led to believe that "partying," or having a party, requires the heavy use of alcohol . . . to the point at which we become party animals. A few examples follow.

1.   More than 40 percent of teenage deaths result from automobile accidents, and more than half of them involve alcohol;
2.   Approximately 10 youths between the ages of 15 and 19 die each day from alcohol-related traffic accidents;
3.   Youths between 15 and 24 years old accounted for 37 percent of all alcohol-related traffic deaths in 1986;
4.   The yearly cost that resulted from teenage drivers who caused automobile accidents following alcohol use amounted to $6 billion in 1986;
5.   By age 18, the average teenager will have seen more than 100,000 beer commercials.[12]

An appropriate social response might be to limit the numbers of individuals harmed by alcohol by determining some general guidelines. Some possible guidelines follow.

1.   Eliminate alcohol promotion to minors, for example, on college campuses.
2.   Strictly enforce drinking laws in places where minors are present.
3.   Teach people methods of responsible drinking for those occasions when people feel it is necessary or socially appropriate to drink.
4.   Enforce drunk driving laws more strictly.

5. Educate judges so they understand the need for harsh penalties and rehabilitation when sentencing intoxicated drivers.[13]

6. Increase education in such a way that people will learn to dissociate drinking from smoking. Relatively few long-term drinkers are nonsmokers and some toxicities are additive.

7. Discourage all advertising that contributes to the automatic association of alcohol use with socializing. In this manner, advertising would become primarily institutional in form.[12]

Comments on Sedative-Hypnotic Drugs

In Chapter 2, psychoactive drugs were organized into several classes (sedatives, stimulants, narcotics, antipsychotics, and psychedelics). Of these, the antipsychotic drugs are seldom (if ever) encountered as drugs of abuse. Of the remaining four classes, the sedative-hypnotic compounds deserve some concluding remarks, primarily because of the number of people who misuse them. This is not to negate the problems associated with stimulants, narcotics, and psychedelics, because serious problems do accompany their misuse. However, the total number of persons affected by these agents is small relative to those affected by sedatives. Our most intense educational efforts should focus on the drugs that exact the greatest societal and personal cost. Recall that there are many sedative compounds and they have diverse chemical structures. They include barbiturates, nonbarbiturate hypnotics, antianxiety agents, ethyl alcohol, bromide, paraldehyde, chloral hydrate, and the general anesthetics. As a group, these compounds comprise the largest category of drugs that are used for recreational effects and are subject to abuse.

My first comment is to remind the reader that the sedative-hypnotics are all virtually identical pharmacologically. They are nonselective general depressants of the central nervous system. They are not magic bullets, love drugs, magic potions or elixirs, nor do they possess any other magical or mystical qualities. Each of these drugs has a potential for harm as well as a potential for certain inherent psychosocial benefits.

My second comment is to emphasize the extent to which compounds are used and the negative health and economic consequences that follow their use. The statistics on alcohol, benzodiazepines, and marijuana have been emphasized throughout this text. Society has not recognized that these compounds are psychoactive drugs—that they have all the positive reinforcing properties and the negative health consequences associated with illegal drugs. We seem to accept the deaths, illnesses, traffic accidents, divorces, social havoc, and dollar costs associated with their use. I would hope that after studying this text, the reader will recognize the health and economic consequences (that is, the risks) as well as the benefits of the widespread ingestion of these agents.

My third comment is that the use and abuse of sedative-hypnotic compounds is not a fad. It will not go away, cannot be legislated away, and will remain a very widespread and serious problem.

Fourth, as stated previously, we must teach people how to use sedative-hypnotic compounds. The time has come to teach people how to drink. For example, we all know that alcohol interferes with one's ability to drive, yet people who drink continue to drive. Few individuals seem to understand blood levels of alcohol and the impairment of driving ability that follows its use.

In many states, a blood alcohol concentration (BAC) of 0.10 percent is considered to be "intoxicating," and an individual driving with a BAC of 0.10 percent or greater may be charged with driving while under the influence of alcohol. Thus, if one is interested only in remaining below a *legally* intoxicating blood level, he or she need only learn how much to drink considering both body weight and the time during which the alcohol is consumed. However, the behavioral effects of alcohol are not "all-or-none"; alcohol (and *all* sedatives) exert a *graded, progressive* impairment of the functioning of the nervous system. Thus, the 0.10 percent blood level is only a *legally established, arbitrary* value. Driving ability is only minimally impaired at a BAC of 0.01–0.04 percent. At 0.05–0.09 percent, judgment and reactions are progressively impaired, a state of disinhibition may be seen, and the risk of accidents doubles or quadruples. The deterioration of driving ability continues at a BAC of 0.10–0.14 percent, with a six- to sevenfold increase in the risk of accidents. At 0.15 percent and higher, one is 25 times more likely to be involved in a serious accident.

Figure 13.2 illustrates the correlation between the amount of alcohol ingested, the resultant BAC, and the impairment of driving performance. To use this figure, first glance at the left margin and find the number closest to your body weight (in pounds). Then, look across the columns to the right and find the column under the number of drinks you have had. Matching your body weight with drinks ingested, find your BAC. From this, subtract the amount metabolized per hour (remember from Chapter 4 that approximately 1 ounce of "hard liquor" is metabolized per hour). The final figure is your approximate BAC. From this number you can predict the degree of impairment of your driving ability.

A few examples will illustrate the use of these data. A 140-pound man takes six drinks in 2 hours. The chart value is 0.125 percent.

Figure 13.2

Relation between blood alcohol concentration, body weight, and the number of drinks ingested. See text for details. Wallet-sized copies of this table are available from the Washington State Liquor Control Board, Capitol Plaza Building, Olympia, Washington 98504. [Data developed by Richard Zylman, Center for Alcohol Studies, Rutgers University, New Brunswick, N.J.]

Blood Alcohol Concentration—a guide

Drinks — One drink equals 1 ounce of 80 proof alcohol; 12 ounce bottle of beer; 2 ounces of 20% wine; 3 ounces of 12% wine.

Weight (lb)	1	2	3	4	5	6	7	8	9	10
100	.029	.058	.088	.117	.146	.175	.204	.233	.262	.290
120	.024	.048	.073	.097	.121	.145	.170	.194	.219	.243
140	.021	.042	.063	.083	.104	.125	.146	.166	.187	.208
160	.019	.037	.055	.073	.091	.109	.128	.146	.164	.182
180	.017	.033	.049	.065	.081	.097	.113	.130	.146	.162
200	.015	.029	.044	.058	.073	.087	.102	.117	.131	.146
220	.014	.027	.040	.053	.067	.080	.093	.106	.119	.133
240	.012	.024	.037	.048	.061	.073	.085	.097	.109	.122
	CAUTION			DRIVING IMPAIRED				LEGALLY DRUNK		

Alcohol is "burned up" by your body at .015% per hour, as follows:

No. hours since starting first drink	1	2	3	4	5	6
Percent alcohol burned up	.015	.030	.045	.060	.075	.090

Calculate your BAC

Example: 180 lb man—8 drinks in 4 hours is .130% on chart.
Subtract .060% burned up in 4 hours. BAC equals .070%—DRIVING IMPAIRED.

Subtract 0.030 percent for metabolism (0.015 percent × 2 hours). The resulting BAC is 0.095 percent—not legally intoxicating but enough to impair driving ability. Next, consider a 120-pound woman taking the same six drinks in the same 2 hours. Chart value is 0.145 percent. Subtract the same 0.030 percent for metabolism. The resulting BAC is 0.115 percent, a legally intoxicating value. Finally, consider a 160-pound man taking four drinks in 4 hours. The chart value is 0.073 percent. Subtract 0.060 percent. The resulting BAC is only 0.013 percent. At this level, driving ability is only minimally impaired. Caution is advised but one can state that such behavior is reasonably responsible.

One final point concerning alcohol and driving is necessary. It is important to remember that the presence of another sedative in the body will potentiate the effects of alcohol. Such drug potentiation is not included in Figure 13.2. While the BAC of Figure 13.2 remains true, when someone has ingested other sedatives with alcohol, the resulting impairment is greatly magnified.

The 1980 edition of the California Vehicle Code, Section 23105, states that "It is unlawful for any person who is under the influence of *any drug* to drive a vehicle upon any highway." Thus, in California, if one is suspected of driving while intoxicated with *any* drug, a blood sample is drawn and chemically analyzed. If psychoactive agents are found upon such analysis, the blood levels are determined and entered into the courtroom record. Thus, individuals can be prosecuted for driving while under the influence of one or more psychoactive drugs, the majority of which are alcohol and other sedatives, either alone or in combination.

My fifth comment is that individuals should understand under what circumstances they should seek or accept tranquilizers prescribed by their physician or given to them by friends. The benzodiazepines (Chapter 3), for example, were never intended to be made available to patients for the long-term management of "coping" with problems associated with day-to-day living. They are intended only for the short-term symptomatic alleviation of extreme anxiety and tension. Yet hundreds of millions are prescribed yearly and we are only now recognizing the extent of their abuse. Since the benzodiazepines have the same pharmacological classification as alcohol, they can somewhat appropriately be referred to as a "martini in a pill." Consumers should be aware of this and recognize the inherent risks and benefits associated with their use.

Sixth, I feel that we should recognize the legal inequities associated with the use of sedative drugs and work to equate the legal penalties with the personal and societal costs that accompany the misuse of each agent. Certainly, there has been a movement in recent years to redefine the legal consequences of possessing marijuana in order to bring penalties more in line with possible dangers to society. On the other hand, sedatives such as alcohol, with higher societal risks and costs, should be handled more seriously. This is not to advocate the reinstitution of prohibition (because such prohibition failed) but to urge stricter enforcement of laws relevant to the use of alcohol and other sedatives when such use might endanger others. Some states, such as Oregon, are lowering the "legal" alcohol levels compatible with vehicle operation (0.08 in this instance) and enforcement is becoming more stringent. Unfortunately, convictions and penalties are slower to reflect these new laws.[14]

Finally, I would advocate establishing strict standards for driving while under the influence of sedatives and THC. The attempts in California are a beginning, but we still have not defined "safe" levels of drugs, under which driving would be considered "legal," even though performance would be somewhat impaired. In addition, in our poly-pharmacy society, we need legal standards relevant to driving while under the influence of *two or more* of these agents (that is, driving while under the combined influence of alcohol and barbiturates, alcohol and tranquilizers, THC and other sedatives, and so on). Perhaps within the next decade, enlightened legislation and enforcement will provide for a more scientific approach to the intoxicated driver.

Drug Abuse and Misuse

The term *drug abuse* is difficult to define. In general, it seems to imply the use of any drug for reasons other than its assigned purposes. However, the concept of assigned purposes is vague. Does it refer to use only in medicine, or to use only according to a doctor's prescription? Does this mean that all uses of drugs for reasons other than the treatment of medically diagnosed disorders is abuse of drugs? Are there no legitimate uses of drugs for recreational pursuits, for relaxation, for experience, or for temporary escape from reality? The history of man's use of psychoactive drugs (including alcohol) clearly indicates that there *is* such a role for psychoactive drugs and that it is not usually considered to be drug abuse. As our society becomes more crowded and more polluted, and as people become more frustrated and more angry, psychoactive drugs may become an acceptable form of recreation, relaxation, or escape *in the absence of any better alternative.* The alternatives should be developed now, before psychoactive drugs do become the only course. Our experiences with alcohol present a discouraging picture of a society whose only form of escape is drug oriented.

Drug use, however, has been the primary recreational alternative for those whose geographical situation or economic status does not allow them enough alternatives. Drugs help one to tolerate confinement when one is unable to escape intolerable limits. When no other alternatives are available, drugs provide an effective means of altering one's mood or achieving altered states of consciousness—changes that are normal, not abnormal, human desires.

Figure 13.3 presents a continuum of use and abuse of psychoactive drugs. This continuum progresses from accepted drug use (both medical and recreational), to drug misuse, compulsive abuse, and drug addiction. Legitimate uses of psychoactive drugs are not all necessarily medical and cannot be dictated by law. Thus, we accept that drugs can be used legitimately for recreation and as a means of experiencing altered states of consciousness.

Compulsive abuse is an extension of misuse and refers to an individual who is no longer flexible in his or her drug behavior and uses the drug despite adverse social or medical consequences. The user has developed an intense reliance on the effects of self-administered drugs. Such reliance deviates from the socially approved and expected pattern of use.[15]

Figure 13.3

A continuum of the use and abuse of psychoactive drugs.

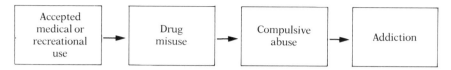

Addiction is a further extension and refers to a person who is overwhelmingly involved with using a drug (compulsive abuse) and securing its supply and who has a high tendency to relapse after withdrawal.[11] Drug use thus pervades the total life activity of the user and controls his or her behavior.

Because drug use can lead to drug abuse, drug education and treatment must include the extent of an individual's behavioral and physiological involvement with psychoactive drugs. Though educational programs and drug alternatives may be useful, formal treatment programs are necessary for those experiencing patterns of compulsive abuse or addiction.

The indications for treatment vary with the drugs being used as well as with the social and cultural factors determining the particular pattern of drug use. Some patterns of drug use, such as the "recreational" (weekly or less frequent) use of marihuana, do not require treatment any more than does the occasional smoking of tobacco or the social use of alcohol. Such casual use is not without hazard, but this does not imply a treatable disorder. It is likely that changing views about drug use will continue to create gray areas where the indications for treatment are unclear. However, there is general agreement that treatment is appropriate for the adverse consequences of drug use and for the compulsive drug user who voluntarily seeks help.[16]

Legitimate use of psychoactive drugs are recognized (Table 13.1), subject to social and legal restrictions. *Medically* legitimate uses include the treatment or prevention of diagnosed diseases or the alleviation of physical or mental discomfort. *Recreationally* legitimate uses generally involve the achievement of altered states of mood or of consciousness, relief from anxiety, induction of euphoria, or escape from uncomfortable or oppressive circumstances.

Drug misuse (step two in Figure 13.3) can, therefore, be described as the use of any drug (legal or illegal) for a medical or recreational purpose *when other alternatives are available, practical, or warranted, or where drug use endangers either the users or others around them.* In medicine, drug misuse applies to the seeking, prescribing, or using of any drug for any purpose other than the pre-

Table 13.1

The medical and recreational uses of psychoactive drugs.

Medical
 1. Treatment or prevention of diagnosed disease
 2. Alleviation of physical or mental discomfort

Recreational
 1. Relief from anxiety
 2. Achievement of a state of disinhibition or euphoria
 3. Achievement of altered states of consciousness
 4. Expansion of creative abilities
 5. Attempt to gain interpersonal or external insight
 6. Escape from uncomfortable or oppressive surroundings
 7. Experience of altered states of mood

vention or treatment of diagnosed disease or the alleviation of physical or mental discomfort. A physician who prescribes a mild sedative-hypnotic tranquilizer for a patient merely because the patient requested it, or to terminate the interview with a patient, may be allowing the patient to misuse a drug. A drug that may properly be used for recreational purposes is misused when it impedes an individual's development outside the use of drugs, when it results in preoccupation with drug use, or when it endangers the physical or mental health of the individual or others.

Alternatives to Drugs

The concept of drug use presented in Table 13.1 leads to the final point of discussion in this book—namely, recognition of the fact that in order to combat drug misuse, *society must provide suitable alternatives*. Consider the following:

Interviewer: Why do you use drugs?
User: Why not?
Interviewer: How could someone convince you to stop?
User: Show me something better.[17]

This terse dialogue is incredibly significant. The recreational use or the medical misuse of drugs, especially psychoactive drugs, will never be stopped (the laws not withstanding) unless suitable alternatives to the drug experience are provided. Drug use and misuse are widespread throughout our society and the individual who uses no drugs at all may be the exception rather than the rule. This is not to say that the use of psychoactive drugs is bad. What is clear is that their use is widespread and will probably become even more widely accepted. Indeed, many segments of our society have accepted the concept of recreational pharmacology.

Recognizing this fact, recognizing the motives of persons who use drugs, and recognizing that it is basic human nature periodically to seek alterations in mood and altered states of consciousness, one can proceed to the active search for alternatives to drug use—alternatives that, if available, might reduce the incidence of drug misuse. As Cohen states, "Alternative is *not* just a synonym for 'substitute' since it implies an orientation which is *more effective* than drugs for giving the person real satisfaction."[18]

Numerous examples of alternatives could be presented. Table 13.2 lists the types of experiences drug users might seek, their motives for seeking that experience, and possible alternatives that

Table 13.2

Motives for, and alternatives to, the use of drugs.

Level of experience	Corresponding motives (examples)	Possible alternatives to drugs (examples)
Physical	Desire for physical satisfaction, physical relaxation, relief from sickness, desire for more energy, maintenance of physical dependence	Athletics, dance, exercise, hiking, diet, health training, carpentry, or outdoor work
Sensory	Desire to stimulate sight, sound, touch, taste; need for sensual-sexual stimulation; desire to magnify sensorium	Sensory awareness training, sky diving, experiencing sensory beauty of nature (lovemaking, swimming, running, mountaineering)
Emotional	Relief from pyschological pain, attempt to solve personal perplexities, relief from bad mood, escape from anxiety, desire for emotional insight, liberation of feeling, emotional relaxation	Competent individual counseling, well-run group therapy, instruction in psychology of personal development (sensitivity training)
Interpersonal	To gain peer acceptance, to break through interpersonal barriers, to "communicate," especially nonverbally, to defy authority figures, to cement two-person relationships, to relax interpersonal inhibitions, to solve interpersonal hangups	Expertly managed sensitivity and encounter groups, well-run group therapy, instruction in social customs, confidence training, social-interpersonal counseling, emphasis on assisting others in distress through education, marriage
Social (including sociocultural and environmental)	To promote social change, to find identifiable subculture, to tune out intolerable environmental conditions, e.g., poverty, changing "awareness" of the "masses"	Social service; community action in positive social change; helping the poor, aged, infirm, young; tutoring handicapped, ecology action

Table 13.2 (*continued*)

Level of experience	Corresponding motives (examples)	Possible alternatives to drugs (examples)
Political	To promote political change, identify with antiestablishment subgroup, to change drug legislation out of desperation with the social-political order, to gain wealth or affluence or power	Political service, political action, nonpartisan projects such as ecological lobbying, field work with politicians and public officials
Intellectual	To escape mental boredom, out of intellectual curiosity, to solve cognitive problems, to gain new understanding in the world of ideas, to study better, to research one's own awareness, for science	Intellectual excitement through reading, discussion, creative games, and puzzles, self-hypnosis, training in concentration, synectics—training in intellectual breakthroughs, memory training
Creative-aesthetic	To improve creativity in the arts, to enhance enjoyment of art already produced, e.g., music, to enjoy imaginative mental productions	Nongraded instruction in producing and/or appreciating art, music, drama, crafts, handiwork, cooking, sewing, gardening, writing, singing, etc.
Philosophical	To discover meaningful values, to grasp the nature of the universe, to find meaning in life, to help establish personal identity, to organize a belief structure	Discussions, seminars, courses in the meaning of life; study of ethics, morality, the nature of reality; relevant philosophical literature; guided exploration of value systems
Spiritual-mystical	To transcend orthodox religion, to develop spiritual insights, to reach higher levels of consciousness, to have Divine visions, to communicate with God, to augment yogic practices, to get a spiritual shortcut, to attain enlightenment, to attain spiritual powers	Exposure to nonchemical methods of spiritual development, study of world religions, introduction to applied mysticism, meditation, yogic techniques
Miscellaneous	Adventure, risk, drama, "kicks," unexpressed motives; prodrug general attitudes	"Outward Bound" survival training, combinations of alternatives listed above, pronaturalness attitudes, brainwave training, meaningful employment

SOURCE: A. Y. Cohen, "The Journey Beyond Trips: Alternative to Drugs," in D. E. Smith and G. R. Gay, eds., *It's So Good, Don't Even Try It Once: Heroin in Perspective* (Englewood Cliffs, N.J.: Prentice-Hall, 1972), pp. 191–192. Examples in brackets added.

might help them attain that experience without drugs. (This table does not state that drugs should *not* be used; it merely lists alternatives for those who wish to reach particular levels of experience without having to resort to a pharmacological intermediary.)

The implementation of these alternatives should not be difficult. Brecher remarked that:

. . . these and other "alternatives to the drug experience" are gaining favor among young people because they are superior to drugs, not because they are safer than drugs. An experienced drug user . . . "often finds that some form of meditation more effectively satisfies his desire to get high. One sees a great many drug takers give up drugs for meditation, but one does not see any meditators giving up meditation for drugs. Once you have learned from a drug what being high really is, you can begin to reproduce it without the drug; all persons who accomplish this feat testify that the nondrug high is superior."[19]

Notes

1. J. H. Jaffe, "Drug Addiction and Drug Abuse," in A. G. Gilman, L. S. Goodman, T. W. Rall, and F. Murad, eds., *Goodman and Gilman's The Pharmacological Basis of Therapeutics*, 7th ed. (New York: Macmillan, 1985), p. 532.
2. E. M. Brecher and *Consumer Reports* editors, *Licit and Illicit Drugs* (Mt. Vernon, N.Y.: Consumers Union, 1972).
3. R. L. Dupont, "The Future of Primary Prevention: Parent Power," *Journal of Drug Education* 10 (1980): 1–5.
4. M. S. Forbes, "Fact and Comment," *Forbes*, December 1, 1986, p. 25.
5. T. J. Glynn, ed., "Drug Abuse Prevention Research," National Institute on Drug Abuse (Washington, D.C.: U.S. Government Printing Office, 1983).
6. "Smoking and Health, a National Status Report—A Report to Congress, 1987," Department of Health and Human Services, Publication Number HHS/PHS/CDC 87-8396 (Washington, D.C.: U.S. Government Printing Office, 1987).
7. J. E. Fielding, "Smoking and Women: Tragedy of the Majority," *New England Journal of Medicine* 317 (Nov. 19, 1987): 1343–1345.
8. W. C. Willett, A. Green, M. J. Stampfer, F. E. Speizer, G. A. Colditz, B. Rosner, R. R. Monson, W. Stason, and C. H. Hennekens, "Relative and Absolute Excess Risks of Coronary Heart Disease Among Women Who Smoke Cigarettes," *New England Journal of Medicine* 317 (Nov. 19, 1987): 1303–1309.
9. R. M. Davis, "Current Trends in Cigarette Advertising and Marketing," *New England Journal of Medicine* 316 (March 19, 1987): 725–732.
10. R. L. Dupont, "The Future of Drug Abuse Prevention," in R. L. Dupont, A. Goldstein, and J. O'Donnell, eds., *Handbook on Drug Abuse*, National Institute on Drug Abuse and Office of Drug Abuse Policy (Washington, D.C.: U.S. Government Printing Office, 1979), pp. 446–452.

11. R. G. Niven, "A Problem in Perspective," *Journal of the American Medical Association* 252 (1984): 1912–1914.
12. N. Postman, C. Nystrom, L. Strate, and C. Weingartner, "Myths, Men and Beer: An Analysis of Beer Commercials on Broadcast Television, 1987" (Falls Church, Va.: AAA Foundation for Traffic Safety, 1988).
13. M. Colquitt, P. Fielding, and J. F. Cronan, "Drunk Drivers and Medical and Social Injury," *New England Journal of Medicine* 317 (Nov. 12, 1987): 1262–1266.
14. K. I. Moull, L. S. Kinning, and J. K. Hickman, "Culpability and Accountability of Hospitalized Injured Alcohol-Impaired Drivers," *Journal of the American Medical Association* 252 (1984): 1880–1883.
15. J. H. Jaffe, "Drug Addiction and Drug Abuse," in A. G. Gilman, L. S. Goodman, T. W. Rall, and F. Murad, eds., *Goodman and Gilman's The Pharmacological Basis of Therapeutics*, 7th ed. (New York: Macmillan, 1985), p. 533.
16. J. H. Jaffe, "Drug Addiction and Drug abuse," in A. G. Gilman, L. S. Goodman, T. W. Rall, and F. Murad, eds., *Goodman and Gilman's The Pharmacological Basis of Therapeutics*, 7th ed. (New York: Macmillan, 1985), pp. 567–568.
17. A. Y. Cohen, "The Journey Beyond Trips: Alternatives to Drugs," in D. E. Smith and G. R. Gay, eds., *It's So Good,Don't Even Try It Once: Heroin in Perspective* (Englewood Cliffs, N.J.: Prentice-Hall, 1972), p. 186.
18. A. Y. Cohen, "The Journey Beyond Trips: Alternatives to Drugs," in D. E. Smith and G. R. Gay, eds., *It's So Good, Don't Even Try It Once: Heroin in Perspective* (Englewood Cliffs, N.J.: Prentice-Hall, 1972), p. 189.
19. E. M. Brecher and *Consumer Reports* editors, *Licit and Illicit Drugs* (Mt. Vernon, N.Y.: Consumers Union, 1972), p. 510.

The Physiology of the Nerve Cell

In studying the nervous system, structure and function are so clearly related that some knowledge of structure is necessary before function can be discussed. To understand the effects of drugs on the nervous system, the principles of the structure and function of the basic element of the nervous system, namely, the *nerve cell* (*the neuron*), must be described.

Nerve cells exhibit two special properties that distinguish them from all other cells of the body. The first is their ability to conduct electrical impulses over long distances. The second is that they have specific input and output relationships both with other nerve cells and with other tissues of the body whose functions the neurons may control (such as muscles and glands). These input-output connections determine the function of a particular neuron and, in turn, the patterns of response that a neuron may elicit.[1]

The Brain

The human brain contains over 20 billion neurons. Most of them share common structural and functional characteristics. Structurally, the typical neuron consists of a cell body that contains the nucleus of the cell and is often referred to as the *soma*. Extending out from the soma are many short fibers called *dendrites*, which respond to the electrical activity of other neurons and conduct such activity to the soma. Also extending from the soma is a fiber called the *axon*, which may be either short or up to 3 feet long (as are the axons projecting down the spinal cord or running from the spinal cord to the muscles). The axon transmits activity from the soma to other neurons or to the muscles or glands of the body. In general, the axon conducts impulses in only one direction: from the soma down the axon to a specialized terminal called the *synapse*. At the synapse, a chemical (the transmitter substance) is released and diffuses across a gap, the synaptic cleft, to the dendrite of the next neuron, thereby transmitting information from one neuron to another. The neurons do not physically touch each other.

Figure I.1 illustrates three neurons and their interactions with one another. Figure I.2 is an illustration of more typical neuronal interactions. Usually, only one axon will arise from the soma but, in its projection, the axon may give off many side branches, sending impulses to a great number of other neurons (causing a divergence of information). Several dendrites arise from one soma. These dendrites branch profusely to form a complex structure sometimes referred to as a *dendritic tree*. This dendritic network receives as many as 50,000 contacts from other cells (resulting in the convergence of information), processes the impulses, and transmits electrical activity to the soma. The soma, in turn, transmits the impulses it receives from the dendrites to as many as 10,000 other neurons. Thus, a great many neurons converge on one neuron, which, in turn, spreads its own impulses to many other neurons. Most cells else-

Figure I.1

Schematic representation of three nerve cells, showing the major subdivisions of such cells and the interactions between them.

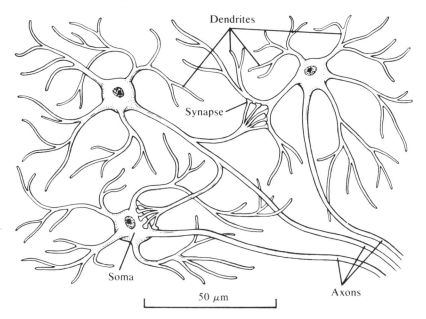

Figure I.2

Diagrammatic representation of neuronal architecture in the cerebral cortex. [Modified from D. H. Hubel, "The Brain," in *The Brain*, a *Scientific American* book (San Francisco: W. H. Freeman and Company, 1979), p. 8.]

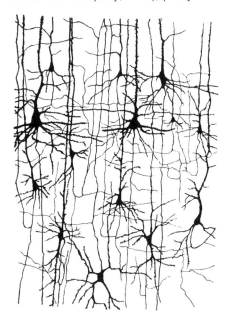

where in the body function as isolated entities; neurons are interconnected in specific manners.

As a consequence of this convergence and divergence of electrical activity, neurons tend to group together and form circuits, and it is the properties of these circuits that determine the way in which information is handled in the nervous system and thus the behavior of the animal. These neural circuits will be discussed in detail in Appendix III. As an overview, however, it can be stated that it is possible to distinguish those areas of the brain where cell bodies and their dendrites are concentrated (these areas are referred to as *nuclei*) from those regions that consist mainly of the axons projecting from one group of neurons to another (these regions are referred to as *fiber tracts*). Thus, axons are sometimes called *fibers* or *nerve fibers*. In the peripheral nervous system (that is, outside the brain and spinal cord), bundles of these axons are commonly referred to as *nerves*.

In the brain, the somas of several thousand neurons group together to form structures called *nuclei*. Further, these nuclei tend to congregate to form yet larger structures, such as the thalamus, hypothalamus, amygdala, and hippocampus.) Each nucleus consists of tens of thousands of individual nerve-cell bodies (somas). The fiber tracts of the brain are often given names indicating the areas of the brain connected by the tracts. For instance, the bundle of axons running from the cortex to the thalamus is referred to as the corticothalamic tract.

In addition to the nerve cells, many other types of cells are found in the brain. The most conspicuous of these are the *glial cells*, one type of which (the astrocyte) we discussed as surrounding the brain capillaries to form part of the blood-brain barrier. Other glial cells provide structural support for the brain or metabolic support for the neurons in an as yet unidentified fashion.

In summary, one neurophysiology text describes the brain as follows:

> The brain, then, is an immense number of spidery nerve cells, interconnected in a complex net, and embedded in a supporting and protecting meshwork of neuroglia. Dendrites spring from the neuron cell body, branch profusely, and along with the soma receive myriads of axon terminals, making it possible for a single nerve cell to gather information from hundreds of others. Furthermore, cell bodies are collected into groups, the nuclei, and these in turn into clusters. Running back and forth between nuclei or between collections of nuclei are fiber tracts, the main channels of communications between one part of the brain and another. Altogether, these structures are arranged in an orderly way to form the brain of the animal and to provide the anatomical basis for neural function.[2]

Psychoactive drugs exert their behavioral effects secondary to alterations in the specific channels of information in specific areas of the brain.

The Axon

The neuron is the primary element of the nervous system and consists of three main divisions: the dendrites, the soma, and the axon. In brief, electrical impulses originate in the dendrites, are integrated in the soma (where the action potentials are formed), and are transmitted down the axon to the synapse. Unlike the dendrites and the soma, the axon is specialized *solely* for the rapid and reliable conduction of electrical activity, which occurs in the form of electrical impulses called *action potentials*. All action potentials conducted down a given axon are essentially identical, and the only manner in which changes in content can be relayed by the axon is by altering the number of action potentials conducted each second.

The axon is, in general, not a major site of action of psychoactive drugs, but it is the site of action of some important drugs, foremost of which are the local anesthetics. Lidocaine (Xylocaine), for example, is a local anesthetic that, when injected into the tissues surrounding the sensory nerves from a tooth, effectively blocks transmission of pain impulses that travel from the nerve endings (specialized dendrites) in the tooth to the brain. The anesthetic does not directly affect the tooth but only blocks the axons in the nerve trunks that are carrying information to the brain.

Most psychoactive drugs exert their effects not on the axon but at the synaptic junction between the axon of one cell and dendrites of another. However, because local anesthetics affect the axon and because the axon is essential for the conduction of action potentials, the properties and functions of the axon are discussed further at the end of this appendix.

The Dendrites

The axon, which specializes in the transmission of action potentials from the soma to the synapse, has the ability to conduct electrical impulses over its full length rapidly and without alteration. Thus, to this point, we have impulses traveling down an axon to the synapse, the functional junction between two separate neurons. How are these impulses then transmitted to the next neuron? In brief, the terminals of the axon align themselves at the synapse in close approximation to the dendrites of the next neuron (Figure I.3). It is this site of connection between the axon terminal and the dendrite that is the point at which impulses are transferred between neurons in the nervous system (see Appendix II).

The dendrites are structures specialized for the receipt of impulses from other neurons. When action potentials have been conducted down the axon of one neuron, the dendrite with which the axon synapses will exhibit an electrical change, the magnitude of which is directly proportional to the frequency at which impulses arrive from the axon (Figure I.4). When the impulses arrive at the synapse, a chemical transmitter is released, diffuses across a small, fluid-filled gap (the synaptic cleft), and alters the dendritic membrane (Figure I.5). If the transmitter chemical affects the membrane in such a manner that the membrane depolarizes, the neuron becomes more excitable (Figure I.4). This depolarization is referred to by physiologists as an *excitatory postsynaptic potential* (EPSP). Note from Figure I.4 that there is a slight delay (approximately 0.5 millisecond) between the arrival of the action potential at the nerve terminal and the EPSP in the dendritic membrane. This time lag is called the *synaptic delay* and is explained by the time required for the transmitter substance released by the axon to reach the dendrite

Figure I.3

A synapse is the relay point where information is conveyed by chemical transmitters from neuron to neuron. A synapse consists of two parts: the knoblike tip of an axon terminal and the receptor region on the surface of another neuron. The membranes are separated by a synaptic cleft some 200 nanometers across. Molecules of chemical transmitter, stored in vesicles in the axon terminal, are released into the cleft by arriving nerve impulses. The transmitter changes the electrical state of the receiving neuron, making it either more likely or less likely to fire an impulse. [From C. F. Stevens, "The Neuron," in *The Brain*, a *Scientific American* book (San Francisco: W. H. Freeman and Company, 1979), p. 11.]

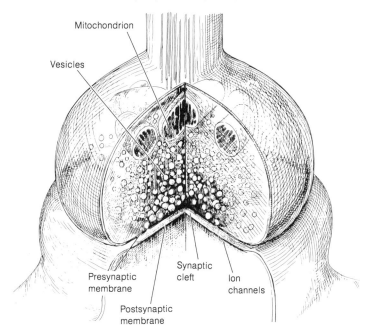

of the next cell. Thus, cells in the brain are connected with one another chemically rather than electrically or physically. The synapse is the primary site of action of most psychoactive drugs.

Thus, the axon is electrically excitable and capable of conducting action potentials rapidly. The dendrite is chemically excitable (by transmitter) and, if the membrane is depolarized, excitatory postsynaptic potentials are induced.

In the central nervous system, all neurons are held in a balance between excitation and inhibition. If *all* synapses were excitatory, we would convulse continuously, because every cell in the brain would continue to discharge at an uncontrolled rate. In order to balance excitation, there must be a process of inhibition. Some transmitter chemicals, instead of depolarizing the dendrites, induce

Figure I.4

Transmission of impulses from one neuron to another at a synapse. Graph *A* is a recording of electrical activity in the axon terminal as an action potential arrives at the synapse. Graph *B* is a recording of electrical activity in the dendrite of the next neuron showing the postsynaptic activity resulting from the transmission of impulses across the synapse. [Modified from C. F. Stevens, *Neurophysiology: A Primer* (New York: John Wiley, 1966), fig. 3.2, p. 35.]

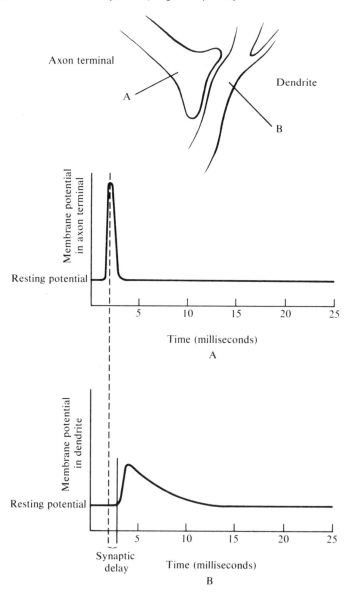

Figure I.5

Transmitter is discharged into the synaptic cleft at the synaptic junctions between neurons by vesicles that open up after they fuse with the axon's presynaptic membrane, a process called exocytosis. This electron micrograph made by Heuser has caught the vesicles in the terminal of an axon in the act of discharging acetylcholine into the neuromuscular junction of a frog. The structures that appear in the micrograph are enlarged some 115,000 diameters. Synaptic vesicles are clustered near the presynaptic membrane. The diagram shows the probable steps in exocytosis. Filled vesicles move up to the synaptic cleft, fuse with the membrane, discharge their contents, and are reclaimed, re-formed, and refilled with transmitter. [From C. F. Stevens, "The Neuron," in "*The Brain*," a *Scientific American* book (San Francisco: W. F. Freeman and Company, 1979), p. 24.]

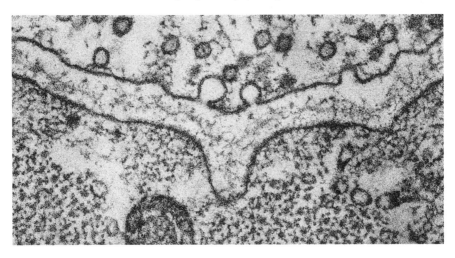

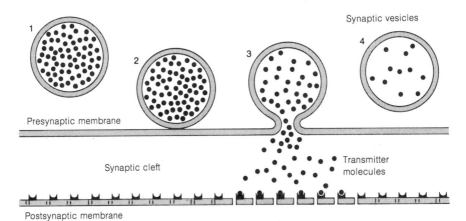

a *hyperpolarization* of the dendritic membrane. This hyperpolarizing potential is referred to as an inhibitory postsynaptic potential (IPSP). This IPSP opposes the action of EPSPs, stabilizes the neuron, and tends to prevent the generation of action potentials.

Thus, although only one type of action potential may be carried down an axon, two types of chemical transmitters can be released, depending upon the neuron: those that depolarize the dendritic membrane or those that hyperpolarize it. All cells in the nervous system receive impulses from both the excitatory and inhibitory synapses. Indeed, the exquisite beauty of the nervous system is maintained by this delicate balance between excitation and inhibition.

The dendrites of a single nerve cell may make as many as 50,000 synapses with axons from other cells. The influence of an individual synaptic connection may be excitatory or inhibitory, and the type of activity seen in the postsynaptic neuron will depend upon the influence exerted by the preponderance of presynaptic neurons. Psychoactive drugs, because they affect synaptic transmission, tend to upset this balance of excitation and inhibition. It is the result of this alteration of excitability within specific areas of the nervous system that leads to drug-induced alterations in behavior.

The Soma

The dendrite and soma (Figure I.6) receive input from other neurons through the synapses and respond by either depolarizing (increasing excitability) or hyperpolarizing (decreasing excitability). All of the impulses received at the dendrites affect the level of excitability of the soma (the cell body), which gives rise to only a single axon and thus to a single channel through which these impulses are transmitted to other neurons. How, then, are the electrical potentials from the dendrites converted into an action potential? It appears that the soma integrates (or averages) the impulses gathered by the dendrites. If the influence of excitatory synapses is greater than the influence of inhibitory synapses, the soma will respond by producing an action potential that spreads into the axon and is conducted to the next synapse. If more inhibitory input is received than excitatory input, the soma will hyperpolarize and the neuron will become less excitable. The soma, therefore, expresses the integration of the dendritic input as depolarization or hyperpolarization (depolarization resulting in the generation of an action potential and hyperpolarization resulting in the blockage of the generation of an action potential).

Concerning the actions of drugs, we have stated that the psy-

Figure I.6

The cell body of a neuron incorporates the genetic material and complex metabolic apparatus common to all cells. Unlike most other cells, however, neurons do not divide after embryonic development; an organism's original supply must serve a lifetime. Projecting from the cell body are several dendrites and a single axon. The cell body and dendrites are covered by synapses, knoblike structures where information is received from other neurons. Mitochondria provide the cell with energy. Proteins are synthesized on the endoplasmic reticulum. A transport system moves proteins and other substances from cell body to sites where they are needed. [From C. F. Stevens, "The Neuron," in *The Brain*, a *Scientific American* book (San Francisco: W. H. Freeman and Company, 1979), p. 17.]

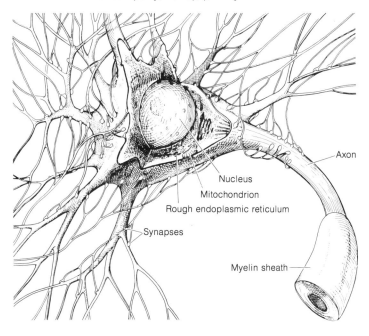

Axon

Nucleus

Mitochondrion

Rough endoplasmic reticulum

Synapses

Myelin sheath

choactive drugs exert their behavioral effects by altering the delicate balance of excitation and inhibition generated by the processes of synaptic transmission.

Properties of Excitable Membranes

All fluid outside the bloodstream is either inside cellular membranes (intracellular fluid) or outside the cells, surrounding them but remaining outside the bloodstream (extracellular fluid). An important difference between extracellular and intracellular fluid is the marked imbalance in the concentration of certain ions (small, electrically charged molecules), which results largely from the varying permeability of the cell membrane to water-soluble, fat-insoluble substances. The cell membranes are structures of protein and fat containing small, water-filled pores. These pores are about 7 Å in diameter. The movement of substances through these pores is limited by the size of the pores. Because of the size of the pores, the membrane is freely permeable to potassium ions (K^+) and chloride ions (Cl^-), which are smaller than 7 Å, relatively impermeable to sodium ions (Na^+), and essentially impermeable to organic anions (A^-), which are present as large protein molecules. The concentrations of sodium (Na^+) and chloride (Cl^-) are much higher in the extracellular fluid than in the intracellular fluid, and the concentrations of potassium (K^+) and organic anions (A^-) are much higher in the intracellular fluid than in the extracellular fluid (Figure I.7).

As a consequence of this ionic imbalance on either side of the cell membrane, there is an electrical potential (difference in voltage) across the membrane. This electrical potential may reach 50 to 90 millivolts, with the inside negative in relation to the outside. Such difference in potential exists in every cell of the body (not only neurons) and is referred to as the *resting potential* of the cell, although

Figure I.7

Distribution of ions across a cell membrane. The cell membrane is a protein-fat barrier (see Figure 1.3) that apparently contains small pores, approximately 7 Å in diameter, and allows the passage of water and of certain small ions: Na^+, sodium ions; Cl^-, chloride ions; K^+, potassium ions; A^-, large protein molecules that contain negative charges. As their relative sizes indicate, potassium and chloride ions are able to diffuse freely though the pores, while sodium ions are less able to do so and protein molecules are largely not able to diffuse.

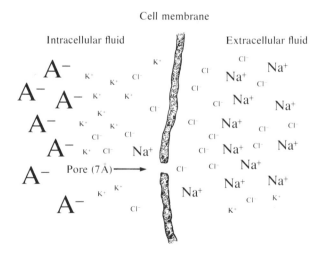

the magnitude of the resting potential varies from one cell type to another. Positive charges tend to move into the cell, and negative charges tend to move out. However, sodium ions (which are positive and are found in high concentrations outside the cell) penetrate the membrane very poorly, and the negatively charged organic proteins (A⁻) on the interior of the cell wall are unable to move out. Such distribution of ions keeps the electrical charges distant from each other and thus maintains the resting potential.

Since *all* cells of the body exhibit this resting potential, what distinguishes nerve cells (which are excitable structures capable of generating action potentials) from all other cells of the body? When the neuron becomes less negative (in relation to the extracellular fluid), the axon is said to be depolarized (Figure I.8). When the axon is depolarized by a few millivolts, the permeability of the membrane is altered so that the membrane becomes rapidly more permeable to Na⁺. Within a fraction of a millisecond, sodium ions traverse the membrane from the outside to the inside of the cell, neutralizing the electrical potential that was formerly maintained across the membrane. So many sodium ions enter the neuron, in fact, that the membrane potential slightly overshoots the neutral potential (0) and the inside of the cell becomes slightly positive in relation to the

Figure I.8

Graph of an action potential. Stimulus was applied at the time indicated by the arrow. [From C. F. Stevens, *Neurophysiology: A Primer* (New York: John Wiley, 1966), fig. 2.3, p. 14.]

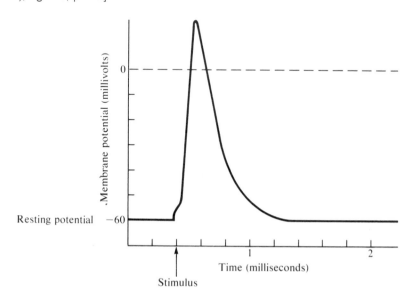

outside. At this point, the membrane loses its increased permeability to sodium ions, no more enter, and potassium ions (which are in high concentrations on the inside of the cell, and which can easily traverse the membrane) leave the cell to restore the difference in potential. Thus, the cell has gone through a brief period during which it has had its resting state upset, and it has become slightly positive on the inside. Through a "pump," the membrane redistributes the ions and restores the original resting potential. All these events, which occur within a period of about one-thousandth of a second, constitute a sequence called an *action potential*.

In addition to electrical excitability, the axon exhibits another important characteristic: the ability to conduct the action potential the length of the axon without being altered or experiencing a decrease in intensity. (The mechanisms by which the ionic gradients are maintained and reestablished after excitation are complicated and beyond the scope of this discussion. Discussions of these topics may be found in the readings listed in the bibliography.)

The axon is capable of conducting impulses at widely varying frequencies, from less than 1 per second to as many as 500 per second, depending upon the degree of depolarization of the soma.

Notes

1. C. F. Stevens, "The Neuron," in *The Brain*, a *Scientific American* book (San Francisco: W. H. Freeman and Company, 1979), pp. 15–25.

Synaptic Transmission and Transmitters

In Appendix I we discussed the electrical phenomena that characterize neurons as unique entities and that are the basis of nervous-system function. We explained that all information transfer in the brain is accomplished by the interaction of neurons with one another. We discussed the dendrite as the recipient of chemical transmitters released by other neurons, the soma as the integrator, and the axon as the structure that transmits action potentials to the synapse. Chemicals released at the synapse then influence the activity of other neurons. We said nothing, however, about how impulses are transmitted from one neuron to another or from neurons to effector organs (muscles or gland cells).

There is now almost universal acceptance of the theory of chemical transmission between neurons. This merely means that transmission across synapses occurs by means of specific agents referred to as *chemical transmitters*. As will be seen, the actions of most psychoactive drugs can be interpreted in terms of their actions on these transmitters, that is, whether they mimic or modify them. This concept of chemical transmission between neurons holds that action potentials conducted down an axon cause the release of specific chemical substances when these potentials reach the axon terminal. These chemicals are, in turn, capable of altering the permeability of the dendritic membrane of the next neuron, resulting in either a depolarization (EPSP) or hyperpolarization (IPSP) of the dendrites of that neuron.

We shall now discuss the steps involved in synaptic transmission and the criteria that a chemical must meet in order to be called a transmitter substance. We shall also discuss specific substances that are thought to function in the central nervous system as synaptic transmitters.

Historical Background

The first suggestion that chemical substances might be involved in the transmission of information between neurons was probably made by Emil DuBois-Reymond in 1877. Subsequent work by such physiologists as Langley (1901), Elliot (1904), Dixon (1907), and Dale (1914) established the foundation for the concept that "excitation of a nerve induces the local liberation of a hormone, which causes specific activity by combination with some constituent of the end-organ, muscle or gland." The work of these early physiologists led to the identification of acetylcholine and epinephrine as transmitter substances in the peripheral nervous system (nerves lying outside the brain and spinal cord).

In 1921, Otto Loewi presented the first definite proof for the chemical mediation of nerve-impulse transmission. Loewi took the hearts out of two frogs and suspended the hearts from a frame. Because the rate at which a heart beats is controlled by nerve fibers (axons) that lead to the heart from the brain, Loewi electrically stimulated the nerve leading to one of the two hearts. He found that such stimulation slowed the rate at which the heart beat. Loewi dripped fluid over the heart that he was stimulating, then took this fluid and dripped it over the second heart (which was not being stimulated); he found that its rate also became slower. This demonstrated that electrical stimulation of the nerve leading to the one heart caused the release of a chemical that could slow the rate of the other heart, the nerves of which were not stimulated, proving that nerves exert their effects by releasing chemicals that act on the structure that the nerves innervate.

Loewi subsequently identified this substance as acetylcholine. He later also discovered that a chemical substance similar to epinephrine was liberated when the accelerator nerve to the heart was stimulated. Epinephrine is a transmitter substance important in the maintenance of many body functions, including heart rate, blood pressure, pupil size, lung function, and sex drive. Since these experiments were performed in cold-blooded animals (frogs), the experiments were repeated in 1927 by Rylant in the perfused rabbit heart. These and other investigations through the 1930s and 1940s established quite conclusively that a chemical mediator is instrumental in the transmission of impulses across synapses. Finally, in 1946 Euler identified norepinephrine as the chemical transmitter in the peripheral sympathetic nervous system. These early developments in studies of neurohumoral transmission are well detailed by Koelle.[1]

Steps in Synaptic Transmission

The synapse is so centrally important to the functioning of the nervous system and to the action of psychoactive drugs that it is useful to examine in more detail its structural features and its process of transferring information from the axon of one cell to the dendrites of another. Figure II.1 shows a schematic representation of a nor-

Figure II.1

Schematic diagram of a norepinephrine (NE) synapse within the central nervous system. The steps in the transmission of information across such a synapse are numbered in this diagram and listed below it.

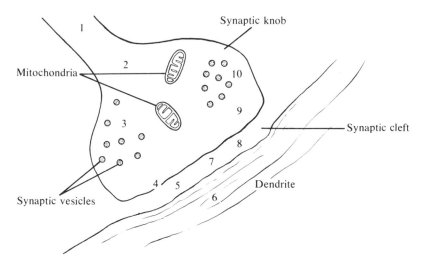

1. Conduction of the action potential down the presynaptic axon.
2. Arrival of the action potential at the nerve terminal.
3. Synthesis of NE (see Figure II.5) and storage of NE in the synaptic vesicles (this may occur before steps 1 and 2).
4. Release of NE from synaptic vesicles into the synaptic cleft upon the arrival of an action potential.
5. Diffusion of NE across the synaptic cleft.
6. Stimulation of the postsynaptic receptors by NE.
7. Release of NE from postsynaptic receptors back into the synaptic cleft.
8. Metabolism of some of the NE in the synaptic cleft by extracellular enzymes.
9. Uptake of some of the NE back into the presynaptic nerve terminal.
10. Uptake of NE in the presynaptic nerve terminal into the synaptic vesicles where it is protected from destruction by the enzyme MAO.

epinephrine synapse (which can be considered a typical synapse). It may be seen that the axon terminal makes close approximation with the dendrite through a narrow space of about 200 Å. This space (the synaptic cleft) separates the presynaptic membrane (the axon and axon terminal) from the postsynaptic membrane of the dendrite. Mitochondria (the metabolic factories of the cell) and numerous small synaptic vesicles are located in the presynaptic terminal. These vesicles are approximately 300 to 600 Å in diameter and in the nervous system are almost universally found in the nerve terminals adjacent to the presynaptic membrane on the presynaptic side of the cleft. In fact, the presence of these synaptic vesicles is considered proof of the presence of a synapse. Transmitter chemical is stored in these vesicles before it is released. The postsynaptic membrane is similar to membranes found elsewhere in the nervous system.

This, then, is the general organization of the synapse. Structure alone, however, does not explain the sequence of events that occurs between the arrival of an action potential at the terminal of one axon and the alterations that are then produced in the postsynaptic membrane of the dendrite of the next neuron. Basically there are 10 steps to consider in the synaptic transmission process (numbered in Figure II.1). Steps 1 through 4 are presynaptic events involving the synthesis, storage, and release of neurotransmitter. Steps 5 through 8 involve the extracellular action of the transmitter; that is, diffusion, receptor activation, and metabolic destruction of transmitter. Steps 9 and 10 involve the reuptake of the chemical transmitter and result in the cessation of information transfer. Step 9 involves the special property of the presynaptic membrane selectively to take up transmitter back into the presynaptic nerve terminal, thus removing it from the synaptic cleft. Finally, step 10 is the active reuptake of the transmitter that is in the intracellular fluid inside the nerve terminal back into the synaptic vesicles where the transmitter is protected from intracellular enzymes that might otherwise destroy it.

Criteria for a Transmitter Substance

Because the evidence for chemical transmission between neurons is virtually conclusive and because the steps in synaptic transmission have been identified, a vigorous search for specific transmitter substances in the central nervous system is currently in progress. A number of criteria must be satisfied in order to prove conclusively that a chemical is in fact an excitatory or inhibitory transmitter at a given synapse (Table II.1).

Common sense would dictate that one criterion would be that

Table II.1

Criteria for a chemical neurotransmitter

1. The proposed compound must be contained within the presynaptic nerve terminal
2. The proposed compound must be released from nerve endings on stimulation of the nerve
3. Injection of the proposed neurotransmitter must mimic the synaptic action that occurs after the normal transmitter is released
4. There must be some mechanism (enzymatic or otherwise) by which transmitter action can be terminated and that fits the time course of transmitter action
5. Drugs that interfere with the actions of the proposed transmitter must exert an identical action upon the effects of nerve stimulation

the transmitter chemical must be contained within the presynaptic terminal or that at least an immediate precursor (a substance that eventually becomes the transmitter) must be present. Strangely enough, for some of the substances that will be discussed in the following text, even this most essential criterion has not been satisfied conclusively. By similar reasoning, it would seem that this transmitter substance in the presynapatic terminal must be released from the synaptic nerve ending in response to the arrival of an action potential. In the peripheral nervous system, this second criterion is relatively easily satisfied, but in the central nervous system it is more difficult, because it is almost impossible to stimulate one axon selectively and to collect any substance that is released from the terminals of that axon. The third criterion is that the injection of a suspected synaptic transmitter must exert an effect on the postsynaptic membrane identical to the effect that follows the release of the normal transmitter. The same technical difficulties hinder the satisfaction of both the second and third criteria. The fourth criterion is that there must be some mechanism (enzymatic or otherwise) by which the action of the transmitter can be terminated and that fits the time course of action of the transmitter substance. This criterion has been more easily satisfied, although there is still difficulty in pinpointing precisely the exact mechanisms involved. The fifth criterion is that drugs that are known to alter the synthesis, release, action, or degradation of a supposed transmitter substance must exert an identical action at the synapse in question.

To date, there are few sites in the brain where any supposed transmitter substance has been shown to meet all these criteria. It is not surprising, however, that more advances have not been made in this area because the technical difficulties of the isolation and study of single synapses in the brain are enormous. In the peripheral nerves, it is often relatively easy to isolate particular types of synapses, which may then be accurately identified.

Specific Transmitter Substances

In this section, we will discuss specific transmitter substances: acetylcholine, norepinephrine and dopamine, serotonin, excitatory and inhibitory amino acids, and the opiate peptides.

Acetylcholine

Acetylcholine was first identified as a transmitter chemical in the peripheral nervous system. We now know that it is present in large amounts in brain tissue. Thus, it is not too surprising that scientists have interpreted this to mean that acetylcholine is also a transmitter chemical in the brain, so we shall discuss the evidence for and against the role of acetylcholine as a transmitter in the central nervous system.

The chemical reactions that take place in the nerve terminal and lead to the synthesis of acetylcholine are illustrated in Figure II.2, and the dynamics of the acetylcholine nerve terminal are portrayed in Figure II.3. Following synthesis, acetylcholine is thought to be stored inside the nerve terminal within synaptic vesicles until it is released into the synaptic cleft upon arrival of an action potential from the axon. The acetylcholine then diffuses across the cleft and attaches itself to receptors on the dendrite of the next neuron, which results in the transmission of information between the two neurons. This attachment is important to the pharmacologist because some psychoactive drugs may either mimic the action of acetylcholine at the dendritic receptor or else block access of the transmitter to the receptor. Drugs that mimic the action of acetyl-

Figure II.2

Chemical reactions in the brain responsible for synthesis of acetylcholine (ACh). The acetylcholine is synthesized from acetyl CoA and choline.

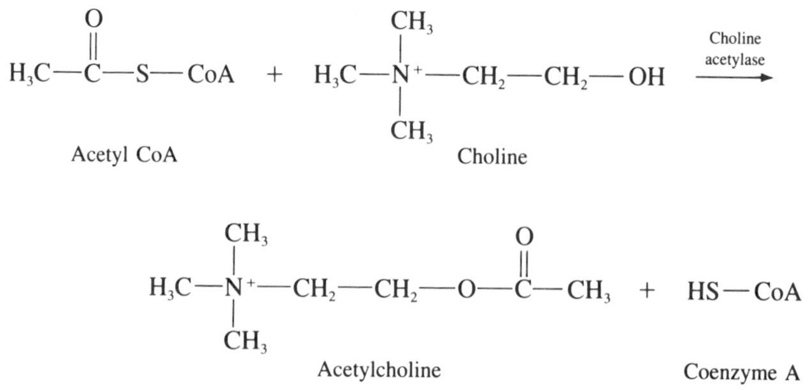

Figure II.3

Schematic diagram of an acetylcholine (ACh) synapse. The steps in transmission of information across such a synapse are numbered in the diagram and listed below it.

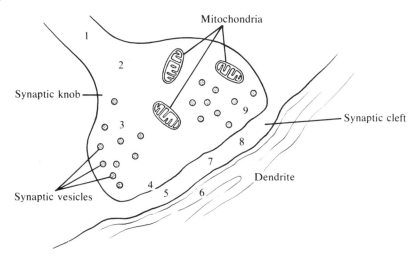

1. Conduction of the action potential down the presynaptic axon.
2. Arrival of the action potential at the nerve terminal.
3. Synthesis of ACh (see Figure II.2) and storage of ACh in the synaptic vesicles (this may occur before steps 1 and 2).
4. Release of ACh from synaptic vesicles into the synaptic cleft upon the arrival of an action potential.
5. Diffusion of ACh across the synaptic cleft.
6. Stimulation of the postsynaptic receptors by ACh.
7. Release of ACh from postsynaptic receptors back into the synaptic cleft.
8. Metabolism of ACh in the synaptic cleft by the enzyme AChE (see Figure II.4).
9. Uptake of choline produced by metabolism of ACh into the presynaptic nerve terminal for the resynthesis of ACh.

choline at the receptor include compounds such as nicotine and muscarine, both of which may alter behavior. Agents thought to block access of acetylcholine to the receptors include atropine and scopolamine.

Once acetylcholine has exerted its effect on the postsynaptic dendritic membrane, its action must somehow be terminated. Acetylcholine is destroyed by an enzyme, acetylcholine esterase (AChE). The process is illustrated in Figure II.4. The reaction that destroys acetylcholine is important to the pharmacologist because many drugs (referred to as AChE inhibitors) will inhibit the destructive enzyme. Such drugs include physostigmine, malathion, parathion, sarin, and soman, all of which may induce nightmares, confusion, hallucinations, feelings of agitation, confusion, and a slowing of intellectual and motor functions.

Figure II.4

Destruction of acetylcholine (ACh) by the enzyme acetylcholine esterase (AChE).

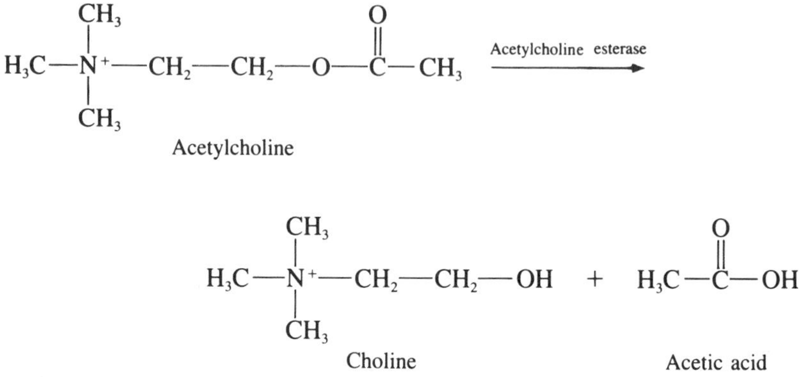

$$H_3C-\overset{\overset{\displaystyle CH_3}{|}}{\underset{\underset{\displaystyle CH_3}{|}}{N^+}}-CH_2-CH_2-O-\overset{\overset{\displaystyle O}{\|}}{C}-CH_3 \xrightarrow{\text{Acetylcholine esterase}}$$

Acetylcholine

$$H_3C-\overset{\overset{\displaystyle CH_3}{|}}{\underset{\underset{\displaystyle CH_3}{|}}{N^+}}-CH_2-CH_2-OH \quad + \quad H_3C-\overset{\overset{\displaystyle O}{\|}}{C}-OH$$

Choline   Acetic acid

The localization of acetylcholine in the brain is poorly delineated. Through indirect evidence it is thought that the highest concentrations of acetylcholine are in the caudate nucleus, certain brainstem nuclei, and the cerebral cortex. Little else is known about the role of acetylcholine in brain function. It is not yet even clear whether acetylcholine is an excitatory transmitter (producing EPSPs) or an inhibitory transmitter (producing IPSPs). It is entirely possible that it may be both excitatory and inhibitory, depending upon the reaction of the postsynaptic membrane to the chemical, because if one takes a microelectrode (a glass pipette with a tip that has a diameter of between 1 and 10 micrometers) and places acetylcholine directly onto individual cells within the brain, one finds that the acetylcholine increases the discharge of some neurons and inhibits the discharge of others.

Norepinephrine and Dopamine

The term *catecholamine* refers to a group of chemically related compounds, the most important of which are epinephrine, norepinephrine, and dopamine. In the peripheral nervous system, epinephrine is a neurotransmitter important in the maintenance of such major body functions as blood pressure and heart rate. Epinephrine is not commonly found in the brain. During the last 10 years, a large body of evidence has accumulated to demonstrate that norepinephrine and dopamine are the catecholamine neurotransmitters in the brain. This evidence appears to be much more substantial than that on acetylcholine, primarily because researchers can locate precisely the catecholamines in the brain. It has also become clear that many drugs that profoundly affect brain function and behavior exert their effects by altering the synaptic action of norepinephrine and dopamine in the brain. In many instances, the effects of new drugs on behavior have been predicted because of knowledge of their effects on the actions of the catecholamine neurotransmitters.

Dopamine and norepinephrine are manufactured within catecholamine neurons by the steps shown in Figure II.5. This synthesis was first proposed in 1939 and has now been confirmed, and the enzymes involved in each step have been identified and intensively studied. We shall not discuss the details of this scheme except to mention the step involving the enzyme tyrosine hydroxylase as a catalyst. Inhibition of this enzyme by drugs such as α-methyl-*p*-

Figure II.5

Synthesis of norepinephrine (NE) from tyrosine. Note the intermediate compounds formed in this reaction: namely, Dopa and dopamine.

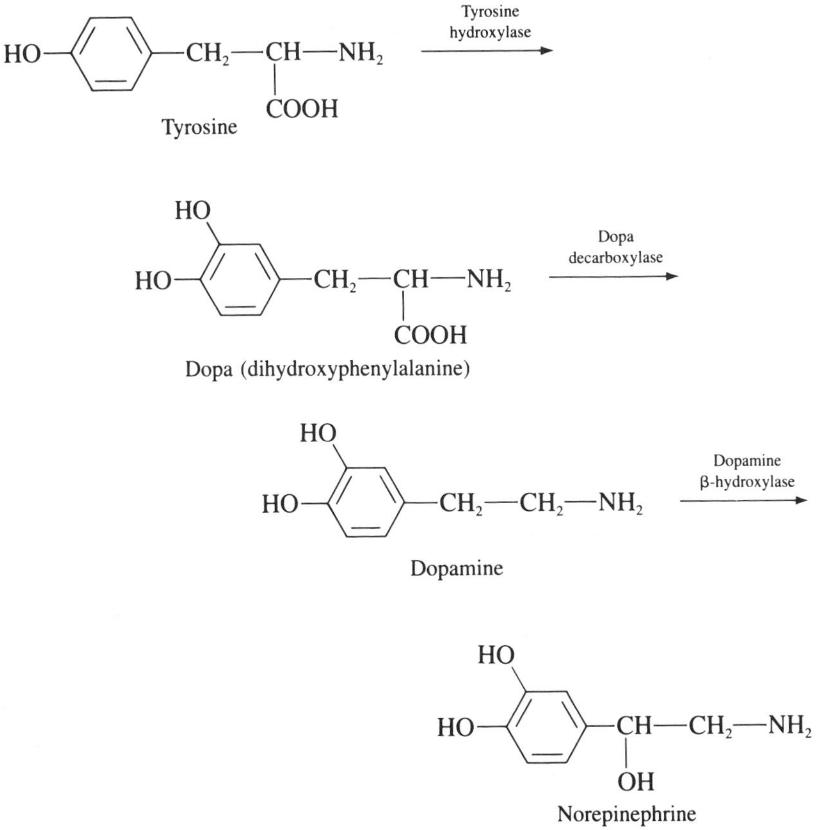

tyrosine results in a reduction in brain catecholamines and induces sedation, apparently secondary to the enzyme's inhibition of NE synthesis, which would indicate that the levels and functioning of neurotransmitters within the brain underlie behavior. By a similar reasoning, one might assume that drugs that alter behavior probably produce their effects secondary to alterations in chemical transmission between neurons. In Parkinson's disease, the dopamine normally present in a part of the brain called the caudate nucleus is reduced in amount. Administration of dopamine into the body is of little therapeutic use because it does not cross the blood-brain barrier. However, the administration of Dopa (the precursor to dopamine) does increase the dopamine levels in the caudate nucleus. What appears to happen is that Dopa is capable of crossing the blood-brain barrier and is converted into dopamine in the brain. This is an example of how knowledge of the chemical synthesis of a tranmitter may be used to clinical benefit.

Metabolic Fate   A transmitter must be synthesized, released, exert a postsynaptic effect, and then be inactivated. Inactivation can occur by either or both of two processes: enzymatic destruction and reuptake of the transmitter from the synaptic cleft back into the presynaptic nerve terminal. Catecholamines are inactivated by the enzymes monoamine oxidase (MAO) and catechol o-methyltransferase (COMT) (Figure II.6). Because these enzymatic inactivations appear to be less important in the termination of dopamine or norepinephrine neurotransmission than is the destruction of acetylcholine by AChE, it is unlikely that the postsynaptic effects of dopamine or norepinephrine are terminated to any significant extent by enzymes. The actions of these transmitters are terminated primarily by an active process—their reuptake across the presynaptic nerve membrane back into the presynaptic nerve ending. Norepinephrine or dopamine, taken up in this way, is then stored again in the synaptic vesicles to be reused later.

The principle of reuptake into the nerve terminal and then into the storage vesicles is crucially important, because there are drugs that may block either the active uptake process into the nerve terminal (thus potentiating the synaptic action of the transmitter) or the uptake of the transmitter from the intracellular fluid in the nerve terminal back into the synaptic vesicles. Reserpine is an example of a drug that blocks this uptake into the vesicle; cocaine is a representative of a class of drugs that blocks reuptake from the synaptic cleft into the nerve terminal. (As stated in Chapters 5 and 8, reserpine and cocaine have nearly opposite effects on the body and the brain.)

Figure II.6

Destruction of dopamine and norepinephrine. The inactivating enzymes are monoamine oxidase (MAO) and catechol *o*-methyltransferase (COMT).

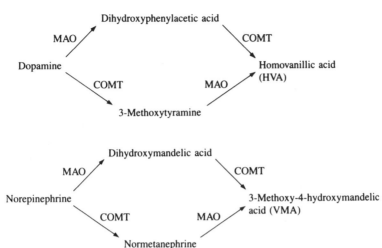

The Catecholamine Synapse   The dynamics of dopamine and norepinephrine are only slightly different from those of other CNS transmitters. A norepinephrine synapse is illustrated in Figure II.1. It is similar to the acetylcholine terminal presented in Figure II.3—that is, the presynaptic nerve terminal contains mitochondria and small vesicles containing stored transmitter. Also, like the acetylcholine terminal, the presynaptic nerve terminal is separated from the postsynaptic dendritic membrane by a distance of approximately 200 Å. The dopamine and norepinephrine terminals, however, contain entirely different chemical products. The amino acid tyrosine (obtained from food) is taken into the presynaptic terminal, where it is transformed to Dopa, dopamine, and, in some terminals, norepinephrine (NE).

In those terminals in which dopamine is not transformed into NE, the dopamine itself serves as the transmitter substance. The transmitter is stored in the synaptic vessels until released. Upon arrival of an action potential at the nerve terminal, the norepinephrine (or dopamine) is released from the vesicles (which cluster close to the cleft) into the synaptic cleft. The transmitter then diffuses across the cleft, reacting with the postsynaptic membrane to transfer information from one neuron to another. The transmission process is terminated by the uptake of NE (or dopamine) back into the nerve terminal, where it is either metabolized by the intracellular enzyme MAO or else taken up into and stored by the vesicles until it is released again.

At present, our knowledge of the functional role of norepinephrine in the brain is limited, in part, by a lack of understanding about which specific behavioral responses are associated with NE neurons. There is circumstantial evidence that the activity of neurons containing norepinephrine is associated with arousal reactions and with mood. This is illustrated by the fact that emotionally intense experiences (such as anxiety, fright, anger, and expectation) are accompanied by release of epinephrine in the peripheral nervous system. It is likely the norepinephrine neurons in the brain act similarly and are a representation of this "sympathetic" nervous system in the rest of the body. This hypothesis was postulated in the early 1950s when reserpine was introduced as a tranquilizing agent and the drug's sedative action was correlated with a depletion of norepinephrine in the brain. Since then, many of the inferences about the functions of NE and dopamine have been drawn from recent work on the location of these substances in the brain.

Localization in Brain   In recent years, much has been learned about the precise localization of dopamine and norepinephrine neurons and synapses within the brain. The cell somas and dendrites are situated in one area of the brain and the axons travel to other sites in the brain, where they synapse with the dendrites of other cells. In discussing the localization of dopamine and norepinephrine in the brain, we have to consider both the sites of the cell bodies (somas) and the sites to which their axons project. Figure II.7 is a schematic diagram of the distribution of norepinephrine in the brain. It appears that most norepinephrine cell bodies are situated in the brainstem and that these cell bodies send axons to certain brain structures. Other cell bodies send axons from the brainstem down to the spinal cord. Because the lower brain and the brainstem appear to be essential to the display of basic instinctual behavior in hunger, thirst, emotion, and sex, norepinephrine may be a neurotransmitter important in the regulation of these functions. More will be said about the physiology and pharmacology of the brainstem in Appendix III.

Dopamine cell bodies are primarily situated in the substantia nigra. These cells send axons to a group of structures called the *basal ganglia*. The dopamine neurons play an important role in movement, and loss of dopamine is associated with the disorder called Parkinson's disease. Thus, dopamine neurons appear to be clearly distinguishable from norepinephrine neurons.

Drug Effects on NE Nerve Terminals   Figure II.1 illustrates the general organization of a nerve terminal, with its process of synthesis,

Figure II.7

Schematic diagram of distribution of NE in rat brain. This illustrates the distribution of the main ascending pathways that contain norepinephrine as the synaptic transmitter. The shaded areas indicate the major nerve-terminal areas. [Modified from U. Ungerstedt, "Adipsia and Aphagia After 6-Hydroxydopamine Induced Degeneration of the Nigro-Striatal Dopamine System," *Acta Physiologica Scandinavica* (Supple.) 367 (1971): fig. 6, p. 110.]

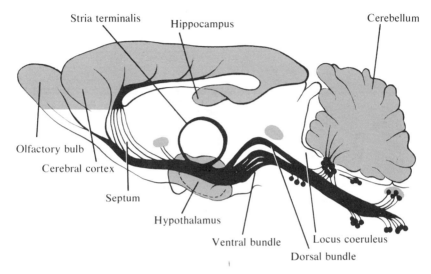

storage, release, metabolism, and reuptake of transmitter, using a norepinephrine terminal as an example. There are many drugs that are capable of inhibiting each of these processes in norepinephrine neurotransmission. Some drugs are capable of interfering with the synthesis of NE—for example, α-methyl-p-tyrosine and α-methyldopa. The latter compound is used clinically as an antihypertensive (the drug lowers blood pressure). Some drugs are capable of blocking the reuptake of norepinephrine from the synaptic cleft back into the nerve terminal, thus increasing the action of NE at the synapse. Such compounds include cocaine and a series of drugs that elevate mood and reverse depression (the tricyclic antidepressants).

Some drugs are capable of blocking the movement of norepinephrine from the intracellular fluid in the presynaptic nerve terminal into the storage granule (synaptic vesicle) where the transmitter is stored and protected from the enzyme MAO. An example of such a drug is reserpine. As a result of this blockage, NE may be metabolized by MAO and the nervous system depleted of the transmitter, with the result being sedation and emotional depression. Some drugs are capable of blocking the enzyme MAO, thereby increasing the NE concentration in the nerve terminal. Tranylcy-promine (Parnate) is one such MAO inhibitor; this action appears to account for the ability of the drug to elevate mood and reverse depression, effects similar to those produced by cocaine. Some compounds (ephedrine, for example) are capable of stimulating the post-synaptic norepinephrine receptor; others (phenoxybenzamine, for example) are capable of blocking the receptor. Some drugs, such as amphetamine, are capable of inducing the release of norepinephrine from the nerve terminal.

Serotonin

Serotonin (also called 5-hydroxytryptamine or 5-HT), like acetyl-choline, norepinephrine, and dopamine, is believed to be a neuro-transmitter in the brain. When 5-HT was first found within the brain, the theory arose that mental illness might be due to bio-chemical abnormalities within the 5-HT system. Current thought holds that this may be partly true, but mental illness is not so simply explained and other neurotransmitters are undoubtedly involved. Reserpine, for example, induces profound mental depression, apparently by depleting both norepinephrine and 5-HT.

More recently, several hallucinogenic compounds (LSD, for example) have been found to resemble 5-HT structurally, and the hypothesis has been advanced that at least some drug-induced hallucinations are due to alterations in the functioning of 5-HT neurons. In the brain, significant amounts of 5-HT are found in the upper brainstem. In the body, large amounts of 5-HT are found in the intestinal tract. The biosynthesis of 5-HT is illustrated in Figure II.8. The drug p-chlorophenylalanine (PCPA) inhibits the enzyme tryptophan hydroxylase, resulting in the depletion of 5-HT, with the concomitant induction of insomnia. An animal given PCPA will not sleep for several days, an effect that has generated much speculation on the role of 5-HT in sleep.

Like norepinephrine and dopamine, 5-HT is destroyed by the enzyme MAO. Metabolism of 5-HT results in formation of 5-hy-droxyindoleacetic acid (5-HIAA). Several hypotheses about a link between levels of 5-HT and mental illness (especially schizophrenia) have followed observations of altered levels of 5-HIAA in the urine of mentally ill patients. In the brain, 5-HT appears to be a neuro-transmitter involved in the regulation of body temperature, sensory perception, and sleep. Its other functions are less clear.

Excitatory and Inhibitory Amino Acids: Benzodiazepine Receptors

Specific roles of excitatory and inhibitory amino acids in behavioral function are now being delineated. Extensive research within the

Figure II.8

Synthesis of 5-hydroxytryptamine (serotonin) from tryptophan.

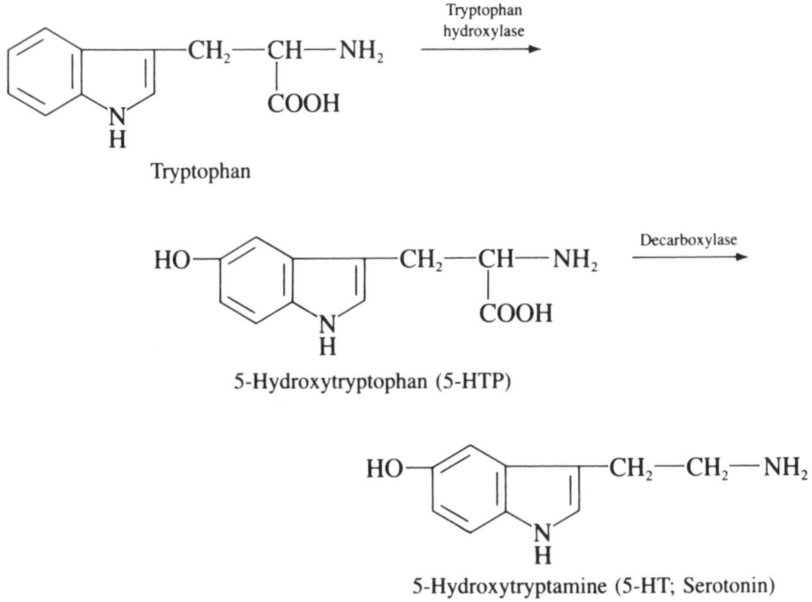

Tryptophan

5-Hydroxytryptophan (5-HTP)

5-Hydroxytryptamine (5-HT; Serotonin)

last few years indicates that certain amino acids may play important roles in the brain as neurotransmitter substances. The brain contains high concentrations of aspartic acid, γ-aminobutyric acid (GABA), and glutamic acid, and the spinal cord contains high concentrations of glycine. The structures of these four compounds are presented in Figure II.9.

Aspartic acid and glutamic acid appear to be universally excitatory; that is, their application to virtually any brain cell results in increased activity of that cell. GABA and glycine appear to be universally inhibitory. Interference with the activity of GABA or glycine synapses usually leads to convulsions. They appear to regulate brain excitability and may have important roles in behavior.[2,3]

GABA is the major inhibitor of neurotransmission in the brain. In drug studies, it has been shown that the antianxiety effects of benzodiazepine tranquilizers such as diazepam (Valium) occur when the synaptic actions of GABA are facilitated. These studies initiated a search for a "natural Valium," which would correspond to the discovery of enkephalins, which we call "natural opiates" (discussed in the next section).

Although no endogenous antianxiety compounds have been identified yet, it is generally agreed that the benzodiazepines po-

Figure II.9

Structures of four possible chemical neurotransmitters within the CNS.

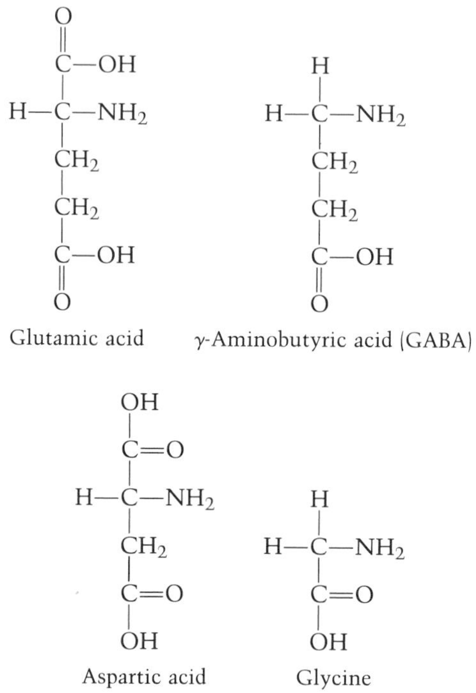

Glutamic acid γ-Aminobutyric acid (GABA)

Aspartic acid Glycine

tentiate the actions of GABA within the brain. There is a close physical approximation of GABA receptors to adjacent benzodiaze-pine receptors, but scientists have not yet been able to physically separate these two types of receptors. It is known that if GABA receptors are blocked (by convulsant drugs), the antianxiety effects of the benzodiazepines are antagonized. Recent research has iden-tified a specific benzodiazepine antagonist (an experimental com-pound called Ro 15-1788), which effectively reverses benzodiazepine overdoses. Should this compound eventually be marketed, it will be a significant advance in the management of patients suffering from benzodiazepine intoxication.

At low doses, the barbiturates (Chapter 3) also bind to benzo-diazepine receptors, but at higher doses they exert a variety of other, nonspecific depressant effects on the nervous system. Thus, the ben-zodiazepines may act by binding to specific benzodiazepine recep-tors that are closely linked with GABA receptors, while the barbi-turates may act on multiple types of synapses, exerting a more generalized depressant effect within the brain.

The Opiate Peptides

In 1967, it was proposed that the opiate narcotics mimic the actions of naturally occurring chemicals within the brain that provide analgesia by acting upon the receptors for those naturally occurring substances. This proposal was based upon three facts. First, opiates are highly specific; that is, certain very minor structural modifications convert an active drug to one that is almost totally inactive. Second, the extreme potency of some narcotics implies that only a specific receptor could account for this potency. For example, a narcotic named etorphine is 500 to 1000 times as potent as morphine. Thus, only a relatively few molecules of etorphine would be necessary for the drug to exert its effects on the brain. Third, pure narcotic antagonists are available (see Chapter 7), and these antagonists exert no other effect but to displace pharmacologically active narcotics from their "receptors."

In 1971, using a potent narcotic (levorphanol) and its inactive mirror-image isomer (dextrophan), researchers demonstrated that only 2 percent of the levorphanol exhibited binding not shared by dextrophan. This 2 percent was postulated to be responsible for the drug's pharmacological actions.

In 1973, three laboratories simultaneously reported finding specific opiate receptors localized in portions of the brain that contained a high concentration of nerve endings. Two years later, a bioassay for opiate receptors was developed. Recalling the fact that opiates exert prominent actions on the gastrointestinal tract (Chapter 7), researchers studied the small intestine of the guinea pig and demonstrated that opiate narcotics inhibited electrically induced muscle contractions and that such inhibition was blocked by the pure narcotic antagonist naloxone. This finding proved the existence of opiate receptors in this preparation.

Once opiate receptors had been identified, attempts were then made to localize them in the brain. It was found that only six areas of the brain have a high concentration of opiate receptors. First, high concentrations are located in the brainstem, lining the wall of the fourth ventricle. In this area, either morphine or electrical stimulation produces analgesia, which is blocked by naloxone. Second, the medial thalamus has a high concentration of opiate receptors. It is this area of the brain that appears to mediate deep pain that is poorly localized and emotionally influenced—the kind of pain most strongly affected by narcotics. Third, opiate receptors are found in specific areas of the spinal cord that are involved with the receipt and integration of incoming sensory information, thus dampening the input of painful stimuli. Fourth, receptors are also located in a specific nucleus of the brainstem that receives pain fibers from the face and the hands. Fifth, receptors are located in those centers of the brainstem involved in the mediation of cough, nausea and vomiting, maintenance of blood pressure, and control of stomach secretions. Finally, the greatest concentration of opiate receptors in the CNS is located in the limbic system, more specifically in the amygdala. Although narcotics are not thought to exert analgesic actions through receptors in the limbic system, such receptors are probably associated with the influences of opiates on emotional behavior (see Chapter 7). Opiate receptors are only rarely found in the cerebral cortex and none have been found in the cerebellum. Opiate receptors have been found in all vertebrates studied, but they have never been found in invertebrates.

In 1976, three types of opiate receptors were postulated. These were termed mu, kappa, and sigma. In 1981, a fourth type of receptor (the delta receptor) was added. More recent postulates focus on subtypes of these receptors.

Mu receptors are located primarily in the brainstem and medial thalamic areas and appear to mediate morphine-induced analgesia and respiratory depression. Kappa receptors are located primarily in the spinal cord and mediate spinal analgesia. In the brainstem, these kappa receptors mediate the sedation and miosis (pupil constriction) induced by opiates. Sigma receptors are located primarily in the limbic system and mediate dysphoria and the psychotomimetic effects produced by certain of the opioids, especially pentazocine (Talwin) and butorphanol (Stadol). The newly described delta receptors are postulated to be involved in alterations of affective behavior and euphoria. These receptors appear to be specific target receptors for the enkephalin peptides. Animal studies indicate that delta receptor stimulation is associated with opioid-induced reductions in respiratory rate.

Some opioid receptors are now being further subdivided. For example, a mu-1 receptor may be associated with analgesia while a mu-2 receptor may be associated with respiratory depression (especially reduced depth of breathing). In the future, perhaps, receptor-specific synthetic opiates might be developed such that specific mu-1 or kappa analgesia can be obtained in the absence of undesirable sigma, delta, or mu-2 side effects. Although this concept may seem to be far-fetched at the present time, it should be remembered that this unfolding story only began in the late 1970s and is proceeding at breakneck speed.

Thus, while receptors for opiates have been localized to specific areas of the brain, this alone does not prove the existence of naturally occurring compounds within the brain that act upon these receptors. Such proof was obtained in 1975, when researchers identified crude extracts from brain that demonstrated actions similar to morphine in the guinea-pig small-intestine preparation (discussed previously); that is, this brain extract inhibited intestinal contractions and this action was blocked by naloxone. Isolated from this crude extract were two proteins, each consisting of fine amino acids. These two proteins were named met-enkephalin and leu-enkephalin. More recently, these proteins have been isolated from pig brain, beef brain, human cerebral spinal fluid, and the pituitary glands of several species. Also isolated from the pituitary gland was a longer protein (called beta-lipotropin), within which was found met-enkephalin and other peptides with opiate activity (Figure II.10).

Beta-endorphin is the amino acid sequence 61–91 of the pituitary peptide, beta-lipotropin. Met-enkephalin is the amino acid sequence 61–65 of the same peptide (Figure II.10). Another pituitary peptide, designated dynorphin, is more potent than either beta-endorphin or met-enkephalin. Several possible functions, including neurotransmission as well as the possible existence of "natural opiates" have been postulated for the endorphins, dynorphins, and enkephalins; but their mechanism of analgesic action is not clear. The question then arises concerning the addictive potential of these compounds. Have we finally found a nonaddicting opiate narcotic? Recent work indicates that the answer to this question is *no*. Physical dependence to these proteins does develop, and there is both cross-tolerance and cross-dependence between these proteins and morphine. Therefore, these compounds probably have the same addiction potential as the opiate narcotics such as morphine. Perhaps laboratory modifications of these proteins may produce synthetic compounds that are nonaddictive. For the present, however, this is only optimistic speculation.

A variety of evidence indicates that the enkephalins are physiological neurotransmitters of specific neuronal systems in the brain that mediate the integration of sensory inputs related to pain, perception, and emotional behavior. Probably, in animals, this system is relatively inactive; otherwise, pure narcotic antagonists such as naloxone would displace the proteins from their receptors and would initiate pain or an increased responsiveness to a painful stimulus. Two studies (one in man and one in animals) into the influence of enkephalins in acupuncture have suggested that these proteins may mediate acupuncture-induced analgesia.

The interesting possibility that enkephalins may play a role in stress responses and in mental illness has been raised. The narcotic antagonist, naloxone, seems to be of some benefit in ameliorating hallucinogenic episodes in chronic schizophrenic patients. Also, in patients with chronic pain, enkephalin levels are altered. Certainly, these reports will stimulate additional attempts to delineate more clearly the role of enkephalins in various emotional states.

Is there a possible role of enkephalins in the tolerance and dependence that develop to opiate narcotics such as morphine? As postulated by A. Goldstein,[4] administration of narcotic analgesics

Figure II.10

The 91 amino-acid sequence (primary structure) of beta-lipotropin. The four structures outlined below beta-lipotropin are fragments known to exert opiatelike activity.

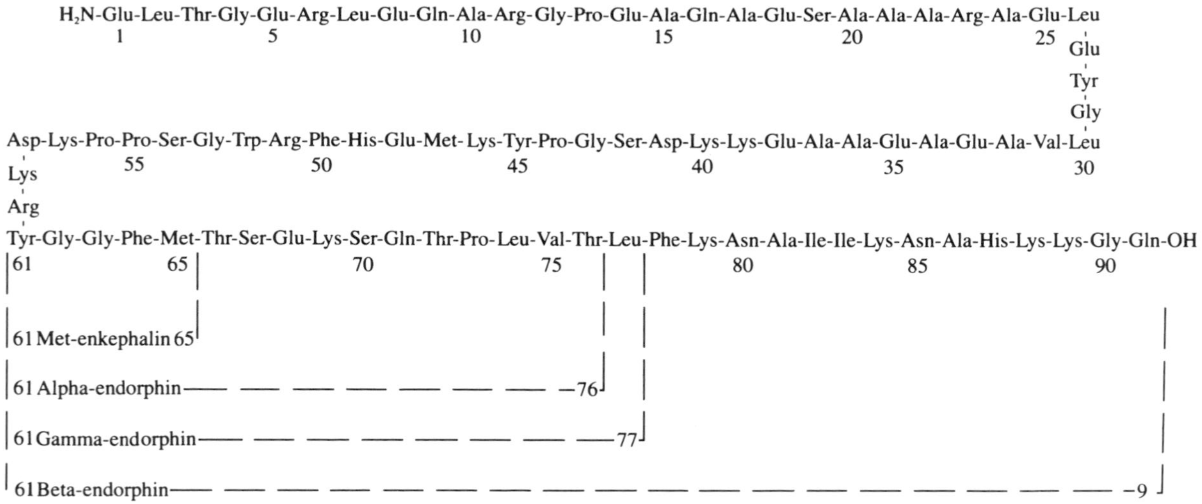

H₂N-Glu-Leu-Thr-Gly-Glu-Arg-Leu-Glu-Gln-Ala-Arg-Gly-Pro-Glu-Ala-Gln-Ala-Glu-Ser-Ala-Ala-Arg-Ala-Glu-Leu
  1   5   10   15   20   25   Glu
                                                                                                                                              Tyr
                                                                                                                                              Gly

Asp-Lys-Pro-Pro-Ser-Gly-Trp-Arg-Phe-His-Glu-Met-Lys-Tyr-Pro-Gly-Ser-Asp-Lys-Lys-Glu-Ala-Ala-Glu-Ala-Glu-Ala-Val-Leu
Lys   55   50   45   40   35   30
Arg

Tyr-Gly-Gly-Phe-Met-Thr-Ser-Glu-Lys-Ser-Gln-Thr-Pro-Leu-Val-Thr-Leu-Phe-Lys-Asn-Ala-Ile-Ile-Lys-Asn-Ala-His-Lys-Lys-Gly-Gln-OH
61   65   70   75   80   85   90

|61   65|
|61 Met-enkephalin 65|
|61 Alpha-endorphin————————————————————76|
|61 Gamma-endorphin——————————————————————77|
|61 Beta-endorphin——9|

such as morphine produces intense stimulation of enkephalin receptors, and the activity of enkephalin neurons is suppressed through a negative-feedback mechanism. As the levels of enkephalins fall, increasing amounts of opiates must be administered in order to achieve the same level of effect (that is, *tolerance* develops). When morphine administration is stopped, neither morphine nor enkephalins are present at the receptor and withdrawal symptoms appear (that is, *physical dependence*). Recovery from withdrawal is achieved only with the return of activity of enkephalin neurons.

In conclusion, exciting evidence has accumulated that has identified endogenous compounds with opiate-like activity.[5-10] The receptors upon which these compounds act appear to be the same receptors as those for the opiate narcotics. Whether opiate addiction can be explained on the basis of these endogenous substances—and the role of these substances in certain emotional states—remains to be delineated more clearly. The next few years will certainly bring an explosion of investigations into this most exciting and fascinating area of pharmacology.

Notes

1. G. B. Koelle, "Neurohumoral Transmission and the Autonomic Nervous System," in L. S. Goodman and A. Gilman, eds., *The Pharmacological Basis of Therapeutics*, 5th ed. (New York: Macmillan, 1975), pp. 410–412.
2. J. R. Cooper, F. E. Bloom, and R. H. Roth, *The Biochemical Basis of Neuropharmacology*, 3d ed. (New York: Oxford University Press, 1978).
3. F. E. Bloom, "Neurohumoral Transmission and the Central Nervous System," in A. G. Gilman, L. S. Goodman, and A. Gilman, eds., *Goodman and Gilman's The Pharmacological Basis of Therapeutics*, 6th ed. (New York: Macmillan, 1980), pp. 246–247.
4. A. Goldstein, "Opioid Peptide (Endorphins) in Pituitary and Brain," *Science* 193 (1976): 1081–1086.
5. A. D. Finck, "Opiate Receptors and Endorphins: Significance for Anesthesiology," *Refresher Courses in Anesthesiology* 7 (1979): 103–114.
6. S. H. Snyder, "Opiate Receptors in the Brain," *New England Journal of Medicine* 296 (1977): 266–271.
7. S. H. Snyder, "Receptors, Neurotransmitters and Drug Responses," *New England Journal of Medicine* 300 (1979): 465–472.
8. S. H. Snyder, "Drug and Neurotransmitter Receptors in the Brain," *Science* 224 (1984): 22–31.
9. E. L. Way, "Sites and Mechanisms of Basic Narcotic Receptor Function Based on Current Research," *Annals of Emergency Medicine* 15 (1986) 1021–1025.
10. M. L. Adams, D. A. Brase, S. P. Welch, and W. L. Dewey, "The Role of Endogenous Peptides in the Action of Opioid Analgesics," *Annals of Emergency Medicine* 15 (1986) 1030–1035.

Basic Anatomy of the Nervous System

In Appendixes I and II, we discussed the neuron—the fundamental unit of the nervous system—and the synapse and chemical neurotransmitters—the means of communication between individual neurons. In this appendix, we will go one step further and discuss the neurons as functional units within specific areas of the brain. It seems logical that we would have a better understanding of the actions of psychoactive drugs after we made an introductory examination of the functions of the nervous system that underlie behavior.

Because the brain is perhaps the most complex of all biological structures, discussion of its anatomy and function is difficult. Still, a number of introductory and straightforward principles can be described that may lead to a relatively uncomplicated outline of the anatomy and physiology of the brain and help explain why different drugs acting at different synapses exert different effects on brain function as well as behavior.

Introductory Terminology

For ease in teaching and in understanding, the nervous system is divided into two major functional systems: the *central nervous system (CNS)* and the *peripheral nervous system*. The central nervous system consists of all the neurons that are situated inside the skull and the spine. The peripheral nervous system consists of all the neurons outside the skull and spine. In turn, the CNS may be subdivided into two major parts: the brain and the spinal cord. The brain is a collection of some 13 billion neurons, with their dendrites and axons, entirely contained within the skull (Figure III.1). The lower part of the brain, which is attached to the upper part of the spinal cord, is referred to as the *brainstem*. The brainstem is situated entirely within the skull. All impulses transmitted (in both directions) between the spinal cord and the brain must of necessity be transmitted through the brainstem, which is also important in the regulation of vital body functions and is a site of action of many psychoactive drugs.

If we divide the brain into its component parts (Figure III.1), we see that the top or front end of the CNS (the *cerebrum*) is considerably larger than the brainstem and the spinal cord. As the upper

Figure III.1

The central nervous system. The situation of the brain and spinal cord within the body (*left*) and the principal components of the central nervous system (*right*).

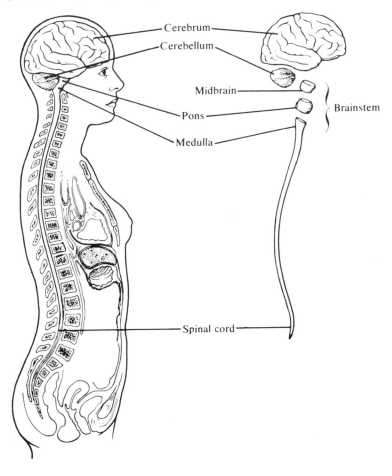

part of the spinal cord enlarges, it separates into three distinct yet completely interconnected segments, referred to as the *medulla*, the *pons* (or bridge), and the *midbrain*. These three segments comprise the brainstem. The area immediately above the brainstem is referred to as the *diencephalon* and includes the hypothalamus, the pituitary gland, the fiber tracts from the eyes (optic tracts), and the thalamus. The region below the thalamus is referred to as the subthalamus. Finally, almost completely covering the brainstem and diencephalon are the two *cerebral hemispheres*, the left and the right.

Although this is not a complete outline of all brain structures (several structures have been omitted), this should suffice as an introduction to the concept that the brain is not a homogeneous structure but may be subdivided anatomically into many functional units.

The Spinal Cord

The spinal cord, in general, handles two types of activities: the spinal reflexes and the channeling of information between the periphery and the brain. If you step on a tack or touch a hot stove, you will immediately withdraw the affected limb. This unconscious reflex withdrawal in response to heat or pain is carried out over an arrangement of neurons called a *reflex arc* set up through the spinal cord. When you step on a tack, sensory receptors are stimulated. These receptors are specialized dendrites of neurons whose sole function is to sense the external environment. In contrast to the typical neuron discussed in Appendix I, the dendrite of this sensory receptor is activated by heat, cold, pain, touch, or pressure rather than by chemically induced synaptic EPSPs. This specialized neuron sends information to the spinal cord, where (through a synapse) a motor neuron is excited (by an EPSP). Excitation of the motor neuron is translated into action potentials that travel to the muscles, which then contract and cause the withdrawal from the painful stimulus.

The motor neurons in the spinal cord are also influenced by information from the brain. For example, certain areas of the brain, when stimulated, will increase the activity of the motor neurons. Many drugs that cause behavioral sedation decrease the flow of information from the brain to the spinal cord. Such drugs are frequently used as muscle relaxants because they decrease the spinal cord's control over muscle tone by indirectly decreasing the activity of the motor neurons. Other drugs can produce just the opposite effect. For example, some convulsant drugs, such as strychnine, block inhibitory controls over the activity of the motor neurons.

Discharges from the motor neurons are increased and convulsions result.

The Brainstem

The brainstem lies inside the skull and connects the spinal cord with the diencephalon and the cerebrum. The major subdivisions of the brainstem are the *medulla, pons,* and *midbrain* (Figure III.1). Behind the midbrain is a large bulbous structure called the *cerebellum.*

Medulla

The medulla is the direct continuation of the spinal cord in the skull. All ascending and descending fiber tracts connecting the brain and the spinal cord pass through the medulla. Also in the medulla are centers largely responsible for the control of respiration (breathing), peripheral vasoconstriction (blood pressure), heart rate, strength of contraction of the heart, functioning of the gastrointestinal tract, and control of sleeping and waking. The medulla also seems to play a fundamental role in behavioral alerting, attention, or arousal. Some depressant drugs (such as the opiates and the barbiturates) depress these centers in the brainstem, and death from an overdose of such drugs may occur as a result of the depression of the centers. Other agents that are clinically used for the treatment of high blood pressure seem to exert at least part of their hypotensive effect by depressing the centers in the medulla that control vascular tone. Drugs that affect the state of arousal of an animal or affect sleeping or wakefulness seem to act in the medulla and in the rest of the brainstem.

All drug actions on the brainstem, however, are not depressant in nature. Some drugs exert both stimulant and depressant effects, depending on the specific area. Morphine, for example, depresses respiratory centers in the medulla, but it also stimulates an area in the medulla called the chemoreceptor trigger zone. Stimulation of this zone may result in vomiting.

The central core of the medulla is a complex network of cell bodies (somas) and fibers (axons) that extends from the medulla up the brainstem almost to the level of the thalamus and is called the *reticular formation.* One portion of this reticular formation is referred to as the *ascending reticular activating system (ARAS).* In 1949, it was demonstrated that electrical stimulation of the ARAS resulted in a transition in the brain-wave activity (the electroencephalogram, or EEG) from that characteristic of sleep to that characteristic of wakefulness. Destruction of the ARAS tended to yield an EEG pattern that is usually associated with drowsiness or sleep. Thus, it would seem, by association, that the ARAS is involved in the control of sleeping and waking (and also behavioral alerting). It was subsequently demonstrated in the mid-1950s that drugs that produce depression (the barbiturates and ether, for example) inhibit activity in the ARAS.

The ARAS is stimulated normally by inputs passing through the brainstem en route from the body to the brain. The resulting activation of the cortex by the ARAS may alert the brain to be ready to receive information. If the ARAS could not be activated by incoming information, the animal would be unaware of its surroundings and would most likely be asleep or not receptive. Barbiturates, for example (see Chapter 3), depress the ARAS so that it is not activated by incoming information and stimuli do not arouse the animal (that is, the animal is asleep or anesthetized).

Drugs that stimulate the ARAS would be expected to arouse the animal and most probably increase behavioral activity. Amphetamine, one such drug, is thought to stimulate behavior by increasing the activity of norepinephrine synapses in the ARAS.

More recently, evidence has been presented that antipsychotic drugs such as chlorpromazine (Chapter 8) may exert their actions by decreasing input into the ARAS and that psychedelic compounds such as LSD (Chapter 9) may exert their actions of intensifying alertness and causing hallucinations by increasing input into the ARAS.

Pons

The pons (or bridge) is the part of the brainstem above the medulla and below the midbrain. The pons contains ascending and descending fiber tracts (axons) connecting the brain, the spinal cord, and the cerebellum and also contains a few structures that control sensory and motor functions to and from the face and head. To date, specific pharmacological actions on the pons have not been clearly delineated.

Midbrain

Above the pons is the midbrain. Toward the cerebrum, the midbrain merges with the thalamus, hypothalamus, and a large number of subthalamic structures. The outstanding features of the midbrain are the relay structures that control vision and hearing. Other structures in the midbrain control eye movement and muscle coordination. On the posterior of the midbrain are two structures called the inferior colliculus and the superior colliculus, which are thought to be possible sites of action of certain psychedelic drugs that induce auditory or visual hallucinations. The ARAS extends forward from the medulla up through the midbrain.

Cerebellum

The cerebellum is a large, highly convoluted structure situated immediately behind the brainstem and connected to it by three large pairs of fiber tracts. The exact functions of the cerebellum are still being studied, but it is quite widely agreed that the cerebellum is necessary for the proper integration of movement. Some drugs exert noticeable effects on cerebellar activity. Drunkenness, characterized by loss of coordination, staggering, loss of balance, and other deficits, appears to be largely due to an alcohol-induced depression of the cerebellum.

The Diencephalon

The diencephalon is a portion of the brain situated above the brainstem, below the cerebral cortex, and buried between the right and left cerebral hemispheres. The diencephalon may be further subdivided into several areas, three of which will be discussed: the thalamus, the hypothalamus, and the subthalamus.

Thalamus

The thalamus is the largest structure of the diencephalon and is actually a group of many smaller structures. Physiologically, the thalamus is often referred to as a way station, where incoming sensory pathways traveling up the spinal cord and through the brainstem synapse before passing into various areas of the cerebral cortex. Thus, the thalamus may be thought of as one of the primary relay stations of the brain.

Various subdivisions of the thalamus receive projections from specific sensory organs and, in turn, the neurons in these subdivisions relay information to specific areas of cerebral cortex. Inputs from vision, hearing, touch, pressure, position, pain, and so on feed into specific regions of the thalamus before being relayed to the areas of the cerebral cortex specifically associated with the senses. Other less well-defined areas of the thalamus are referred to as association areas. These areas do not receive sensory information directly but somehow integrate incoming information and relay it to the so-called association areas of the cerebral cortex. There are certain other areas of the thalamus that do not project directly into the cerebral cortex but connect the ARAS and the rest of the reticular formation with other thalamic regions, with the hypothalamus, and with the limbic system. These areas appear to form what is called the diffuse thalamic projection system, which has been implicated as a site of action of several psychoactive drugs. Electrical stimulation of the diffuse thalamic projection system yields behavioral alerting and EEG arousal reactions similar to those that follow stimulation of the ARAS. This diffuse thalamic projection system may therefore be an extension of the ARAS.

Subthalamus

The subthalamus is a small area underneath the thalamus and above the midbrain containing a variety of small structures that, in general, constitute one of our motor systems, the extrapyramidal system. Patients with Parkinson's disease, a disorder characterized by exaggerated motor movements, have a deficiency of the neurotransmitter dopamine in the terminals of their nerve axons, which originate from cell bodies in the substantia nigra (one of the subthalamic structures). Administration of Dopa to these patients replaces the dopamine and ameliorates the symptoms (see Appendix II). Thus, in humans, as well as in lower mammals and birds, the subthalamic structures, together with the cerebellum, seem to be important in the control and coordination of motor activity.

Hypothalamus

The hypothalamus consists of a collection of structures in the lower portion of the brain near the junction of the midbrain and the thalamus. The hypothalamus has important centers for the control of such vegetative functions as eating, drinking, sleeping, the regulation of body temperature, sexual behavior, and water balance. (More intensive discussions of the functional anatomy of the hypothalamus and limbic system may be found in textbooks of physiological psychology listed in the bibliography. The structures are mentioned here, albeit briefly, because their functions are altered by many psychoactive drugs.) In addition, activity of the pituitary gland (Chapter 11) is under the close control of the hypothalamus. The hypothalamus also appears to be important in the modulation of emotion and behavior and is a site of action of many psychoactive drugs, either as a site of the drug's primary action or as a site responsible for side effects associated with the use of the drug. It is pertinent to mention the so-called reward centers in the hypothalamus, the self-stimulation centers, especially the posterior hypothalamus and other areas of the median forebrain bundle and the limbic system, which appear to contain norepinephrine neurons and to modulate what are referred to, in operant conditioning, as approach and avoidance behavior.

Limbic System

Closely associated with the hypothalamus is the limbic system, the major components of which are the amygdala, the hippocampus, the mammillary bodies, and a variety of other smaller structures. Recently, considerable attention has been drawn to the study of the effects of drugs on the hypothalamus and the limbic system. Because the limbic system and hypothalamus interact in the regulation of emotion and emotional expression, these structures are logical sites in which to study drugs that alter emotion or responses to emotional experiences. It is felt that some tranquilizers such as chlordiazepoxide (Librium) or diazepam (Valium) may depress limbic functions at doses below those that depress other functions in the brain. Such actions would result in "tranquilization" or "relief from anxiety" at doses lower than those that result in behavioral depression. The classical notion that the limbic system is important in learning and memory has prompted investigations of this structure and the hypothalamus as sites of action of compounds that affect learning and memory. Atropine and scopolamine (Chapter 9) impair learning and memory and cause prominent alterations in electrical activity that may be recorded from the limbic system's structures. Certain structures of the limbic system have extremely low thresholds for seizure activity. It has been postulated (and in some cases demonstrated) that certain convulsant drugs act rather specifically upon structures of the limbic system.

The hypothalamus influences five categories of function: emotional behavior, eating and drinking behavior, sexual behavior, control of body functions (homeostasis), and control of the pituitary gland. It appears that the hypothalamus integrates emotional behavioral patterns. In the 1940s, W. R. Hess found that electrical stimulation of certain areas of the hypothalamus induced the sorts of responses usually encountered in expressions of rage. He suggested that these responses were part of the mechanisms in the brain and body that are normally involved in the mediation of the fight/flight/fright response. The fight/flight/fright reaction may be seen after the administration of such sympathomimetic drugs as amphetamine, which, for instance, increases activity apparently as a result of its action on the centers in the hypothalamus and the limbic system.

A satiety center is situated in one part of the hypothalamus, and a feeding center exists in another part. If the satiety center is destroyed, an animal will feed excessively and become obese; if the feeding and drinking centers are destroyed, an animal will neither eat nor drink. Amphetamine is a potent appetite suppressant and the drug has often been used clinically (although improperly) for this purpose. It is thought that amphetamine stimulates the neurons in the satiety center so that the animal stops eating because it feels full.

The hypothalamus is an important structure for both the neural and the humoral control of sexual behavior. If the front part of the hypothalamus is destroyed, an animal will not mate. Electrical stimulation of this part of the hypothalamus usually leads to an increase in sexual behavior. Since most of the patterns observed during periods of sexual arousal are sympathetic in origin (for example, increased heart rate, increased blood pressure, and behavioral excitement), it is not surprising that this emotion would arise from a center in the brain that is involved in the control of the sympathetic nervous system. Much of the sex drive appears to result from an action of neurons in the hypothalamus.

The hypothalamus is also important in the hormonal control of sex. Neurons in the hypothalamus produce and secrete substances called releasing factors, which travel to the nearby pituitary gland. There, they cause the production and secretion of hormones that act on the sex organs to cause sexual development, menstrual cycling, ovulation, and sperm formation. (The hypothalamus and pituitary gland are so active in the regulation of body hormones that Chapter 11 of this book was devoted entirely to this topic and to the action of drugs that affect fertility.)

We stated previously that the hypothalamus is involved in a process of homeostasis. This merely means the hypothalamus is involved in the control of vital body functions such as temperature regulation and water balance. It appears that the hypothalamus contains discrete areas for the control of body temperature, one area being responsible for increasing body temperature and the other for decreasing it. If body temperature is increased, the anterior portion of the hypothalamus is activated and induces sweating and dilatation of cutaneous blood vessels, to aid the body in lowering its temperature. If body temperature (or skin temperature) drops, the posterior portion of the hypothalamus is activated and induces shivering and constriction of the cutaneous blood vessels in an effort to conserve heat.

Certain cells of the hypothalamus are osmoreceptors. This means that these cells are capable of responding to the osmolarity (salinity, saltiness) of the blood. These cells, by releasing antidiuretic hormone (ADH), control the ability of the body to retain fluids. If the osmolarity of the blood increases above normal, this is sensed by the osmoreceptor cells of the hypothalamus, ADH is released, and the kidneys respond by conserving rather than excreting body fluids. The hypothalamus is closely involved in the functioning of the pituitary gland, which may be regarded as the master gland of the body because, under the influence of the hypothalamus, it releases a number of hormones that control body function (see Chapter 11).

The Cerebral Cortex

In humans, the cerebral cortex makes up the largest portion of the brain. The cerebral cortex is separated into two distinct hemispheres, the left and the right. Numerous fiber tracts interconnect the two hemispheres both at a level above the thalamus and through multisynaptic pathways in the brainstem. In humans, because skull size is limited and the cerebral cortex has grown so large, the cortex is deeply convoluted and fissured. We will not discuss the functions of the cerebral cortex at length, but it is important to mention that, like the portions of the brain discussed previously, the cerebral cortex is divided functionally—that is, it contains distinct centers for vision, hearing, speech, sensory perception, emotion, and so on.

The nervous system is extremely complex in structure and function and the cerebral cortex represents the ultimate development of this complexity. Volumes have been devoted to the structure and function of even small parts of the cerebral cortex, and only now are we beginning to understand something of the brain's precise functioning and interrelations. At present, little is known about the action of psychoactive drugs on the cerebral cortex. Undoubtedly, many psychoactive drugs will ultimately be found to affect the cerebral cortex, but our present knowledge of cortical function limits the precise delineation of such actions.

Drug Transport

The absorption, distribution, metabolism, and excretion of drugs involve the passage of drugs across cell membranes. When we consider the passage of drugs out of the stomach and into the blood, we must take into account the fact that most drugs exist as a *mixture* of forms that are either water soluble or fat soluble. In the water-soluble form, the drug molecule exists in an electrically charged form called an ion and is therefore referred to as being ionized. The extent to which any given drug exists in either the water-soluble or the fat-soluble form depends on the drug itself and on the relative acidity of the fluid in which it is dissolved.

As we stated in Chapter 1, the body may be divided, theoretically, into several compartments, each with a different pH. The gastric juice is very acid (about pH 1.0), whereas the intestinal contents vary from about pH 2.0 to pH 6.6. Blood is slightly alkaline (pH 7.4), while the urine in the kidneys is acidic (usually between pH 4.5 and pH 7.0). These pH differences among blood, gastric juice, intestine, and kidney play a major role in determining whether a drug will be absorbed from an area of low pH to an area of higher pH or vice versa.

Most drugs are weak acids or bases and are presented in solution in both un-ionized and ionized forms; the proportion of ionized drug to un-ionized drug depends upon the pK_a of the drug (the pH at which the drug is 50 percent ionized) and upon the acidity of the medium in which the drug is dissolved. The un-ionized portion is usually fat soluble and can readily diffuse across cell membranes, but the ionized fraction is less able to penetrate most body membranes. The rate of equilibration of the un-ionized portion of a drug across the membrane is directly related to the drug's fat solubility because that is the limiting factor in determining passage through the membrane.

If a pH difference exists across the membrane (as for example, between stomach and blood), the fraction of ionized drug will be considerably greater on one side of the membrane than on the other. At equilibrium, the concentration of the un-ionized drug will be equal on both sides of the membrane; but the quantity of drug will be higher on the side where the degree of ionization is greater. This is illustrated in Figure IV.1, in which a weakly acidic drug is shown to exist in the gastric juice largely in the un-ionized (fat-soluble) form. Approximately 1000 times as much of this particular drug exists in the un-ionized form as exists in the ionized form at this pH. In the blood, however, this weakly acidic drug exists largely in the ionized form, because it is now in an alkaline medium, so that approximately 1000 times as much drug exists in the ionized form as exists in the un-ionized form at this pH. Since un-ionized molecules are in equilibrium across the membrane, the concentrations of un-ionized drug will be the same in both compartments. However, as may be seen from Figure IV.1, there is a considerably larger quantity of drug in the blood than in the gastric juice because, in blood, the drug exists largely in the ionized form. Because these ionized drug molecules are unable to traverse the membrane back into the

Figure IV.1

Compartmentalization of weakly acidic drug (*HA*) across cellular membrane separating stomach from blood. Note that in compartments of different pH, more or less of a drug will exist in an ionized or un-ionized form. Note also that only the un-ionized portion of the drug is in equilibrium across the membrane. [After L. Z. Benet and L. B. Sheiner, "Pharmacokinetics: The Dynamics of Drug Absorption, Distribution and Elimination," in A. G. Gilman, L. S. Goodman, T. W. Rall, and F. Murad. eds., *Goodman and Gilman's The Pharmacological Basis of Therapeutics*, 7th ed. (New York: Macmillan, 1985), fig. 1.2, p. 4.]

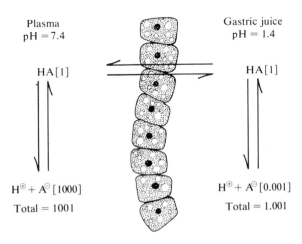

Fatty cellular membrane

Plasma
pH = 7.4

Gastric juice
pH = 1.4

HA[1]

HA[1]

$H^{\oplus} + A^{\ominus}$ [1000]

Total = 1001

$H^{\oplus} + A^{\ominus}$ [0.001]

Total = 1.001

stomach, the drug is *absorbed* through this process of ion trapping. The ratio of un-ionized to ionized drug at each pH (and therefore in each compartment) can be calculated from the Henderson-Hasselbalch equation: pH = pK_a + log [base/acid].[1-2]

Many drugs, however, are not weak acids but are weak *bases* (that is, they are slightly alkaline). In acidic compartments, such as the stomach, these weak bases are highly ionized and therefore do not pass through cell walls. In a basic (or alkaline) medium, however, such drugs are less ionized and exist largely in a fat-soluble form. A weak base is poorly absorbed from the stomach because it is highly ionized in gastric fluid and is ion-trapped in the stomach. In the intestine, however, the drug becomes less ionized and thus is better able to cross the membrane separating intestine from blood. This is illustrated in Figure IV.2, in which, in the intestine (pH 6.6), a weak base exists in both un-ionized and ionized forms. Slightly more of the drug is un-ionized. In the blood (pH 7.4), this same drug is more ionized than un-ionized (predictable from the Henderson-Hasselbalch equation). Thus, because only the un-ionized drug is in equilibrium across the membrane, there is a higher concentration of drug in the blood than in the intestine and the drug is absorbed. The absorption of weak bases from the intestine is much less complete than the absorption of weak acids from the stomach because

Figure IV.2

Compartmentalization of weak base drug (*HA*) across cellular membrane separating intestne from blood. Compare with Figure IV.1, which illustrates the distribution of a weak acid between the stomach and the blood. The difference of pH values in stomach and intestine allows for greatly different rates and degrees of absorption.

Fatty cellular membrane

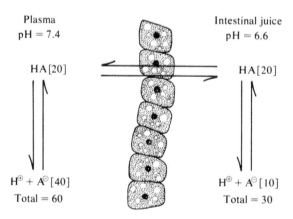

Plasma		Intestinal juice
pH = 7.4		pH = 6.6
HA[20]		HA[20]
$H^{\oplus} + A^{\ominus}$[40]		$H^{\oplus} + A^{\ominus}$[10]
Total = 60		Total = 30

there is a much smaller pH difference across the membrane. There-fore, absorption of drugs that are weak bases (compounds such as reserpine, codeine, morphine, or atropine) is much less efficient than absorption of weak acids and such drugs are often administered by injection.

The anatomy of the gastrointestinal tract is illustrated in Figure IV.3. Food (and drugs) must first pass through the stomach before they reach the intestine. Because weak acids are well absorbed from the stomach, large amounts frequently do not reach the intestine. Weak bases, however, are not absorbed from the stomach and must survive several hours exposure to stomach acids before they are passed into the intestine where they may be absorbed. This pro-longed exposure to stomach acids tends to destroy many drugs and

Figure IV.3

Schematic illustration of gastrointestinal tract.

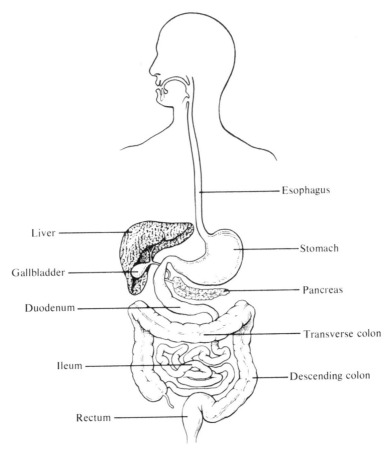

is another reason for the poor and incomplete absorption of weak bases that have been administered orally.

Notes

1. L. Z. Benet and L. B. Sheiner, "Pharmacokinetics: The Dynamics of Drug Absorption, Distribution and Elimination," in A. G. Gilman, L. S. Goodman, T. W. Rall, and F. Murad, eds. *Goodman and Gilman's The Pharmacological Basis of Therapeutics*, 7th ed. (New York: Macmillan, 1985).
2. R. R. Levine, *Pharmacology: Drug Actions and Reactions*, 3rd ed. (Boston: Little, Brown), 1983.

The Dose-Response Relationship

As demonstrated in Chapter 1, there is little selectivity of distribution of drugs in the body. Psychoactive compounds are usually found fairly equally distributed to all tissues of the body (for example, there is usually as much drug in the liver or heart as there is in the brain). Thus, the selectivity of the compound (if any) is not dependent upon selective distribution of the drug but upon a selective distribution of receptors for the drug: the drug will act only where its receptors are situated. At different doses, the drug may interact with a variety of receptors. A drug, therefore, cannot be completely characterized by a single action because different effects are observed at different doses. Few drugs exert only one effect.

One of the basic principles of pharmacology is that drug effects cannot be specifically delineated unless one considers the amount (or dose) of the drug.[1-2] The relation between the dose of the drug and the intensity of a response is referred to as the *dose-response relation*. In Figure V.1 two types of dose-response curves are illustrated. In one case, the dose of the drug is plotted against the percentage of individuals exhibiting a characteristic effect. In the other example, the dose of the drug is plotted against the intensity or the magnitude of the response in a single individual. Both of these curves indicate that for each drug there is a dose low enough to produce no noticeable effect.

At the opposite extreme, there is a dose beyond which no greater response can be elicited. This dose-response relation is valid for only a single effect of the drug. Because every drug is capable of producing many effects, each drug will have a different dose-response curve for each observable effect that the drug induces. For example, for a sedative compound, a dose-response curve could be drawn for the

Figure V.1

Two types of dose-response curves. *Left*, the curve obtained by plotting the dose of drug against the percentage of subjects showing a given response at any given dose. *Right*, the dose of drug against the intensity of the response observed in any single individual at a given dose. The intensity of response is plotted as a percentage of the maximum obtainable response.

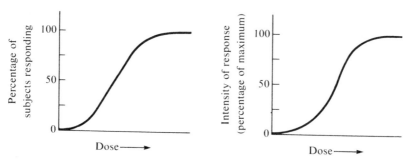

amount of sedation induced. We could equally well draw a dose-response curve for the relation between the dose of a drug and the number of animals put to sleep at each dose. Finally, we could draw a dose-response curve comparing the dose of the drug and the number of animals that died after the drug was administered (Figure V.2).

Figure V.2

A particular dose-response curve. This is the sort that would be obtained by plotting various doses of a drug against the deaths induced by progressive increases in dosage. Each point represents the number of deaths that occur in each group of 10 animals.

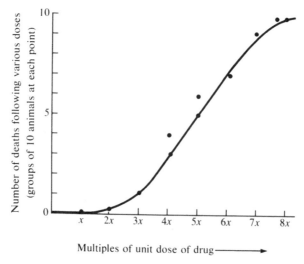

Figure V.3

Three principal components of dose-response curve: potency, slope, and maximum effect. [After E. M. Ross and A. G. Gilman, "Pharmacodynamics: Mechanisms of Drug Action and the Relationship Between Drug Concentration and Effect," in A. G. Gilman, L. S. Goodman, T. W. Rall, and F. Murad, eds. *Goodman and Gilman's The Pharmacological Basis of Therapeutics*, 7th ed. (New York: Macmillan, 1985), fig. 2-5, p. 44.]

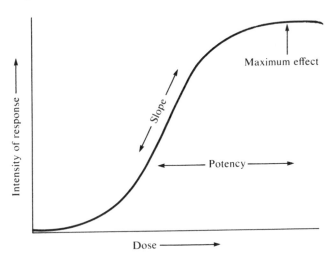

For each comparison, however, the curve demonstrates three pertinent characteristics of the drug: its *potency* (from the position of the curve on the horizontal axis or the abscissa), its *slope* (the degree of intensification of response with a given increase in dose), and the dose required to produce the maximum effect. These three characteristics are illustrated in Figure V.3.

Potency

The situation of the dose-response curve along the dose axis is an expression of the potency of the drug. We have all heard the statement that one drug is more potent than another, but what does this mean? Potency would obviously be influenced by the factors already discussed in this book—that is, absorption, distribution, metabolism, and excretion. For example, if two drugs are studied for their sedative effects but only one passes the blood-brain barrier, that drug would be the more potent. If both drugs were capable of producing sedation but one was capable of exerting this action at half the dose level of the other, the first drug would be considered as the more potent drug.

Potency, however, is a relatively unimportant characteristic of a drug, because it makes little difference whether the effective dose of a drug is 0.1 gram or 10 grams as long as the drug is administered in an appropriate dose and undue toxicity is not observed at that dose (a factor called *safety*, to be discussed in the following section). Thus, there is little justification for the concept that the more potent the drug, the better it is. High potency, in fact, may be more of a disadvantage than an advantage, because an extremely potent drug may also be much more toxic (or dangerous) and therefore require much more careful handling.

Slope

Slope refers to the more or less linear, central portion of the dose-response curve. A steep dose-response curve (for a CNS depressant) implies that there is a smaller difference between the dose that produces death and the dose that causes mild sedation than would be observed with a depressant that had a lower slope. The steeper the slope, the smaller the increase in dose required to go from a minimal response to a maximal effect. The slope of the dose-response curve is one of the variables that must be considered in determining the relative safety of a drug.

Maximum Effect

The peak of the dose-response curve indicates the maximum effect produced by a drug. Not all stimulant drugs, for example, are capable of exerting the same level of CNS stimulation. Caffeine, even in massive doses, is incapable of exerting the same intensity of CNS stimulation that is induced by amphetamine. Thus, the maximum effect is an inherent property of a drug. Some drugs may be used to the point of maximum effect. However, with most pharmacological agents, undesired side effects limit the upper range of dosage. Thus, the usefulness of a compound is correspondingly limited, even though the drug is inherently capable of producing a greater effect. Another example of differences in maximum effect may be found in the analgesic effects of morphine and aspirin. Morphine has sufficient efficacy to provide relief from intense pain that aspirin, even at massive doses, is incapable of relieving. Note that potency and maximum effect of the drug are two separate considerations and, although one compound may be less potent than another, it may still be capable of exerting a greater maximal effect.

Variability

The final factor to be considered in a dose-response curve is variability. The dose of a drug that will produce a given response in a number of animals will vary considerably. Figure V.4 illustrates a Gaussian (bell-shaped) distribution of drug variability in a population of animals. Note that, although the *average* dose required to elicit a given response in this population of animals may be easily calculated (illustrated by the dotted line), some animals will respond to a drug at a dose very much lower than the average and some animals will not respond until extremely large doses have been administered. Because of this variation in susceptibility to a drug, it is *extremely important* that the dose of any drug be individualized. Generalizations about "average doses" are risky at best. This Gaussian distribution, however, allows us to estimate the dose of the drug that will produce the desired effect in 50 percent of the subjects. This dose is considered to be the ED_{50} for the drug (the effective dose for 50 percent of the subjects).

Closely related to the ED_{50} is the LD_{50} (lethal dose for 50 percent of the subjects). The LD_{50} is calculated exactly like the ED_{50} except that the dose of the drug is plotted against the number of subjects (usually mice) that die following various doses of the compound. Pharmacologists feel that delineation of both the ED_{50} and LD_{50} is necessary for public safety in order to prevent accidental drug-induced deaths in humans. Both the ED_{50} and the LD_{50} are usually determined in laboratory mice, and the ratio of the LD_{50} to the ED_{50}

Figure V.4

Biological variation in susceptibility to drugs. This curve is a Gaussian distribution, with the dose of drug plotted against the number of subjects requiring a given dose for a given response to occur. Note that, for a given response, some individuals will require only a small amount of the drug while others will require much more than what is considered normal.

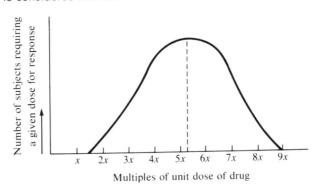

Multiples of unit dose of drug

is an index of the relative *safety* of the drug. The higher the ratio, the greater the difference between the lethal and effective doses of the compound.

The relation between the ED_{50} and the LD_{50} for a depressant drug is illustrated in Figure V.5, in which two dose-response curves are shown: the one on the left illustrates the dose of drug necessary to induce sleep in the population of mice and the one on the right illustrates the dose of drug necessary to kill a similar population. If one extrapolates across the 50-percent point (dotted lines), and determines the doses necessary to induce sleep in 50 percent and death in another 50 percent, one could determine a ratio between the median toxic dose and the median effective dose (LD_{50} : ED_{50}). In this case, the ratio would be 100:10, or 10. This figure is referred to as the *therapeutic index* of the drug—that is, the dose necessary to kill 50 percent of the mice is 10 times that necessary to induce sleep in another 50 percent. This may sound like a rather large margin, but note the 50-milligram point on the abscissa. It may be observed that, at a dose of 50 milligrams, 95 percent of the mice would be put to sleep while 5 percent of the mice would die. This overlap demonstrates the difficulty encountered in assessing the relative safety of drugs for use in large populations and serves as an excellent example of biological variation in individual responses to drugs. With this particular compound, a dose could not be administered that would guarantee that 100 percent of the mice would sleep and none would die.

Because the ED_{50} and LD_{50} refer to the means of a population's response to a drug and these terms do not account for biological variation on the tails of the curves, it has been suggested by some pharmacologists that a more meaningful index of a drug's safety

Figure V.5

Two dose-response curves. *Left*, the dose of a drug required to induce a given response. *Right*, the lethal dose of the compound.

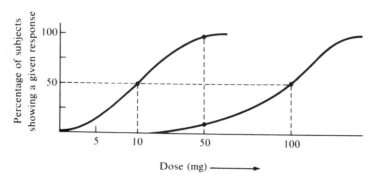

would be a ratio of the lethal dose for 1 percent of the population to the effective dose for 99 percent of the population ($LD_1 : ED_{99}$). A pharmacologist would determine the dose that would be effective for 99 percent of the mice and the dose that would be lethal to only 1 percent. A sedative drug with a $LD_1 : ED_{99}$ of 1 would be a safer compound than the drug illustrated in Figure V.5. Thus, these therapeutic ratios offer an index of the relative *safety* of a compound.

It is important to note, however, that a drug does not have a single therapeutic index, but many, because drugs exert more than one effect. Ideally, a therapeutic ratio should be drawn for each observed effect of the drug. For example, the margin of safety for aspirin for relief of headache is greater than its margin of safety for relief of the pain of arthritis because much higher therapeutic doses are used for arthritic pain than for a simple headache. The use of such indices obtained from data in laboratory mice is limited. A drug might be found to have an adequate margin of safety in mice, and it might be safe for a majority of patients. But these therapeutic indices seldom consider the patient who for some reason (such as allergy) will exhibit an unusual and unexpected response to the drug. It is important for consumers to realize that, within tolerable limits, a risk/benefit ratio can be calculated for all drugs.

Notes

1. L. Z. Benet and L. B. Sheiner, "Introduction, General Principles," in A. G. Gilman, L. S. Goodman, T. W. Rall, and F. Murad, eds., *Goodman and Gilman's The Pharmacological Basis of Therapeutics*, 7th ed. (New York: Macmillan, 1985), pp. 1–48.
2. R. R. Levine, *Pharmacology: Drug Actions and Reactions*, 3rd ed. (Boston: Little, Brown, 1983).

Oral Contraceptives

Patient Instructions

Author's Note: *The U.S. government requires that instruction material be included with all oral contraceptives dispensed by a pharmacist. Such material is an attempt to increase patient awareness by advising patients of the risks, benefits, and alternatives to the use of oral contraceptives. This information is included here as a supplement to the material presented in Chapter 12.*

What You Should Know about Oral Contraceptives

Oral contraceptives ("the pill") are the most effective way (except for sterilization) to prevent pregnancy. They are also convenient and, for most women, free of serious or unpleasant side effects. Oral contraceptives must always be taken under the continuous supervision of a physician.

It is important that any woman who considers using an oral contraceptive understand the risks involved. Although the oral contraceptives have important advantages over other methods of contraception, they have certain risks that no other method has. Only you can decide whether the advantages are worth these risks. This appendix will tell you about the most important risks. It will explain how you can help your doctor prescribe the pill as safely as possible by telling him about yourself and being alert for the earliest signs of trouble. It will also tell you how to use the pill properly, so that it will be as effective as possible.

Who Should Not Use Oral Contraceptives

A. If you have any of the following conditions, you should not use the pill:
1. Clots in the legs or lungs
2. Angina pectoris
3. Known or suspected cancer of the breast or sex organs
4. Unusual vaginal bleeding that has not yet been diagnosed
5. Known or suspected pregnancy

B. If you have had any of the following conditions, you should not use the pill:
1. Heart attack or stroke
2. Clots in the legs or lungs

C. Cigarette smoking increases the risk of serious adverse effects on the heart and blood vessels from oral-contraceptive use. This risk increases with age and with heavy smoking (15 or more cigarettes per day) and is quite marked in women over 35 years of age. If you use oral contraceptives you should not smoke.

D. If you have scanty or irregular periods or are a young woman with an irregular cycle, you should use another method of contraception because, if you use the pill, you may have difficulty becoming pregnant or may fail to have menstrual periods after discontinuing use of the pill.

Deciding to Use Oral Contraceptives

If you do not have any of these conditions and are thinking about using oral contraceptives, you need to know the advantages and risks of all contraceptive methods before you choose one. This appendix describes the advantages and risks of oral contraceptives. Except for sterilization, the IUD, and abortion, which have their own exclusive risks, the only risks or other methods of contraception are those due to pregnancy should the method fail. Your doctor can answer your questions about other methods of contraception. He can also answer any questions you may have after reading this appendix on oral contraceptives.

What Oral Contraceptives Are and How They Work   Oral contraceptives are of two types. The most common, often simply called "the pill," is a combination of an estrogen and a progestogen, the two kinds of female hormones. The amount of estrogen and progestogen can vary, but the amount of estrogen is most important because it relates to both the effectiveness and some of the dangers of oral contraceptives. This kind of oral contraceptive works principally by preventing release of an egg from the ovary. When the amount of estrogen is 50 micrograms or more, and the pill is taken as directed, oral contraceptives are more than 99 percent effective (that is, there would be less than one pregnancy if 100 women used the pill for 1 year). Pills that contain 20 to 35 micrograms of estrogen vary slightly in effectiveness, ranging from 98 percent to more than 99 percent effective.

The second type of oral contraceptive, often call the "mini-pill," contains only a progestogen. It works in part by preventing release of an egg from the ovary but also by keeping sperm from reaching the egg and by making the uterus (womb) less receptive to any fertilized egg that reaches it. The mini-pill is less effective than the combination pill—about 97 percent effective. In addition, the progestogen-only pill has a tendency to cause irregular bleeding, which may be quite inconvenient, or cessation of bleeding entirely. The progestogen-only pill is used despite its lower effectiveness in the hope that it will not have some of the serious side effects of the estrogen-containing pill, though the seriousness of its side effects are not fully known. The following information about the combination pill applies to the mini-pill as well.

Other Nonsurgical Ways to Prevent Pregnancy   Other methods of contraception have lower risks than oral contraceptives or none at all. They are also less effective than oral contraceptives, but, used properly, may be effective enough for many women. Table 11.2 reported pregnancy rates (the number of women out of 100 who would become pregnant in 1 year) that occur when using these methods.

The figures (except for the IUD) vary widely because people differ in how well they use each method. Very faithful users of the various methods obtain very good results, except for those practicing the calendar method of periodic abstinence (rhythm). Except for the IUD, effective use of these methods requires somewhat more effort than simply taking a pill every day, but it is an effort that many couples undertake successfully.

The Dangers of Oral Contraceptives
Circulatory disorders (abnormal blood clotting and stroke due to hemorrhage). Blood clots (in various blood vessels of the body) are the most common of the serious side effects of oral contraceptives. A clot can result in a stroke (if the clot is in the brain), a heart attack (if the clot is in a blood vessel of the heart), or a pulmonary embolus (a clot that forms in the legs or pelvis, then breaks off and travels to the lungs). Any of these can be fatal. Clots also occur rarely in the blood vessels of the eye, resulting in blindness or impairment of vision in that eye. There is evidence that the risk of clotting

increases with higher estrogen doses. It is therefore important to keep the dose of estrogen as low as possible, so long as the oral contraceptive used has an acceptable pregnancy rate and does not cause unacceptable changes in the menstrual pattern. Furthermore, cigarette smoking by oral-contraceptive users increases the risk of serious adverse effects on the heart and blood vessels. This risk increases with age and with heavy smoking (15 or more cigarettes per day) and begins to become quite marked in women over 35 years of age. For this reason, women who use oral contraceptives should not smoke. The risk of abnormal clotting increases with age in both users and nonusers of oral contraceptives, but the increased risk from the contraceptive appears to be present at all ages. For oral-contraceptive users in general, it has been estimated that in women between the ages of 15 and 34 the risk of death due to a circulatory disorder is about 1 in 12,000 per year, whereas for nonusers the rate is about 1 in 50,000 per year. In the age group 35 to 44, the risk is estimated to be about 1 in 2,500 per year for oral-contraceptive users and about 1 in 10,000 per year for nonusers.

The risk of heart attack increases naturally with age and is also increased by such heart attack risk factors as high blood pressure, high cholesterol, obesity, diabetes, and cigarette smoking. In the absence of any other risk factors, the use of oral contraceptives alone may double the risk of heart attack. However, the combination of cigarette smoking, especially heavy smoking, and oral-contraceptive use greatly increases the risk of heart attack. Oral-contraceptive users who smoke are about five times more likely to have a heart attack than users who do not smoke and about 10 times more likely to have a heart attack than nonusers who do not smoke. It has been estimated that users between the ages of 30 and 39 who smoke have about a 1 in 10,000 chance each year of having a fatal heart attack compared to about a 1 in 50,000 chance in users who do not smoke, and about a 1 in 100,000 chance in nonusers who do not smoke. In the age group 40 to 44, the risk is about 1 in 1,700 per year for users who smoke compared to about 1 in 10,000 for users who do not smoke and to about 1 in 14,000 per year for nonusers who do not smoke. Heavy smoking (about 15 cigarettes or more a day) further increases the risk. If you do not smoke and have none of the other heart attack risk factors described, you will have a smaller risk than listed. If you have several heart attack risk factors, the risk may be considerably greater than listed. In addition to blood-clotting disorders, it has been estimated that women taking oral contraceptives are twice as likely as nonusers to have a stroke due to rupture of a blood vessel in the brain.

Formation of tumors. Studies have found that when certain animals are given estrogen continuously for long periods, cancers may develop in the breast, cervix, vagina, and liver. These findings suggest that oral contraceptives may cause cancer in humans. However, studies to date in women taking currently marketed oral contraceptives have not confirmed that oral contraceptives cause cancer in humans. Several studies have found no increase in breast cancer in users, although one study suggested oral contraceptives might cause an increase in breast cancer in women who already have benign breast disease (for example, cysts). (The reader is referred to page 245 for further comments on cancer risk and oral contraceptive use.)

Women with a strong family history of breast cancer or who have breast nodules, fibrocystic disease, or abnormal mammograms or who were exposed to DES (diethylstilbestrol), an estrogen, during their mother's pregnancy must be followed very closely by their doctors if they choose to use oral contraceptives. Many studies have shown that women taking oral contraceptives have less risk of getting benign breast disease than those who have not used oral contraceptives. Recently, strong evidence has emerged that estrogens, when given for periods longer than 1 year to postmenopausal women, increase the risk of uterine cancer. There is also some evidence that a kind of oral contraceptive that is no longer marketed, the sequential oral contraceptive, may increase the risk of cancer of the uterus. There remains no evidence, however, that the oral contraceptives now available increase the risk of this cancer.

Oral contraceptives can cause, although rarely, a benign (nonmalignant) tumor of the liver. These tumors do not spread, but they may rupture and cause internal bleeding, which may be fatal. A few causes of cancer of the liver have been reported in women using oral contraceptives, but it is not yet known whether the drug caused them.

Dangers to a developing child if oral contraceptives are used during or immediately preceding pregnancy. Oral contraceptives should not be taken by pregnant women because they may damage the developing child. An increased risk of birth defects, including heart defects and limb defects, has been associated with the use of sex hormones, including oral contraceptives, in pregnancy. In addition, the developing female child whose mother has received DES during pregnancy has a risk of getting cancer of the vagina or cervix in her teens or young adulthood. This risk is estimated to be about 1 in 1000 exposures or less. Abnormalities of the urinary and sex organs have been reported in male offspring so exposed. It is possible that other estrogens, such as those in oral contraceptives, could have the same effect on the child if the mother took them during pregnancy.

If you stop taking oral contraceptives to become pregnant, your doctor may recommend that you use another method of contraception for a short while. There is evidence from studies in women who have had miscarriages soon after stopping the pill that the lost fetuses are likely to be abnormal. Whether there is an overall increase in miscarriage in women who become pregnant soon after stopping the pill as compared with women who do not use the pill is not known, but it is possible. If, however, you do become pregnant soon after stopping oral contraceptives, and you do not have a miscarriage, there is no evidence that the baby has an increased risk of being abnormal.

Gallbladder disease. Women who use oral contraceptives have a greater risk than nonusers of developing gallbladder disease requiring surgery. The increased risk may first appear within 1 year of use and may double after 4 or 5 years of use.

Other side effects of oral contraceptives. Some women using oral contraceptives experience unpleasant side effects that are not dangerous and are not likely to damage their health. Some of these may be temporary. Your breasts may feel tender, nausea and vomiting may occur, you may gain or lose weight, and your ankles may swell. A spotty darkening of the skin, particularly of the face, is possible and may persist. You may notice unexpected vaginal bleeding or changes in your menstrual period. Irregular bleeding is frequently seen when using the mini-pill or combination oral contraceptives containing less than 50 micrograms of estrogen.

More serious side effects include worsening of migraine, asthma, epilepsy, and kidney or heart disease because of a tendency for water retention. Other side effects are growth of preexisting fibroid tumors of the uterus, mental depression, and liver problems with jaundice (yellowing of the skin). Your doctor may find that levels of sugar and fatty substances in your blood are elevated; the long-term effects of these changes are not known. Some women develop high blood pressure; this ordinarily returns to original levels when the oral contraceptive is discontinued. Other reactions, although not proved to be caused by oral contraceptives, are occasionally reported. These include more frequent urination and some discomfort when urinating, nervousness, dizziness, some loss of scalp hair, an increase in body hair, an increase or decrease in sex drive, appetite changes, cataracts, and a need for a change in contact lens prescription or an inability to use contact lenses.

After you stop using oral contraceptives, it may take a while before you are able to become pregnant or before you resume having menstrual periods. This is especially true of women who had irregular menstrual cycles before using oral contraceptives. As discussed previously, your doctor may recommend that you wait a short while after stopping the pill before you try to become pregnant. During this time, the doctor may suggest that you use another form of contraception. You should consult your physician before resuming use of oral contraceptives after childbirth, especially if you plan to nurse your baby. Drugs in oral contraceptives are known to appear in the milk, and the long-range effect on infants is not known at this time. Furthermore, oral contraceptives may reduce your milk supply and affect its quality.

Comparison of the Risks of Oral and Other Contraceptive Methods
The many studies on the risks and effectiveness of contraceptive methods have been analyzed to estimate the risk of death associated with each. This risk has two parts: (1) the risk of the method itself (for example, the risk that oral contraceptives will cause death due to abnormal clotting), and (2) the risk of death due to pregnancy or abortion in the event the method fails. The results of this analysis are shown in Figure VI.1. The height of the bars represents the number of deaths per 100,000 women each year. There are six sets of bars, each set referring to a specific age group of women. Within each set of bars, there is a single bar for each of the different contraceptive methods. For oral contraceptives, there are two bars— one for smokers and the other for nonsmokers. The analysis is based on present knowledge, and new information could, of course, alter it. The analysis shows that the risk of death from all methods of birth control is low and less than that associated with childbirth, except for oral contraceptives in women over 40 years old who smoke. It shows that the lowest risk of death is associated with the traditional condom or diaphragm when it is backed up by early abortion in case of failure to prevent pregnancy. Also, at any age the risk of death (due to unexpected pregnancy) from the use of traditional contraception, even without a backup of abortion, is generally the same as, or less than, that from the use of oral contraceptives.

How to Use Oral Contraceptives as Safely and Effectively as Possible

What to Tell Your Doctor
You can make use of the pill as safely as possible by telling your doctor if you have any of the following:
    1. Conditions that mean you should not use oral contraceptives:
        Clots in the legs or lungs
        Clots in the legs or lungs in the past
        A stroke, heart attack, or angina pectoris
        Known or suspected cancer of the breast or sex organs
        Unusual vaginal bleeding that has not yet been diagnosed
        Known or suspected pregnancy

Figure VI.1

Estimated annual number of deaths associated with control of fertility and no control per 100,000 nonsterile women, by regimen of control and age of woman.

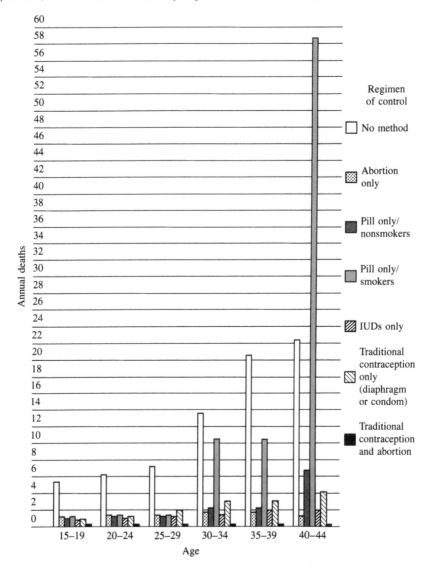

2. Conditions that your doctor will want to watch closely or that might cause him or her to suggest another method of contraception:
A family history of breast cancer

Breast nodules, fibrocystic disease of the breast, or an abnormal mammogram

Diabetes

High blood pressure

High cholesterol

Cigarette smoking

Migraine headaches

Heart or kidney disease

Epilepsy

Mental depression

Fibroid tumors of the uterus

Gallbladder disease

3. Once you are using oral contraceptives, you should be alert for signs of a serious adverse effect and call your doctor if any occur:

Sharp pain in the chest, coughing blood, or sudden shortness of breath (indicating possible clots in the lungs)

Pain in the calf (possible clot in the leg)

Crushing chest pain or heaviness (indicating possible heart attack)

Sudden severe headache or vomiting, dizziness or fainting, disturbance of vision or speech, or weakness or numbness in an arm or leg (indicating a possible stroke)

Sudden partial or complete loss of vision (indicating a possible clot in the eye)

Breast lumps (you should ask your doctor to show you how to examine your own breasts)

Severe pain in the abdomen (indicating a possible ruptured tumor of the liver)

Severe depression

Yellowing of the skin (jaundice)

How to Take the Pill so that It Is Most Effective

To achieve maximum contraceptive effectiveness, oral contraceptives must be taken exactly as directed and at intervals not exceeding 24 hours. It is recommended that tablets be taken at the same time each day, preferably after the evening meal or at bedtime. Taking them on a definite schedule will decrease the chance of forgetting a tablet and will also help to keep the proper amount of medication in your system.

Dosage Schedule   The dosage is one tablet daily for 21 days in a row per menstrual cycle. Tablets are than discontinued for 7 days. The basic schedule is 21 days on—7 days off.

During the first month, you should begin taking medication on Day 5 of your menstrual cycle whether or not you still have your period. (Day 1 is the first day of menstruation, even if it is almost midnight when you start.) Note: During your first month, if you start taking tablets later than Day 5 of your menstrual cycle, you should protect yourself by also using another method of birth control until you have taken a tablet daily for seven consecutive days. Thereafter, if you follow directions carefully you will obtain the full contraceptive benefit. If you begin taking tablets later than the proper day, the possibility of ovulation and pregnancy occurring before beginning medication should be considered. Take one tablet every day until you finish all 21 tablets. No tablets are then taken for 1 week (7 days). Your period will usually begin about 3 days after you take the last tablet. Do not be alarmed if the amount of bleeding is not the same as before. On Day 8, start a new series, even if you still have your period. If, for example, you took tablets for the first time on a Tuesday, Day 8 will also be a Tuesday. Thus, you will always begin a new cycle on the same day of the week as long as you do not interrupt your original schedule. If you start taking tablets later than Day 8, you should protect yourself by also using another method of birth control until you have taken a tablet daily for seven days in a row.

The 28-day dosage schedule is virtually the same: one active tablet daily for 21 consecutive days followed by one inactive tablet daily for seven consecutive days. You should begin taking tablets on the first Sunday after your menstrual period begins, whether or not you are still bleeding. If your period begins on a Sunday, take your first tablet that very same day.

Spotting or Breakthrough Bleeding   Spotting is slight staining between menstrual periods that may not even require a pad. Breakthrough bleeding is a flow much like a regular period, requiring sanitary protection. Spotting is more common than breakthrough bleeding, and both occur more often in the first few cycles than in later cycles. These types of bleeding are usually temporary and without significance. It is important to continue taking your pills on schedule. If the bleeding persists for more than a few days, consult your doctor.

Forgotten Pills   The chance of becoming pregnant is probably quite small if you miss only one tablet in a cycle. Of course, with each additional one you skip, the chance increases. If you miss one or two tablets you are still protected against pregnancy as long as you begin taking your next tablet on the proper day.

It is important to take a missed tablet as soon as it is remembered. If two consecutive tablets are missed, they should both be taken as soon as remembered. The next tablet should then be taken at the usual time. Any time you miss one or two tablets, or begin a new series after the proper starting day, you should also use another method of birth control until you have taken a tablet daily for seven consecutive days. If breakthrough bleeding occurs following missed tablets, it will usually be temporary and of no consequence. Although there is little likelihood of pregnancy occurring if only one or two tablets are missed, the possibility of pregnancy increases with each successive day that scheduled tablets are missed.

If you forget to take three tablets in a row, do not take them when you remember. Wait four more days—which makes a whole week without tablets. Then begin a new series on Day 8 after the last tablet was taken. During the seven days without tablets, and until you have taken a tablet daily for seven consecutive days, you should protect yourself from pregnancy by also using another method of birth control. If you are on a 28-day product and forget to take three active tablets in a row, do not take them when you remember. Stop taking all medication until the first Sunday following the last missed tablet. Then, whether or not you have had your period, and even if you are still bleeding, start a new series. During the days without tablets and until you have taken an active tablet daily for seven consecutive days, you should protect yourself from pregnancy by also using another method of birth control.

At times there may be no menstrual period after a cycle of pills. Therefore, if you miss one menstrual period but have taken the pills *exactly as you were supposed to,* continue as usual into the next cycle. If you have not taken the pills correctly and miss a menstrual period, or if you are taking mini-pills and it is 45 days or more from the start of your last menstrual period, you may be pregnant and should stop taking oral contraceptives until your doctor determines whether or not you are. Until you can get to your doctor, use another form of contraception. If two consecutive menstrual periods are missed, you should stop taking pills until it is determined whether you are pregnant. If you do become pregnant while using oral contraceptives, you should discuss the risks to the developing child with your doctor.

Periodic Examination

Your doctor will take a complete medical and family history before prescribing oral contraceptives. At that time and about once a year thereafter, he or she will generally examine your blood pressure, breasts, abdomen, and pelvic organs, including a Papanicolaou (Pap) smear, a test for cancer.

Summary

Oral contraceptives are the most effective method, except sterilization, for preventing pregnancy. Other methods, when used conscientiously, are also very effective and have fewer risks. The serious risks associated with oral contraceptives occur infrequently, and the "pill" is a very convenient method of contraception. The presence or past existence of certain conditions greatly increases the risks of oral contraceptives; such patients should use another method of birth control. Those who decide to use the "pill" should read the appendix carefully so that they can use it safely and effectively.

Based on his or her assessment of your medical needs, your doctor has prescribed this drug for you. Do not give the drug to anyone else.

Glossary

Absorption, drug—mechanisms by which a drug reaches the bloodstream from the skin, lungs, stomach, intestinal tract, or muscle.

Abstinence syndrome—a state of altered behavior observed following cessation of drug administration.

Acetaminophen (Tylenol)—a nonnarcotic, nonsalicylate analgesic and antipyretic drug devoid of anti-inflammatory effects.

Acetylcholine (Ach)—a neurotransmitter in the central and peripheral nervous systems.

Additive effect—an increased effect observed when two drugs having similar biological actions are administered. The net effect is the sum of the independent effects exerted by each drug.

Administration, drug—procedures through which a drug gains entrance into the body (oral administration of tablets or liquids, inhalation of powders, injection of sterile liquids, and so on).

Affective disorder—a type of mental disorder characterized by recurrent episodes of mania and/or depression.

Agonist—a drug that attaches to a receptor and produces actions that mimic or potentiate those that resemble the effects of an endogenous transmitter.

Alcohol (ethyl alcohol, ethanol)—a widely used sedative-hypnotic drug.

Aldehyde dehydrogenase—an enzyme that carries out a specific step in alcohol metabolism: the metabolism of acetaldehyde to acetate. This enzyme may be blocked by the drug disulfiram (Antabuse).

Amantadine (Symmetrel)—an antiviral drug that is useful in the treatment of Parkinson's disease.

Amphetamine—a behavioral stimulant.

Anesthetic drug—a sedative-hypnotic compound used primarily in doses capable of inducing a state of general anesthesia involving both loss of sensation and loss of consciousness.

Antagonist—a drug that attaches to a receptor and blocks the action of either an endogenous transmitter or an agonist drug.

Antianxiety agent—a sedative-hypnotic compound used in subhypnotic doses.

Antidepressant—A drug useful in treating mental depression in depressed patients without producing stimulant effects in normal individuals.

Antipsychotic drugs—a class of psychoactive drugs, all of which have the ability to calm psychotic states and make the psychotic patient more manageable.

Ascending reticular activating system (ARAS)—a network of neurons in the brainstem thought to function in arousal mechanisms.

Aspirin—a nonnarcotic analgesic and anti-inflammatory drug.

Baclofen (Lioresal)—a GABA derivative that is useful in the treatment of spasticity.

Barbiturate—a class of chemically related sedative-hypnotic compounds, all of which share a characteristic six-membered ring structure.

Benzodiazepine—a class of chemically related sedative-hypnotic agents of which chlordiazepoxide (Librium) and diazepam (Valium) are examples.

Bromocriptine (Parlodel)—a stimulant of dopamine receptors occasionally used in the treatment of Parkinson's disease.

Brain syndrome, organic—pattern of behavior induced when neurons are either reversibly depressed or irreversibly destroyed. Behavior is characterized by clouded sensorium; disorientation; shallow and labile affect; and impaired memory, intellectual function, insight, and judgment.

Bufotenin—a psychoactive drug found in cohoba snuff, the skin and parotid gland of the toad, and in small amounts in the mushroom *Amanita muscaria*.

Caffeine—a behavioral and general cellular stimulant found in coffee, tea, cola drinks, and chocolate.

Carbamazepine (Tegretol)—an antiepileptic drug.

Carbidopa (in Sinemet)—a drug that inhibits the enzyme DOPA-decarboxylase, allowing increased availability of DOPA within the brain.

"China White"—street term for illicit derivatives of fentanyl-type narcotics.

Chlordiazepoxide (Librium)—a benzodiazepine, sedative-hypnotic drug.

Chlorpromazine (Thorazine)—a phenothiazine, antipsychotic drug.

Citalopram—a drug that selectively blocks the active reuptake of serotonin into presynaptic nerve terminals.

Clomiphene (Clomid)—an ovulation-inducing agent thought to act by blocking the inhibitory (negative-feedback) effect that estrogens exert on the hypothalamus.

Clonidine (Catapres)—an antihypertensive drug that is useful in ameliorating the symptoms of narcotic withdrawal.

Cocaine—a behavioral stimulant.

Codeine—a sedative and pain-relieving agent found in opium, structurally related to morphine but less potent, and constituting approximately 0.5 percent of the opium extract.

Convulsant—a drug that produces convulsions by blocking inhibitory neurotransmission.

Cross-dependence—a condition in which one drug can prevent the withdrawal symptoms associated with physical dependence on a different drug.

Cross-tolerance—a condition in which tolerance of one drug results in a lessened response to another drug.

Dantrolene (Dantrium)—a drug that acts to limit the release of calcium ions in muscle, thereby reducing muscle spasticity.

Delirium tremens (DTs, "rum fits")—a syndrome of tremulousness, with hallucinations, psychomotor agitation, confusion and disorientation, sleep disorders, and other associated discomforts, lasting several days after alcohol withdrawal.

Dementia—a general designation for nonspecific mental deterioration.

Dependence, drug—state in which the use of a drug is necessary for either physical or psychological well-being.

Depo-Provera—a long-acting, injectable preparation of progesterone, useful as a long-acting female contraceptive.

"Designer drug"—street term for illicit derivatives of fentanyl-type narcotics.

Diazepam (Valium)—a benzodiazepine, antianxiety drug.

Dicarbamates—a class of chemically related sedative-hypnotic agents of which meprobamate (Equanil, Miltown) is an example.

Diethylstilbestrol—a synthetically produced estrogen occasionally used in high doses as a postcoital contraceptive.

Diisopropyl fluorophosphate (DFP)—an irreversible acetylcholine esterase (AChE) inhibitor.

Dimethyltryptamine (DMT)—a psychedelic drug found in many South American snuffs, such as yopo (prepared from the beans of the tree *Piptadenia peregrina*).

Disinhibition—a physiological state within the central nervous system characterized by decreased activity of inhibitory synapses, which results in a net excess of excitatory activity.

Droperidol (Inapsine)—an antipsychotic drug chemically classified as a butyrophenone.

Drug—any chemical substance used for its effects on bodily processes.

Drug interaction—the modification of the action of one drug by the concurrent or prior administration of another drug.

Drug misuse—the use of any drug (legal or illegal) for a medical or recreational purpose when other alternatives are available, practical, or warranted, or when drug use endangers either the user or others with whom he or she may interact.

Drug receptor—the specific molecular substance in the body with which a given drug interacts in order to produce its effect.

Drug tolerance—a state of progressively decreased responsiveness to a drug.

Endorphins—term referring to naturally occurring proteins with *endogenous morphine*-like activity.

Enkephalin—a naturally occurring protein with morphine-like activity.

Enzyme induction—the increased production of drug-metabolizing enzymes in the liver stimulated by certain drugs, such that use of these drugs increases the rate at which the body can metabolize them. It is one mechanism by which pharmacological tolerance is produced.

Epilepsy—a neurological disorder characterized by occasional, sudden, and uncontrolled discharge of neurons.

Estrogen—a body hormone secreted primarily from the ovaries of females in response to stimulation by follicle-stimulating hormone (FSH) from the pituitary gland.

Fentanyl—a potent narcotic analgesic.

Fetal alcohol syndrome—a symptom complex of congenital anomalies seen in newborns of women who ingested high doses of alcohol during critical periods of pregnancy.

Gamma-aminobutyric acid (GABA)—an inhibitory amino acid neurotransmitter in the brain.

Haloperidol (Haldol)—an antipsychotic drug chemically classified as a butyrophenone.

Harmine—a psychedelic agent obtained from the seeds of *Peganum harmala*.

Hashish—an extract of the hemp plant (*Cannabis sativa*) with a higher concentration of THC than marijuana.

Heroin—a semisynthetic opiate produced by a chemical modification of morphine.

Ibotinic acid—a psychedelic agent found in *Amanita muscaria*.

Ibuprofen (Advil, Motrin)—a nonnarcotic, nonsalicylate analgesic and anti-inflammatory drug.

Ketamine (Ketalar)—a psychedelic surgical anesthetic.

Levo-DOPA—a precursor substance to the transmitter Dopamine, useful in ameliorating the symptoms of Parkinson's disease.

β-Lipotropin—a 91-amino acid protein containing amino acid sequences with morphine-like activity.

Lithium—an alkali metal effective in the treatment of mania and depression.

Local anesthetic—a drug that reversibly blocks nerve conduction.

Lysergic acid diethylamide (LSD)—a semisynthetic psychedelic drug.

Major tranquilizer (antipsychotic tranquilizer)—a drug used in the treatment of psychotic states.

Mania—a mental disorder characterized by an expansive emotional state, elation, hyperirritability, excessive talkativeness, flight of ideas, and increased behavioral activity.

MAO inhibitor—a drug that inhibits the activity of the enzyme monoamine oxidase.

Marijuana—a mixture of the crushed leaves, flowers, and small branches of both male and female individuals of the hemp plant (*Cannabis sativa*).

MDA—a synthetically produced derivation of amphetamine.

Meperidine (Demerol)—a synthetically produced opiate narcotic.

Meprobamate (Equanil)—a sedative-hypnotic agent frequently used as an antianxiety drug.

Mescaline—a psychedelic drug extracted from the peyote cactus (*Lophophora williamsii*).

Methadone (Dolophine)—a synthetically produced opiate narcotic.

Methaqualone (Quaalude)—a sedative-hypnotic compound of relatively low potency.

Methylphenidate (Ritalin)—a CNS stimulant chemically and pharmacologically related to amphetamine.

Minor tranquilizer—any sedative-hypnotic drug promoted primarily for use in the treatment of anxiety.

Mixed agonist-antagonist—a drug that attaches to a receptor, producing weak agonist effects but displacing more potent agonists, precipitating withdrawal in drug-dependent individuals.

Monoamine oxidase (MAO)—an enzyme capable of metabolizing norepinephrine, dopamine, and serotonin to inactive products.

Monoamine oxidase inhibitor (MAOI)—an antidepressant drug that acts through inhibition of the enzyme monoamine oxidase.

Morphine—the major sedative and pain-relieving drug found in opium, being approximately 10 percent of the crude opium exudate.

Muscarine—a drug extracted from the mushroom *Amanita muscaria* that directly stimulates acetylcholine receptors.

Muscimol—a psychedelic agent found in *Amanita muscaria.*

Myristin—a psychedelic agent obtained from nutmeg and mace.

Naloxone (Narcan)—a pure narcotic antagonist.

Naltrexone (Trexan)—a long-acting narcotic antagonist.

Nicotine—a behavioral stimulant found in tobacco.

Norepinephrine (NE)—a synaptic transmitter in both the central and peripheral nervous systems.

Ololiuqui—a psychedelic drug obtained from the seeds of the morning glory.

Opiate—any natural or synthetic drug that exerts actions on the body similar to those induced by morphine, the major pain-relieving agent obtained from the opium poppy (*Papaver somniferum*).

Opiate narcotic—a drug that has both sedative and analgesic actions.

Opium—a crude resinous exudate from the opium poppy.

Parkinson's disease—a disorder of the motor system characterized by involuntary movements, tremor, and weakness.

Pentylenetetrazol (Metrazol)—a convulsant drug.

Pergonal—a preparation of follicle-stimulating hormone extracted from the urine of postmenopausal females.

Pharmacodynamics—study of the interactions of drugs with the receptors responsible for the action of a drug in the body.

Pharmacokinetics—study of the factors that influence the absorption, distribution, metabolism, and excretion of a drug.

Pharmacology—the branch of science that deals with the study of drugs and their actions on living systems.

Phencyclidine (Sernyl)—a psychedelic surgical anesthetic.

Phenothiazine—a class of chemically related compounds useful in the treatment of psychosis.

Phenytoin (Dilantin)—an antiepileptic drug.

Physical dependence—a state in which the presence of a drug is required in order for an individual to function normally. Such a state is revealed by withdrawing the drug and noting the occurrence of withdrawal symptoms (abstinence syndrome). Characteristically, withdrawal symptoms can be terminated by readministration of the drug.

Physostigmine—an acetylcholine esterase (AChE) inhibitor.

Picrotoxin—a convulsant drug.

Placebo—a pharmacologically inert substance that may elicit a significant reaction largely because of the mental "set" of the patient or the physical setting in which the drug is taken.

Potency—a measure of drug activity expressed in terms of the amount required to produce an effect of given intensity. Potency varies inversely with the amount of drug required to produce this effect—that is, the more potent the drug, the lower the amount required to produce the effect.

Progesterone—a hormone secreted from the ovaries in response to stimulation by luteinizing hormone (LH) from the pituitary gland.

Progestins—a group of synthetically produced progesterones, most frequently found in oral contraceptive tablets.

Psilocybin—a psychedelic drug obtained from the Mexican mushroom *Psilocybe mexicana*.

Psychedelic drug—any drug with the ability to alter sensory perception.

Psychoactive drug—any chemical substance that alters mood or behavior as a result of alterations in the functioning of the brain.

Psychological dependence—a compulsion to use a drug for its pleasurable effects. Such dependence may lead to a compulsion to misuse a drug.

Reserpine (Serpasil)—an antipsychotic drug.

Risk/benefit ratio—an arbitrary assessment of the risks and benefits that may accrue from administration of a drug.

Scopolamine—an anticholinergic drug that crosses the blood-brain barrier to produce sedation and amnesia.

Sedative-hypnotic drug—any chemical substance that exerts a nonselective general depressant action upon the nervous system.

Serotonin (5-Hydroxytryptamine, 5-HT)—a synaptic transmitter both in the brain and in the peripheral nervous system.

Side effect—any drug-induced effect that accompanies the primary effect for which the drug was administered.

Spasticity—a state of abnormal increases in muscle tension, resulting in increased resistance of the muscle to stretching.

Strychnine—a convulsant drug.

Teratogen—any chemical substance that may induce abnormalities of fetal development.

Testosterone—a hormone secreted from the testes that is responsible for the distinguishing characteristics of the male.

Tetrahydrocannabinol (THC)—a major psychoactive agent found in marijuana, hashish, and other preparations of hemp (*Cannabis sativa*).

Tolerance, drug—state of progressively decreasing responsiveness to a drug.

Toxic effect—any drug-induced effect that is either temporarily or permanently deleterious to any organ or system of an animal or patient to which the drug is administered. Drug toxicity includes both the relatively minor side effects that invariably accompany drug administration and the more serious and unexpected manifestations that occur in only a small percentage of individuals taking a drug.

Bibliography

Textbooks of Pharmacology

American Medical Association *Drug Evaluations*, 6th Ed. Philadelphia: Saunders, 1986.

Barchas, J. D., P. A. Berger, R. D. Ciaranello, and G. R. Elliott, eds. *Psychopharmacology: From Theory to Practice*. New York: Oxford, 1977.

Bevan, J. A., and J. H. Thompson *Essentials of Pharmacology: An Introduction to the Principles of Drug Action*, 3d ed. Philadelphia: Lippincott, 1983.

Carlton, P. L. *A Primer of Behavioral Pharmacology*. New York: W. H. Freeman and Co., 1983.

Csaky, T. Z., and B. A. Barnes *Cutting's Handbook of Pharmacology*, 7th ed. Norwalk, Conn.: Appleton-Century-Crofts, 1984.

DiPalma, J. R. *Basic Pharmacology in Medicine*, 2d ed. New York: McGraw-Hill, 1981.

Gilman, A. G., L. S. Goodman, T. W. Rall, and F. Murad, eds. *Goodman and Gilman's The Pharmacological Basis of Therapeutics*, 7th ed. New York: Macmillan, 1985.

Goth, A. *Medical Pharmacology*, 11th ed. St. Louis: Mosby, 1984.

Hollister, L. E. *Clinical Pharmacology of Psychotherapeutic Drugs*, 2d ed. New York: Churchill-Livingstone, 1983.

Katzung, B. G., ed. *Basic and Clinical Pharmacology*, 3d ed. Norwalk, Conn.: Appleton and Lange, 1987.

Levine, R. R. *Pharmacology: Drug Actions and Reactions*, 3d ed. Boston: Little, Brown, 1983.

Melmon, K. L., and H. F. Morrelli (eds.) *Clinical Pharmacology: Basic Principles in Therapeutics*, 2d ed. New York: Macmillan, 1978.

Meltzer, H. Y., ed. *Psychopharmacology: The Third Generation of Progress*. New York: Raven Press, 1987.

McKim, W. A. *Drugs and Behavior: An Introduction to Behavioral Pharmacology*. Englewood Cliffs, N.J.: Prentice-Hall, 1986.

Alcohol and Alcoholism

Cohen, S. *The Alcoholism Problems: The Selected Issues*. New York: Haworth Press, 1983.

Edwards, G., and J. Littleton, eds. *Pharmacological Treatments for Alcoholism*. New York: Methuen, 1984.

Estes, N. J., and M. E. Heinemann *Alcoholism: Development, Consequences and Intervention*. St. Louis: Mosby, 1986.

Goldstein, D. P. *Pharmacology of Alcohol*. New York: Oxford, 1983.

Health Technology Case Study 22, *The Effectiveness and Costs of Alcoholism Treatment*. Office of Technology Assessment. Washington, D.C.: U.S. Government Printing Office, 1983.

Israel, Y., and J. Mardones *The Biological Basis of Alcoholism*. New York: Wiley-Interscience, 1971.

Jellinek, E. M. *The Disease Concept of Alcoholism*. New Haven, Conn.: Hillhouse Press, 1960.

Knott, D. H. *Alcohol Problems: Diagnosis and Treatment*. Elmsford, N.Y.: Pergamon, 1986.

Light, W. H. *Neurobiology of Alcohol Abuse*. Springfield, Ill.: C. C. Thomas, 1986.

Majchrowicz, E., and E. P. Noble, eds. *Biochemistry and Pharmacology of Ethanol*. New York: Plenum, 1979.

Mann, M. *New Primer on Alcoholism*, 2d ed. New York: Holt, 1968.

Mendelson, J. H. "The Biochemical Pharmacology of Alcohol," in D. H. Efron, ed., *Psychopharmacology: A Review of Progress, 1957–1967*. Washington, D.C.: U.S. Government Printing Office, 1968.

Pattison, E. M., ed. *Selection of Treatment for Alcoholics*. New Brunswick, N.J.: Rutgers Center for Alcohol Studies, 1982.

Pattison, E. M., M. B. Sobell, and L. C. Sobell *Emerging Concepts of Alcohol Dependence*. New York: Springer-Verlag, 1977.

Seixas, F. A., K. Williams, and S. Eggleston, eds. "Medical Consequences of Alcoholism," *Annals of the New York Academy of Sciences* 252 (25 April 1975).

Sobell, M. B., and L. C. Sobell *Individualized Behavioral Treatment of Alcohol Problems*. New York: Plenum, 1977.

U.S. Department of Health and Human Services. *Fourth Special Report to the United States Congress on Alcohol and Health.* Washington, D.C.: U.S. Government Printing Office, 1981.

U.S. Department of the Treasury and U.S. Department of Health and Human Services. *Report of the President and the Congress on Health Hazards Associated with Alcohol and Methods to Inform the General Public of these Hazards.* Washington, D.C.: U.S. Government Printing Office, 1981.

Heroin and Opiate Narcotics

Biernacki, P. *Pathways from Heroin Addiction: Recovery without Treatment.* Philadelphia: Temple University Press, 1986.

Brecher, E. M., and *Consumer Reports* editors *Licit and Illicit Drugs: The Consumers Union Report on Narcotics, Stimulants, Depressants, Inhalants, Hallucinogens, and Marihuana—Including Caffeine, Nicotine, and Alcohol.* Mount Vernon, N.Y.: Consumers Union, 1972.

DeLong, J. V. "Treatment and Rehabilitation," in *Dealing with Drug Abuse—A Report to the Ford Foundation,* prepared by the Drug Abuse Survey Project, P. M. Wald and P. B. Hutt, cochairmen. New York: Praeger, 1972.

Goldstein, A., ed. *The Opiate Narcotics: Neurochemical Mechanisms of Analgesia and Dependence.* Elmsford, N.Y.: Pergamon, 1976.

Jaffe, J. H., and W. R. Martin "Opioid Analgesics and Antagonists," in A. G. Gilman, L. S. Goodman, T. W. Rall, and F. Murad, eds., *Goodman and Gilman's The Pharmacological Basis of Therapeutics,* 7th ed. New York: Macmillan, 1985.

National Institute on Drug Abuse *Research Monograph No. 28: Narcotic Antagonists.* Washington, D.C.: U.S. Government Printing Office, 1981.

Smith, D. E., and G. R. Gay *It's So Good, Don't Even Try It Once: Heroin in Perspective.* Englewood Cliffs, N.J.: Prentice-Hall, 1972.

Cigarettes and Smoking

Jarvik, M. E., J. W. Cullen, E. R. Gritz, T. M. Vogt, and L. J. West, eds. *Research on Smoking Behavior,* National Institute on Drug Abuse, Research Monograph No. 17. Washington, D.C.: U.S. Government Printing Office, December 1977.

Krasnegor, N. A., ed. *Cigarette Smoking as a Dependence Process,* National Institute on Drug Abuse, Research Monograph No. 23. Washington, D.C.: U.S. Government Printing Office, January 1979.

Mangan, G. L., and J. F. Golding *The Psychopharmacology of Smoking.* New Rochelle, N.Y.: Cambridge University Press, 1984.

U.S. Department of Health, Education, and Welfare *Smoking and Health: Report of the Surgeon General.* Washington, D.C.: U.S. Government Printing Office, 1979.

U.S. Department of Health, Education, and Welfare *The Health Consequences of Smoking for Women: Report of the Surgeon General.* Washington, D.C.: U.S. Government Printing Office, 1980.

U.S. Department of Health and Human Services *The Health Consequences of Smoking: Cancer.* Washington, D.C.: U.S. Government Printing Office, 1982.

U.S. Department of Health and Human Services *The Changing Cigarette: Health Consequences of Smoking.* Washington, D.C.: U.S. Government Printing Office, 1981.

Antipsychotic Tranquilizers

Clark, W. G., and J. del Giudice *Principles of Psychopharmacology.* New York: Academic Press, 1970.

Klawans, H. L., ed. *Clinical Pharmacology,* vol. 1. New York: Raven Press, 1976.

Lickey, M. E., and B. Gordon *Drugs for Mental Illness.* New York: W. H. Freeman and Co., 1983.

Longo, V. G. *Neuropharmacology and Behavior.* San Francisco: W. H. Freeman and Co., 1972.

Schou, M. "Pharmacology and Toxicology of Lithium," in H. W. Elliott, ed., *Annual Review of Pharmacology and Toxicology,* vol. 16, pp. 231–243. Palo Alto, Calif.: Annual Reviews, 1976.

Simpson, L. L., ed. *Drug Treatment of Mental Disorders.* New York: Raven Press, 1976.

Snider, S. H., S. P. Banerjee, H. I. Yamamura, and D. Greenberg "Drugs, Neurotransmitters, and Schizophrenia." *Science* 184 (24 June 1974): 1243–1253.

Von Brucke, F. T., O. Hornykiewicz, and E. B. Sigg *The Pharmacology of Psychotherapeutic Drugs.* New York: Springer-Verlag, 1969.

Cannabis

Government Reports *Cannabis: A Report of the Commission of Inquiry into the Non-Medical Use of Drugs,* Gerald LeDain, chairman. Ottawa: Information Canada, 1972.

Final Report of the Commission of Inquiry into the Non-Medical Use of Drugs, Gerald LeDain, chairman. Ottawa: Information Canada, 1973.

National Commission on Marihuana and Drug Abuse, Raymond P. Shafer, chairman. *Drug Use in America: The Problem in Perspective.* Washington, D.C.: U.S. Government Printing Office, 1973.

National Commission on Marihuana and Drug Abuse, Raymond P. Shafer, chairman. *Marihuana: A Signal of Misunderstanding.* New York: New American Library, 1972.

The President's Commission on Law Enforcement and Administration of Justice. *Task Force Report: Narcotics and Drug Abuse.* Washington, D.C.: U.S. Government Printing Office, 1967.

Secretary of Health, Education, and Welfare   *Marihuana and Health: Seventh Annual Report to the U.S. Congress.* Washington, D.C.: U.S. Government Printing Office, 1977.

Other Recommended References   Braude, M. C., and S. S. Szara, eds.   *Pharmacology of Marihuana* (2 vols.). New York: Raven Press, 1976.

Brecher, E. M., and *Consumer Reports* editors   *Licit and Illicit Drugs: The Consumers Union Report on Narcotics, Stimulants, Depressants, Inhalants, Hallucinogens, and Marihuana—Including Caffeine, Nicotine, and Alcohol.* Mount Vernon, N.Y.: Consumers Union, 1972.

Brecher, E. M., and *Consumer Reports* editors   "Marihuana: The Health Questions," *Consumer Reports* 40 (March 1975): 143–149.

Dornbush, R. L., A. M. Freedman, and M. Fink, eds.   "Chronic Cannabis Use," *Annals of the New York Academy of Sciences* 282 (1976): 1–430.

The Indian Hemp Drugs Commission Report, 1893–94. Contained in 7 volumes and 2 supplements. Simla: Government Central Printing Office. Reprinted in 1971 by Johnson Reprint Corp., New York.

Maykut, M. O.   *Health Consequences of Acute and Chronic Marijuana Use.* Elmsford, N.Y.: Pergamon, 1981.

Mikuriya, T. H., ed.   *Marijuana: Medical Papers, 1839–1972.* Oakland, Calif.: Medi-Comp Press, 1973.

New York Academy of Sciences   "Marihuana: Chemistry, Pharmacology and Patterns of Social Use," *Annals of the New York Academy of Sciences* 191 (31 December 1971).

The Mayor's Committee on Marihuana   *The Marihuana Problem in the City of New York.* Lancaster, Pa.: The Mayor's Committee on Marihuana, 1944. Reprinted in 1973 by Scarecrow Reprint Corp., Metuchen, N.J., and published under the auspices of the Library of the New York Academy of Medicine.

Paton, W. D. M.   "Pharmacology of Marijuana," in H. W. Elliott, ed., *Annual Review of Pharmacology,* vol. 15, pp. 191–220. Palo Alto, Calif.: Annual Reviews, 1975.

Nerve Physiology and Neuroanatomy

Cooper, J. R. and F. E. Bloom   *The Biochemical Basis of Neuropharmacology,* 5th ed. New York: Oxford University Press, 1986.

Eccles, J. C.   *The Understanding of the Brain.* New York: McGraw-Hill, 1973.

Eyzaguirre, C.   *Physiology of the Nervous System.* Chicago: Year Book Medical Publishers, 1985.

Gluhbegovic, N., and T. H. Williams *The Human Brain: A Photographic Guide.* Hagerstown, Md.: Harper & Row, 1980.

Grossman, S. P. *A Textbook of Physiological Psychology.* New York: Wiley, 1967.

Guyton, A. C. *Basic Human Neurophysiology,* 3d ed. Philadelphia: Saunders, 1981.

Isaacson, R. L., R. J. Douglas, J. F. Lubar, and L. W. Schmaltz *A Primer of Physiological Psychology.* New York: Harper & Row, 1971.

Iverson, S. D., and L. L. Iverson *Behavioral Pharmacology,* 2d ed. New York: Oxford University Press, 1980.

Netter, F. H. *The Nervous System* (the Ciba Collection of Medical Illustrations, vol. 1). Summit, N.J.: Ciba Pharmaceutical Products, 1962.

Rech, R. A., and K. W. Moore *An Introduction to Psychopharmacology.* New York: Raven Press, 1971.

Ruch, P. C., and H. D. Patton *Physiology and Biophysics.* Philadelphia: Saunders, 1965.

Schmidt, R. F. *Fundamentals of Neurophysiology,* 3d ed., New York: Springer-Verlag, 1985.

Scientific American, The Brain. San Francisco: W. H. Freeman and Company, 1979.

Somjen, G. *Neurophysiology: The Essentials.* Baltimore: Williams & Wilkins, 1983.

Smith, C. G. *Basic Neuroanatomy.* Toronto: University of Toronto Press, 1961.

Stein, J. F. *An Introduction of Neurophysiology.* Oxford: Blackwell, 1982.

Stevens, C. F. *Neurophysiology: A Primer.* New York: Wiley, 1966.

Stratton, D. B. *Neurophysiology.* New York: McGraw-Hill, 1981.

Thompson, R. F. *The Brain: An Introduction to Neuroscience.* New York: W. H. Freeman and Co., 1984.

Drug Education

Bennett, G., C. Vourakis, and D. S. Woolf *Substance Abuse: Pharmacologic Developments and Clinical Perspectives.* New York: Wiley, 1983.

Califano, J. A., Jr. *Report on Drug Abuse and Alcoholism.* New York: Warner Books, 1982.

Cohen, S. *The Substance Abuse Problems: New Issues for the 1980s.* New York: Haworth Press, 1985.

Cohen, S., and J. F. Callahan, eds. *The Diagnosis and Treatment of Drug and Alcohol Abuse.* New York: Haworth Press, 1986.

The Drug Abuse Survey Project *Dealing with Drug Abuse: A Report to the Ford Foundation.* New York: Praeger, 1972.

DuPont, R. L., A. Goldstein, and J. O'Donnell, eds. *Handbook on Drug Abuse.* National Institute on Drug Abuse. Washington, D.C.: U.S. Government Printing Office, 1979.

Hoffman, F. G. *Handbook on Drug and Alcohol Abuse: The Biomedical Aspects.* New York: Oxford University Press, 2d ed., 1983.

Jones, C. L., and R. Battjes "Etiology of Drug Abuse, Implications for Prevention," NIDA Research, Monograph No. 56. Washington, D.C.: U.S. Government Printing Office, 1985.

Kirsch, M. M. *Designer Drugs.* Minneapolis: CompCare Publications, 1986.

Lennard, H. L., L. J. Epstein, A. Bernstein, and D. C. Ransom *Mystification and Drug Misuse.* San Francisco: Jossey-Bass, 1971.

Marin, P., and A. Y. Cohen *Understanding Drug Use.* New York: Harper & Row, 1971.

National Institute on Drug Abuse *Doing Drug Education: The Role of the School Teacher.* Washington, D.C.: U.S. Government Printing Office, 1975.

National Institute on Drug Abuse *Drug Abuse Prevention Research.* Washington, D.C.: U.S. Government Printing Office, 1983.

National Institute on Drug Abuse *Why Evaluate Drug Education? Task Force Report.* Washington, D.C.: U.S. Government Printing Office, 1975.

Petersen, R. C., ed. *The International Challenge of Drug Abuse.* Washington, D.C.: U.S. GOvernment Printing Office, 1978.

Schuckit, M. A. *Drug and Alcohol Abuse,* 2d ed. New York: Plenum, 1985.

U.S. Department of Health and Human Services, "Alcohol and Drug Abuse Among Adolescents," No. 1. Washington, D.C.: U.S. Government Printing Office, April 1986.

Weil, A. *The Natural Mind.* Boston: Houghton Mifflin, 1973.

Index